Pollution and Environmental Health

Pollution and Environmental Health

Edited by Michelle Randall

MURPHY & MOORE
www.murphy-moorepublishing.com

Published by Murphy & Moore Publishing,
1 Rockefeller Plaza,
New York City, NY 10020, USA
www.murphy-moorepublishing.com

Pollution and Environmental Health
Edited by Michelle Randall

International Standard Book Number: 978-1-63987-440-8 (Hardback)

Cataloging-in-Publication Data

Pollution and environmental health / edited by Michelle Randall.
p. cm.
Includes bibliographical references and index.
ISBN 978-1-63987-440-8
1. Pollution. 2. Environmental health. 3. Health risk assessment.
I. Randall, Michelle.
TD174 .P65 2022
363.73--dc23

TABLE OF CONTENTS

PREFACE

This book aims to highlight the current researches and provides a platform to further the scope of innovations in this area. This book is a product of the combined efforts of many researchers and scientists, after going through thorough studies and analysis from different parts of the world. The objective of this book is to provide the readers with the latest information of the field.

The process of introducing materials that are harmful in nature, into the environment is termed as pollution. These materials are also known as contaminants or pollutants. They are released into the environment through various mechanisms such as smokes from automobiles, burning of coal, use of pesticides, etc. Pollution is broadly classified into air pollution, water pollution, land pollution, noise pollution and light pollution. Environmental health is a sub-discipline of public health which focuses on the impact of natural and built environment on human health. It is further divided into environmental and occupational medicine, epidemiology, toxicology, and environmental science. Some of the major health concerns addressed by this discipline are air quality, climate change and solid waste management. The book aims to shed light on some of the unexplored aspects of pollution and environmental health, and the recent researches in this field. There has been rapid progress in this field and its applications are finding their way across multiple industries. This book on pollution and environmental health is a collective contribution of a renowned group of international experts.

I would like to express my sincere thanks to the authors for their dedicated efforts in the completion of this book. I acknowledge the efforts of the publisher for providing constant support. Lastly, I would like to thank my family for their support in all academic endeavors.

Editor

1

Evaluation of factors affecting on lipid extraction for recovery of fatty acids from *Nannochloropsis oculata* micro-algae to biodiesel production

Mohammad Malakootian[1*], Behnam Hatami[2], Shidwash Dowlatshahi[3], Ahmad Rajabizadeh[3]

[1]Professor, Environmental Health Engineering Research Center, Department of Environmental Health, Kerman University of Medical Sciences, Kerman, Iran
[2]MSc, Department of Environmental Health, Kerman University of Medical Sciences, Kerman, Iran
[3]Instructure, Environmental Health Engineering Research Center, Department of Environmental Health, Kerman University of Medical Sciences, Kerman, Iran

Abstract
Background: This study aimed at determining the appropriate method for dewatering and drying biomass and selecting a suitable organic solvent for lipid extraction.
Methods: *Nannochloropsis Oculata* was cultured in Gillard F/2 medium and after reaching the end of the stationary growth phase, algal biomass was separated from aqueous by centrifuge and dried through three methods: Oven, Air-dried and Lyophilized. Soxhlet apparatus achieved lipid extraction of all samples: diethyl ether, n-hexane and n-pentane using three solvents. At each stage, the quantity and quality of the extracted lipids were determined by Gas Chromatography.
Results: In all three drying methods, palmitic acid and palmitoleic acid, and most significantly fatty acid composition of microalgae were extracted. The fatty acid composition of palmitic acid extracted by Diethyl ether was significantly more than the other two solvents. Maximum production of triglyceride was observed in Lyophilized and air-dried microalgae where lipid extraction was performed with diethyl ether solvents and are 75.03% and 76.72% of fatty acid.
Conclusion: The use of Lyophilized method for dewatering and drying of biomass and Diethyl ether as solvent for the extraction of lipids from biomass, studied in this paper, as compared to other methods, had higher yields and researches proved that the production of biodiesel from microalgae's lipid was more efficient.
Keywords: Nannochloropsis oculata, Lipid, Solvent, Biomass, Biodiesel

***Correspondence to:**
Mohammad Malakootian
Email: m.malakootian@yahoo.com

Introduction

Rapid depletion of fossil fuels with increasing energy consumption and global warming have resulted in a move towards alternative energy sources with less emissions (1,2). In recent years, biodiesel as a renewable, biodegradable, and nontoxic energy has received considerable attention (3-5). The raw materials for biodiesel production now mainly include vegetable seed oil, soybean oil, some recovered animal fats and microalgae (3). Due to high growth rate, short growth time, high biomass production and low land use, microalgae have certain advantages compared to other biodiesel sources (1,4). The application of microalgae to economical production of biodiesel requires that a high percentage of microalgal biomass be composed of fatty acid containing compounds that can be converted to Fatty Acid Methyl Esters (FAME) (6). Microalgae are theoretically capable of producing much more lipids than any conventional crop and depending on the species; microalgae produce many different kinds of lipids (4,7).

The key processes involved in biodiesel production using microalgae are cultivation, biomass harvesting, dewatering and drying of biomass, lipid extraction from biomass, and conversion of lipid to biodiesel (1). Each one of these steps is important in the economic production of biodiesel from microalgae. Meanwhile, researches continue in this field to achieve the optimal condition for each step. For example, different studies are being conducted on the quality and quantity of microalgae cellular lipid as the result of variety of growth condition (temperature and light

intensity) or type of the medium (nitrogen, phosphate and iron concentration) (8-10). Furthermore, some studies are being done on the methods of microalgae extraction from medium by centrifuge, chemical coagulation and electrical coagulation or converting lipid to biodiesel using various catalysts (11-14).
Drying and lipid extraction from oleaginous microalgae are important steps in biodiesel production. The diversities of composition and structure of lipids from various kinds of microalgae call for different methods of extraction, thereby affecting the cost of operations (2). Lipid extraction from microalgae biomass is done through various means: mechanical, organic solvent, enzymatic extraction, osmotic shock, supercritical fluid extraction, and microwave/ultrasound assisted extraction (5,7,15). In spite of recently developed extraction methods including supercritical fluid extraction or microwave/ultrasound assisted extraction, lipid extraction from biomass by organic solvents was still found superior in comparison to other because of simplicity, relatively low cost and the non-requirement for special equipment. This method is nowadays used extensively in researches related to biodiesel (5). In studies conducted so far, only the effect of solvent on the quantity of lipid has been surveyed while quality of extracted lipid has an important role in biodiesel production and its correspondence with standards. The purpose of this study was to investigate the effect of solvent type on fatty acids composition extracted from microalgae. Taking into consideration the temperature's effect on fatty acids composition, three common methods of drying microalgae biomass were studied, and the quality of fatty acid attained from each method was determined in biodiesel production.

Methods

The study was conducted in the first half of 2012 at the Environmental Health Engineering Research Center of Kerman University of Medical Science using pilot in laboratory scale.

Culture conditions of Nannochloropsis oculata

Stock culture of *Nannochloropsis oculata* was obtained from the Research Institute for Aquaculture in the south of the Iran. This microalga is a eukaryotic photosynthetic microorganism and given its simple structure, it had a fast growth rate (8). Stock culture was cultivated on liquid of F/2 Gillard medium in bubble column photobioreactors. Column photobioreactors were made of Pyrex glass tubes (650 mm in height and 35 mm of internal diameter). Fluorescent lamps (FL20D, OSRAM, Korea) were used as the light source for their growth. According to the study of Banerjee *et al* (16) and Sen *et al* (17) continuously illuminated 70 $\mu E\ m^{-2}\ s^{-1}$ and the photoreactors were operated at 20 °C on the basis of data reported in the literature (8). Sterile-air containing 2% (v/v) CO2 by filtering using glassfiber was aerated into the column through an air sparger at the bottom of the column at 0.5 v/v flow rate.

Dewatering and drying of biomass

After the microalgae reached the end of the stationary growth phase, the algal biomass was extracted from medium by centrifuge (8000 rpm, 20 minutes) (1,5) and was dried by the three different methods. Drying in oven (105 °C for 4 hours), drying in ambient temperature (20 to 25 °C for one week) and Lyophilization (by freeze dryer machine, model of EYELA and temperature of -69 °C) were some of the methods of study (7).

Extracting lipid from biomass by the method of soxhlet

20 g of every sample of dried biomass, unified gently by mortar and lipid extraction from it was done by soxhlet model of Soxtee 2050 in this way: Each cycle entailed boiling for 25 minutes, lipid extraction for 40 minutes, and solvent recovery for 15 minutes. The extraction of all the samples was done in 5 cycles. For the extraction process, 3 common solvents, Diethyl ether, N-hexane and N-pentane with different boiling temperatures having purity levels were used. The extracted lipid by 0.45 μm filter, was smoothed to remove microalgae leftovers (8). The drying and extracting lipid steps were repeated three times, and the results were reported on averages. After determining the amount of lipid, the dried lipid was solved in 0.4 ml Isopropyl alcohol, and the amount of triglycerides in lipid was measured according to Xin *et al* (18).

Analyzing and determining the fatty acid characteristics

To determine the compositions of fatty acid, 150 mg of each sample of extracted lipid was derived by BF3 according to the EN Iso5509 standard (6). The organic phase, attained by Gas chromatography machine model Technologies (7890 A-5975c Agilent) equipped with DB-wax pole (30 m length, 0.25 mm internal diameter, 0.25 μm thickness) and Flame Ionization Detector (FID), was analyzed. The temperature of injector and detector was fixed at 250 °C. The temperature attained 180 °C within 5 minutes and 220 °C at the speed of 4 °C/min and was maintained at this degree for 25 minutes. Helium was also used as carrier gas in the amount of 1.5 ml/min. The compositions of fatty acid were calculated on the basis of the percentage of total fatty acid and according to the peak attained from analyzing (9,19).

Statistical analysis

Data were analyzed using one-way ANOVA, and Tukey test was used to determine the statistical difference between media. A value of $P<0.05$ was considered statistically significant (20,21).

Results

The results of important fatty acid compositions extracted using different organic solvents in *Nannochloropsis oculata* microalgae that dried in oven, in the vicinity of open air, and through the lyophilization method are presented in Figures 1 to 3. The results showed that in all of these methods, the highest percentage of compositions was related to palmitic and palmitoleic acids. The results related to the quantity of extracted compositions also showed that in lyophilization and open-air methods, the Diethyl ether was more suitable than the two other solvents. The results of triglyceride extracted using different

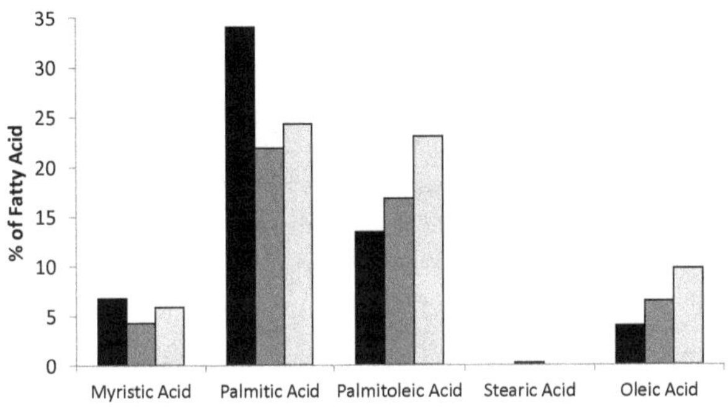

Figure 1. Fatty acid compositions in dried microalgae by oven and using different organic solvents (% of total fatty acids)

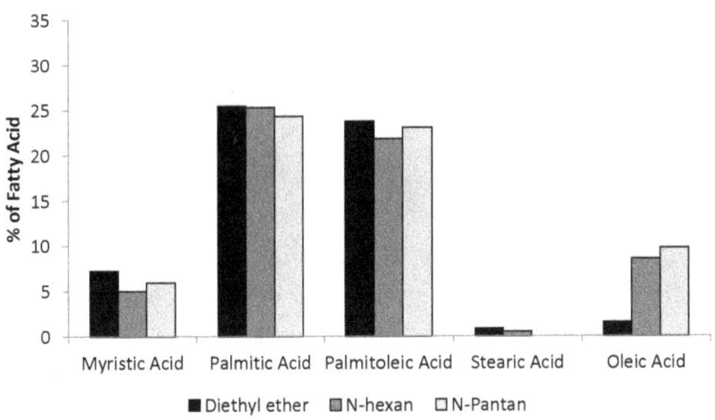

Figure 2. Fatty acid compositions in dried microalgae by open air and using different organic solvents (% of total fatty acids)

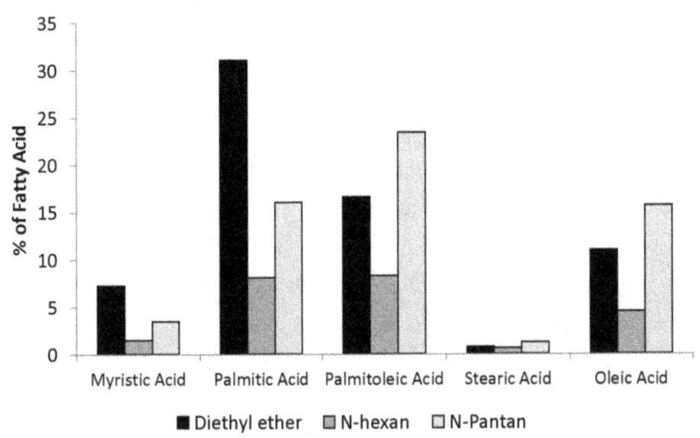

Figure 3. Fatty acid compositions in dried microalgae by lyophilization and using different organic solvents (% of total fatty acids)

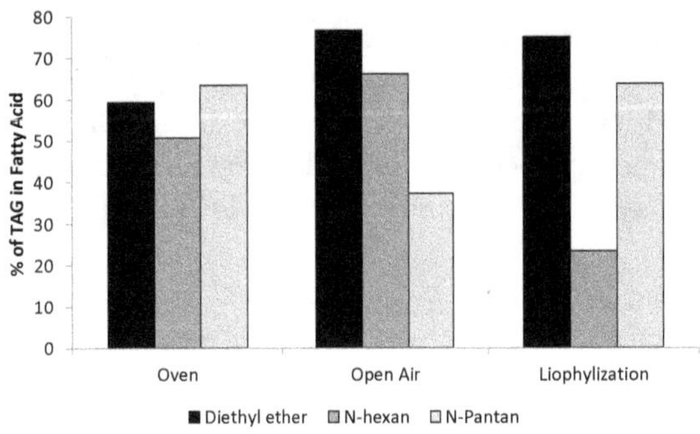

Figure 4. Triglyceride extracted by using different organic solvents in *Nannochloropsis oculata* microalgae that dried by different methods (% of TAG in total fatty acids)

organic solvents in *Nannochloropsis oculata* microalgae dried by different methods are presented in Figure 4.

Discussion

Effect of biomass drying on fatty acid extracted from microalgae

Vegetable oils currently used for biodiesel production are mainly C16 and C18. Olofsson *et al* proposed myristic acid, palmitic acid, palmitoleic acid, stearic acid, and oleic acid as important fatty acids for biodiesel production (22). In this study, the one-way ANOVA results and Tukey test showed that in all three methods of biomass drying, the highest composition of microalgae fatty acid are palmitic and palmitoleic acids ($P<0.05$). Comparison of these two compositions among the three methods of drying microalgae also showed that the amount of palmitic acid in lyophilization and oven methods is more than its amount in the other method. But the amount of palmitoleic acid in dried microalgae in open air is more than its amount in the two other methods. The comparison between Figures 1 to 3 showed that the proportion of palmitoleic acid to palmitic acid is decreased by increasing temperature as in the biomass dried in open air than biomass dried in oven. This proportion is decreased because of increasing temperature and reached 0.66% from 1.398% that is according to Kleinschmidt *et al* results (23). Also Widjaja *et al* (5) in a study on the effect of drying temperature on the lipid extracted from Chlorella vulgaris concluded that the temperature of 60 °C caused the quantity in the amount of extracted lipid to decrease. But by increasing temperature to 80 °C or more, the amount of lipid decreased substantially. The temperature can affect the pattern, route and metabolism activity of microalgae cell and, as a result, affect the cellular composition (24). The result further showed that the highest percentage of fatty acid in dried microalgae was attained in open air and that the prolixity of drying time was one weakness in this method that made it uneconomical. Whereas the preparation of microalgae by lyophilization method is done in a shorter time, does not require special storage conditions, and dewatering is done easily (9).

The lyophilization method leads to better extraction of lipid by increasing the sample's contact area (25). Microalgae further consist of special cellular environment that is thick. It needs the suitable method of defeat cell before lipid extraction. Hence the lyophilization method is considered as one of the important methods in this field (2).

The effect of solvent's type on fatty acid extracted from microalgae

There are two major steps in lipid extraction from microalgae using solvent: one is the full extraction and solving lipid in organic solvent and the other is the omission of non-lipid components in extracted solvent. The retrieval of used solvent and the type of solvent have crucial roles in determining the efficiency of lipid extraction and economic performance of the process (2).

Different solvents solve different kinds of lipid in themselves that regarding the relationship between microorganism lipid and other cellular components the relationship between lipid environment and solvent coexistence and also specifications of solvent, such as polarity and molecular chain length is different (2). The one-way ANOVA test results and Tukey test results between case study solvents showed that the amount of palmitic acid and myristic acid in extracted fatty acid composition by Diethyl ether was more than the two other solvents ($P<0.05$). Also, the amount of palmitoleic acid, stearic acid and oleic acid in fatty acid composition extracted by N-Pentane was more than the two other solvents ($P<0.05$).

These results showed that the used solvent polarity had an important effect on yield and composition of lipid extracted from microalgae. In this study, three different organic solvents were used; Diethyl ether is being a solvent with high polarity and N-hexane and N-pentane being non-polar solvents. The results showed, like the study of Widjaja *et al* (5) and the study of Ryckebosch *et al* (7) on Nannochloropsis salina, that N-hexane is not a suitable solvent to extract lipid from it, whereas in the study on the types of Botryccous, Chlorella vulgaris, and Scenedesmos the solvent of hexane mixture/iso propanol showed better results as compared to other solvents in different temperatures and pressures (26). Also in the study of McNichol *et al* (6), the result of the survey relating to extraction by the method of soxhlet and solvent polarity's effect on lipid yields showed that polar solvents like Chloroform/Methanol, Ethanol, and Acetone had higher lipid yield than non-polar solvents like N-hexane. The spot welding of solvent is another factor that influences the choice of a solvent in biomass lipid extraction. Among the case study of solvents, Diethyl ether has the lowest spot welding and has advantage over the two other solvents.

Effect of biomass drying method and solvent's kind on biodiesel production from microalgae

According to the interpretation of different results attained from fatty acid compositions as the result of different methods of drying biomass and the type of solvent, biodiesel production in the amount of attained triglyceride in each method is meaningful because the oil extracted from microalgae in the form of triglyceride is convertible to biodiesel (21). The triglyceride in Nannochloropsis oculata includes saturated fatty acids and monounsaturated fatty acids stored in cell vacuoles (22)and in some of the microalgae kinds consist of 40 to 70% of biomass dry weight (21).

According to Figure 4 and the results of one-way ANOVA test and Tukey test, the amount of triglyceride in the dried microalgae fatty acid composition in open air and lyophilization method in which lipid extraction is done by Diethyl ether solvent, are more and equal to 76.72% and 75.03% of fatty acid. In this study, three temperatures of high (oven method), average (open air) and low (liphilization) were used. The temperature was one important factor in the amount of triglyceride in the composition of microalgae fatty acid and in the production of biodiesel (27,28). By increasing extraction temperature in oven method, the amount of triglyceride decreased. It was because of triglyceride oxidation in high temperature, and as the result of formation of Hydroproxid (-OOH) by Aldehydes, Ketones and fatty acids, showed more reactions (5).

Conclusion

Because of the temperature effects on microalgae cellular structure and solvent type effects on fatty acid composition, method of biomass drying is one of the determining factors in the extraction of microalgae biomass lipid. The results of this study showed that using lyophilization method in order to dewater and dry biomass and also Diethyl ether as solvent in order to extract lipid from Nannochloropsis oculata biomass had higher yield as compared to other study methods of this research and in researches related to biodiesel production from microalgae lipid.

Acknowledgements

The work was financially supported by the Research and Technology Assistance Division of Kerman University of Medical Sciences, Iran. This work was also partially supported by the Environmental Health Engineering Research Center of Kerman University of Medical Sciences, Iran.

Competing interests

Authors declare that they have no competing interests.

Authors' contributions

SD and BH conceived and designed the study. MM and AR performed the literature search and wrote the manuscript. All authors participated in the data acquisition, analysis and interpretation. All authors critically reviewed, refined and approved the manuscript.

References

1. Lee JY, Yoo C, Jun SY, Ahn CY, Oh HM. Comparison of several methods for effective lipid extraction from microalgae. Bioresour Technol 2010; 101(1): 75-7.
2. Wang C, Chen L, Rakesh B, Qin Y, Lv R. Technologies for extracting lipids from oleaginous microorganisms for biodiesel production. Frontiers in Energy 2012; 6(3): 266-74.
3. Xue F, Zhang X, Luo H, Tan T. A new method for preparing raw material for biodiesel production. Process Biochem 2006; 41(7): 1699-702.
4. Tran HL, Hong SJ, Lee CG. Evaluation of extraction methods for recovery of fatty acids from Botryococcus braunii LB 572 and Synechocystis sp. PCC 6803. Biotechnol Bioprocess Eng 2009; 14(2): 187-92.
5. Widjaja A, Chien CC, Ju YH. Study of increasing lipid production from fresh water microalgae Chlorella vulgaris. Journal of the Taiwan Institute of Chemical Engineers 2009; 40(1): 13-20.
6. McNichol J, MacDougall KM, Melanson JE, McGinn PJ. Suitability of soxhlet extraction to quantify microalgal fatty acids as determined by comparison with in situ transesterification. Lipids 2012; 47(2): 195-207.
7. Ryckebosch E, Muylaert K, Foubert I. Optimization of an analytical procedure for extraction of lipids from microalgae. J Am Oil Chem Soc 2012; 89(2): 189-98.
8. Converti A, Casazza AA, Ortiz EY, Perego P, Del Borghi M. Effect of temperature and nitrogen concentration on the growth and lipid content of nannochloropsis oculata and chlorella vulgaris for biodiesel production. Chemical Engineering and Processing: Process Intensification 2009; 48(6): 1146-51.
9. Huerlimann R, de Nys R, Heimann K. Growth, lipid content, productivity, and fatty acid composition of tropical microalgae for scale-up production. Biotechnol Bioeng 2010; 107(2): 245-57.
10. Srinivas R, Ochs C. Effect of UV-A irradiance on lipid accumulation in Nannochloropsis oculata. Photochem Photobiol 2012; 88(3): 684-9.
11. Umdu ES, Tuncer M, Seker E. Transesterification of Nannochloropsis oculata microalga's lipid to biodiesel on Al2O3 supported CaO and MgO catalysts. Bioresour Technol 2009; 100(11): 2828-31.
12. Arai S, Nakashima K, Tanino T, Ogino C, Kondo A, Fukuda H. Production of biodiesel fuel from soybean oil catalyzed by fungus whole-cell biocatalysts in ionic liquids. Enzyme Microb Technol 2010; 46(1): 51-5.
13. Tan T, Lu J, Nie K, Deng L, Wang F. Biodiesel production with immobilized lipase: a review. Biotechnol Adv 2010; 28(5): 628-34.
14. Uduman N, Qi Y, Danquah MK, Forde GM, Hoadley A. Dewatering of microalgal cultures: A major bottleneck to algae-based fuels. Journal of Renewable and Sustainable Energy 2010; 2(1): 012701.
15. Araujo GS, Matos LJ, Fernandes JO, Cartaxo SJ, Gonçalves LR, Fernandes FA, *et al.* Extraction of lipids from microalgae by ultrasound application: prospection of the optimal extraction method. Ultrason Sonochem 2013; 20(1): 95-8
16. Banerjee S, Hew WE, Khatoon H, Shariff M, Yusoff FM. Growth and proximate composition of tropical marine Chaetoceros calcitrans and Nannochloropsis oculata cultured outdoors and under laboratory conditions. African Journal of Biotechnology 2011; 10(8): 1375-83.
17. Sen B, Koser M, Alp M, Erbas H. Studies on growth of marine microalgae in batch cultures: III. Nannochloropsis Oculata (Eustigmatophyta). Asian J Plant Sci 2005; 4(6): 642-4.
18. Xin L, Hong-ying H, Jia Y, Yin-hu W. Enhancement effect of ethyl-2-methyl acetoacetate on triacylglycerols production by a freshwater microalga, Scenedesmus sp. LX1. Bioresour Technol 2010; 101(24): 9819-21.
19. Gouveia L, Oliveira A. Microalgae as a raw material for biofuels production. J Ind Microbiol Biotechnol 2009; 36(2): 269-74.
20. Durmaz Y. Vitamin E (α-tocopherol) production by the marine microalgae Nannochloropsis oculata (Eustigmatophyceae) in nitrogen limitation. Aquaculture 2007; 272(1–4): 717-22.
21. Pal D, Khozin-Goldberg I, Cohen Z, Boussiba S. The effect of light, salinity, and nitrogen availability on lipid production by Nannochloropsis sp. Appl Microbiol Biotechnol 2011; 90(4): 1429-41.
22. Olofsson M, Lamela T, Nilsson E, Bergé JP, Pino VD, Uronen P, *et al.* Seasonal variation of lipids and fatty acids of the microalgae Nannochloropsis oculata grown in outdoor large-scale photobioreactors. Energies 2012; 5(5): 1577-92.
23. Kleinschmidt MG, McMahon VA. Effect of growth temperature on the lipid composition of cyanidium caldarium: i. class separation of lipids. Plant Physiol 1970; 46(2): 286-9.
24. Huang X, Huang Z, Wen W, Yan J. Effects of nitrogen supplementation of the culture medium on the growth, total lipid content and fatty acid profiles of three microalgae (Tetraselmis subcordiformis, Nannochloropsis oculata and Pavlova viridis). J Appl Phycol 2013; 25(1): 129-37.

25. Abu-Rezq TS, Al-Musallam L, Al-Shimmari J, Dias P. Optimum production conditions for different high-quality marine algae. Hydrobiologia 1999; 403: 97-107.
26. Boselli E, Velazco V, Caboni MF, Lercker G. Pressurized liquid extraction of lipids for the determination of oxysterols in egg-containing food. J Chromatogr A 2001; 917(1-2): 239-44.
27. Sandnes JM, Källqvist T, Wenner D, Gislerød HR. Combined influence of light and temperature on growth rates of Nannochloropsis oceanica: linking cellular responses to large-scale biomass production. Journal of Applied Phycology 2005; 17(6): 515-25.
28. Juneja A, Ceballos RM, Murthy GS. Effects of environmental factors and nutrient availability on the biochemical composition of algae for biofuels production. Energies 2013; 1(6): 4607-38.

2

Biodegradation of high concentrations of phenol by baker's yeast in anaerobic sequencing batch reactor

Ali Asghar Najafpoor[1], Abbas Sadeghi[2], Hossein Alidadi[1], Mojtaba Davoudi[2], Batoul Mohebrad[3], Ahmad Hosseinzadeh[4], Salman Jafarpour[4], Asma Zarei[4*]

[1]Associate Professor, Health Sciences Research Center, Department of Environmental Health Engineering, School of Health, Mashhad University of Medical Sciences, Mashhad, Iran
[2]Assistant Professor, Health Sciences Research Center, Department of Environmental Health Engineering, School of Health, Mashhad University of Medical Sciences, Mashhad, Iran
[3]Educated Student of Environmental Health Engineering, School of Health, Mashhad University of Medical Sciences, Mashhad, Iran
[4]MSc Student of Environmental Health Engineering, Student Research Committee, School of Health, Mashhad University of Medical Sciences. Mashhad, Iran

Abstract
Background: Phenol, as a pure substance, is used in many fields because of its disinfectant, germicidal, local anesthetic, and peptizing properties. Aqueous solutions of phenol are produced as waste in industries and discharged into the environment. Therefore, elevated concentrations of phenol may be found in air or water because of industrial discharge or the use of phenolic products.
Method: The strains of *Saccharomyces cerevisiae* used in this project were natural strains previously purchased from Razavy company. They were grown at 30°C on Petri plates containing yeast extract glucose (YGC) and then purified by being spread onto new plates, and isolated colonies were obtained. These colonies provided the basis of selection. Prepared strains were applied in anaerobic sequencing batch reactors (ASBRs) as first seed. The experiment conditions were optimized using response surface methodology (RSM). After the determined runs were performed using Design-Expert software, data were analyzed using mentioned software as well.
Results: This study evaluated the capability of baker's yeast to remove phenol in high concentrations. The tested strains showed excellent tolerance to phenol toxicity at concentrations up to 6100 mg/L. Study of the batch degradation process showed that the phenol removal rate could exceed 99.9% in 24 hours at a concentration of 1000 mg/L. The results showed catechol is the first intermediate product of phenol degradation. In survey results of the Design–Expert software, R2 and Adeq precision were 0.97 and 25.65, respectively.
Conclusion: The results demonstrated that ASBR performs robustly under variable influent concentrations of inhibitory compounds. The high removal performance despite the high phenol concentration may be a result of reactor operating strategies. Based on the progressive increase of inlet phenol concentration, allowing for an enhanced biomass acclimation in a short time, results at the microbiological levels showed that the increase of phenol concentration was accompanied by a decrease in the microbial community and a progressive selection of the most adapted phenotypes.
Keywords: Yeast, Phenol, ASBR, Biotransformation, Synthetic solutions, Design of experiments software

***Correspondence to:**
Asma Zarei
Email: Asiranuniv@yahoo.com

Introduction

As a result of industrialization, mankind has encountered vast environmental concerns, despite improvements to the quality of life. Rapid accumulation of recalcitrant chemicals in the biosphere severely endangers the environment and human health (1). Phenol and its derivatives are released into the environment through wastewater discharges from industries such as oil refineries, coke ovens, coal conversion, the synthesis of chemicals, steel mills, pulp and paper, textile and pharmaceutical factories. Phenol concentrations in these effluents vary from 10 to 17500 mg/L.

Phenol has acute and chronic effects on human health. Inhalation and dermal exposure to phenol are considered acute effects (less than 14 days of exposure) and are highly irritating to skin, eyes, and mucous membranes. Other acute health effects are headache, dizziness, fatigue, fainting, weakness, nausea, vomiting, and lack of appetite at high levels of phenol exposure. Effects from chronic exposure (longer than 365 days) include irritation of the gastrointestinal tract. Phenol can change blood pressure and cause liver and kidney damage, and the nervous system is also negatively affected by long-term exposure. The Environmental Protection Agency (EPA) has classified phenol as a group D, not classifiable as to human carcinogenicity. Animal studies have not shown tumors resulting from oral exposure to phenol, but dermal studies have reported that phenol applied to the skin may be a tumor promoter and/or a weak skin carcinogen in mice (2-4).

It is necessary to develop highly efficient techniques for the removal of these pollutants from wastewater to protect the environment. Several methods have been developed for phenol removal, such as precipitation, coagulation, ion exchange, and ultrafiltration; however, each of these methods suffers from one or more limitations (5). Biodegradation has been highly appreciated as the most versatile promising approach. Indeed, bioprocesses have been proven to be efficient approaches for the complete mineralization of organic compounds (6). Additionally, biological methods are preferred over physicochemical methods because of their economical aspects as well as nontoxic by-products. The anaerobic degradation of phenol offers the advantages of requiring no oxygen, producing low waste-biomass, and generating a valuable waste product - methane gas (7-10). In the available literature, no report on the treatment of phenol using an anaerobic sequencing batch reactor (ASBR) was found. Different anaerobic technologies have been implemented to cope with the presence of phenol because of the advantages they offer over other biological unit operations, eg., high organic loading rates, low sludge production, and energy production. Among them are ASBRs, given their various advantages such as operational simplicity, efficient quality control of the effluent, flexibility of use, and high biogas yield (4,11). Accordingly, understanding the various aspects of this process is essential to improve the efficiency of the system. Among microorganisms, yeasts have high capabilities in the degradation of recalcitrant compounds such as phenol. Thus, the primary objective of this study was to investigate the performance of the ASBR when treating a synthetic wastewater containing high concentrations of phenol.

Methods

2.1 Preparation of yeast

The *Saccharomyces cerevisiae* strains tested in this project are natural strains previously purchased from Razavy company. They were grown at 30°C on Petri plates containing yeast extract glucose (YGC) and then purified by spreading them onto new plates to obtain isolated colonies (Figure 1). These colonies provided the basis of selection.

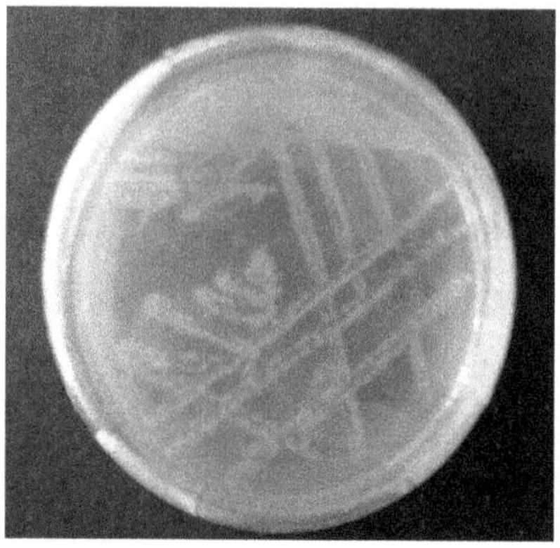

Figure 1. Image of the yeast culture in yeast extract glucose (YGC) medium under a temperature of 30°C.

Bioreactor and culture conditions

The optimal design of feeding is a very important aspect in developing the fermentation process. For the biodegradation studies feeding carried out in the bioreactor contained phenol at different concentrations in the range of (1000-6100 ppm) and was sterilized. Among the aromatic hydrocarbons, phenol is considered to be the principal component that inhibits cell growth (1), particularly when its concentration exceeds 500 mg/L. Moreover, high concentrations of phenol are converted to carbon dioxide at a lower rate than low concentrations (12). It has been reported that some strains of bacteria (6,13-15) or fungi (16,17), especially certain strains of yeast, are capable of converting phenol to carbon dioxide and water and are tolerant of phenol toxicity at concentrations of 500 mg/L or higher. A conventional ASBR to form high density polyethylene cylinders with a working volume of 4 L, an internal diameter of 15 cm, and a working height of 30 cm was operated under anaerobic conditions in 24-, 18.75-, 13.25-, 8.25-, and 3-hour cycles with nearly 95% of cycle time to reaction, about 2% of reaction time to feeding and withdrawal, and the rest to settling. The corresponding hydraulic retention time (HRT) varied between 3 hours and 24 hours depending on the cycle length. Solid retention time (SRT) was set at 10 h.

The initial biomass concentration was 0.01 g/L. Triplicate assays were carried out with 2 different types of carbon sources: only phenol and phenol + glucose. The initial phenol and glucose concentrations were 500 mg/L and 5 g/L, respectively. To avoid excess loss of sludge, the reactor was initially operated at the high settling time of 30 minutes. In the initial stage, feeding time was kept high was and then decreased gradually as the operation proceeded. The reactor was fed with synthetic wastewater containing phenol at different concentrations and sodium bicarbonate to maintain alkalinity in the range requirement.

For microbial community characterization, samples were taken from the reactor at the end of the last operation cycle under each phenol concentration tested. The reaction time increased exponentially with inlet concentration, probably due to an inhibitory effect which required increasing the reaction period and operating the ASBR at a lower organic loading rate (OLR) (Figure 2).

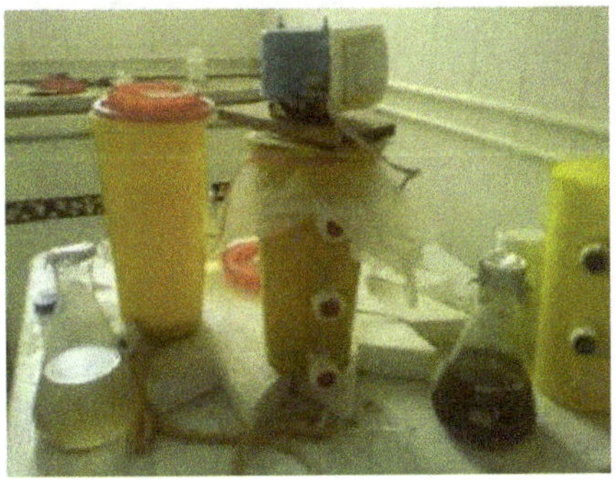

Figure 2. Flow diagram of the anaerobic sequencing batch reactor (ASBR) experimental setup.

Batch biodegradation assay

Optical density (OD) measurement is a common procedure usually used in predictive microbiology to follow microbial growth. It is easily applicable, rapid, and inexpensive compared with plate count methods. Growth curves were obtained based on OD at 600 nm, and the growth rates for the cells grown on each phenol concentration were simultaneously calculated. Cells were incubated at 37°C, centrifuge rate of 200 rpm, and pH of 7.5.

During 90 days of experiments, samples were collected at proper time intervals, centrifuged, and analyzed for pH, biomass, residual phenol, and glucose concentrations. Supernatants of the drawn samples were used for analysis.

Estimation of phenol concentration

To measure the residual phenol concentration, samples were centrifuged in a centrifuge for 5 minutes. Phenol concentration was detected by a direct photometric method based on the rapid condensation of 4-aminoantipyrene followed by oxidation with alkaline potassium ferricyanide and resulting in red coloration which can be measured by a spectrophotometer UV-VIS +T80. The developed procedure was in accordance with standard methods (18).

Estimation of biomass concentration

The biomass concentration was estimated using the dry weight method. A 50 ml sample of culture broth was withdrawn from the bioreactor and centrifuged at 4000 rpm for 5 minutes in plastic centrifuge tubes. The supernatant was decanted into small bottles and stored at 40°C for subsequent phenol estimation. The pellets were rinsed off the tube into a preweighed 1.2 millipore filter paper (Whatman GF/C). The filter paper was then dried in an oven at 105°C for 12- 24 hours, cooled in a desiccator at room temperature, and reweighed until a constant dry weight was obtained. The difference between the preweighed filter paper and the second weight was used to estimate the dry weight of the biomass (19).

Measurement of catechol

To obtain the chromatogram of catechol, the concentration of the phenolic compound was determined by high performance liquid chromatography (HPLC). The gradient elution of 2 solvents was used – mobile phase solvent A (20 mM phosphoric acid [pH 2.0 unadjusted]) and solvent B (acetonitrile) (75:25, A:B). Column Ascentis® RP-Amide 15 cm × 4.6 mm I.D., 5 μm particles (565324-U) was used. Flow rate was 1.5 ml/min. The temperatures of the injector and detector were fixed at 30°C and the sample was injected at a rate of 25 μl. The biotransformation compounds formed by phenol were monitored by the detector UV, 270 nm.

Design of experimental methodology

A design of experiments was applied using Design-Expert 6.0 (trial version). Design study was performed with 4 variables at 2 levels to explore the effects of variables on the response in the investigated region. Biomass concentration, phenol concentration, HRT, and pH were considered the most effective independent variables. A total of 30 experiments with 4 variables was performed and augmented with 8 replications at the center points to evaluate the pure error. The experiments were conducted in an ASBR reactor as described in the Methods section. Percentage of phenol removed was taken as the response. Experiments were performed according to the experimental design matrix given in Table 1 and within the ranges indicated.

The matrix for five variables was varied at 5 levels ($-\alpha$, -1, $+1$, $+\alpha$). The higher level of variable was designed as "+1," the lower level was designed as "−1," and star points were designed as "$-\alpha$ and $+\alpha$." In the optimization process the response can be related to the chosen variables by linear or quadratic models (Table 1).

Results

The results of model statistical analysis

In this part explanations of the study results obtained by analysis design of experimental software are presented (Table 2).

Table 1. Points selected for RSM design

Parameter	Code	-1 Level	+1 Level	- Alpha	+ Alpha
Phenol concentration	A	2275	4825	1000	6100
pH	B	4.38	7.125	3	8.5
Biomass concentration	C	0.50	1.50	0.01	2
HRT	D	8.25	18.75	3	24

Abbreviations: RSM, response surface methodology; HRT, hydraulic retention time.

Table 2. Results of ANOVA for response surface reduced quadratic model

Source	Sum of squares (SS)	Degrees of freedom (DF)	Mean square (MS)	F value	P value, Prob > F
Model	0.061	14	4.348	40.48	<0.0001
A	0.053	1	0.053	493.55	<0.0001
B	3.504	1	3.504	32.62	<0.0001
C	5.042	1	5.042	4.69	0.046
D	3.750	1	3.750	0.35	0.563
AB	1.562	1	1.562	1.45	0.246
AC	3.062	1	3.062	2.85	0.112
AD	5.625	1	5.625	0.52	0.480
BC	1.056	1	1.056	9.83	0.006
BD	3.063	1	3.063	2.85	0.112
CD	1.563	1	1.563	1.45	0.246
A2	8.048	1	8.048	7.49	0.015
B2	6.519	1	6.519	0.61	0.448
C2	2.333	1	2.333	0.022	0.884
D2	1.174	1	1.174	10.93	0.0048
Residual	1.611	15	1.074		
Lack of fit	1.011	10	1.011	0.84	0.619
Pure error	6.000	5	1.200		
Core total	0.062	29			

Mean = 0.91; SD = 0.010; R-squared = 0.97; adjusted R-squared= 0.95.

Optimization of reaction conditions with response surface methodology

As mentioned in the Methods section, the pH and phenol concentrations were crucial parameters together with biomass concentrations and HRT. Design study was performed based on these parameters and obtained results are given in Table 3.

As a result of the analysis, the following model for coded factors was obtained (Equation 1).

$$|\% \text{ Removal} = 0.92 - (0.047*A) - (0.012*B) + (4.583*C) - (1.250*D) - (3.125*A*B) - (4.375*A*C) - (1.875*A*D) - (8.125*B*C) + (4.375*B*D) + (3.125*C*D) - (5.417*A^2) - (1.542*B^{2)}) - (2.917*C^2) - (6.542*D^2)$$

The statistical optimization results were quite promising. Statistical analysis determined that approximately 92% removal was achieved under optimum conditions. According to experimental design method, pH, and phenol concentrations were found to be statistically significant because their *P* values were lower than 0.0001. The positive coefficient value of the biomass concentration indicated that it has a positive effect on phenol removal in contrast to phenol concentration which has a negative coefficient. The effects of phenol and biomass concentrations showed that the percentage of phenol removal increased with increasing biomass concentrations and decreased with increasing phenol concentrations. Time was found to be statistically non-significant because of a high *P* value. When the graph showing the interaction between the phenol concentration and contact time is analyzed; however, it can be seen that phenol removal shows a slight improvement between 3 hours and 24 hours as if it has an optimum value somewhere in-between.

The conditions of the optimum point predicted by the program can be seen in Table 4. In order to verify this prediction, confirmation experiments were performed in the same way as the optimization experiments (Table 5).

The results were between the confidence levels (Table 4) of the predicted percentage of phenol removal. This indicates that the model is useful within the given range of conditions, verifying the reliability of the model. The results clearly showed that parameters influence each other, and the ideal value for one depends on the values of others. This is a unique feature of the experimental design methodology compared with traditional methods in which the simultaneous observation of two parameters is very difficult.

The effects of considered parameters (pH, phenol concentration, HRT and biomass concentration) on phenol removal efficiency are given in Figures 3, 4, 5 and 6, respectively.

Optical density and growth measurement

A previous calibration curve was developed to obtain correlations between OD and growth time of yeast. Therefore, in this work, the area under the OD/time curve was considered an appropriate indicator of the overall yeast growth due to the fact that this value showed a clear proportionality (direct or inverse) with the kinetic growth parameters. As a graphic example, Figure 7 shows the plot of OD versus time for growing yeast under constant glucose

Table 3. Experimental design matrix and responses

Phenol concentration (ppm)	pH	Biomass concentration (g/l)	Hydraulic retention time (h)	Removal efficiency (%)
4825	4.38	0.51	18.75	85
3550	5.75	1.01	18.50	91
3550	8.50	1.01	13.50	90
1000	5.75	1.01	13.50	99.9
2275	4.38	0.51	18.75	94
2275	7.13	0.51	18.75	94
3550	5.75	1.01	13.50	92
4825	7.13	0.51	8.25	86
3550	5.75	2.00	13.50	93
4825	7.13	1.50	18.75	83
2275	4.38	1.50	18.75	97
3550	4.38	0.51	13.50	91
4825	7.13	0.51	18.75	85
3550	5.75	1.01	24.00	90
4825	7.13	1.50	8.25	83
3550	5.75	1.01	13.5	92
2275	7.13	1.01	18.75	95
3550	3.00	1.01	13.5	93
4825	4.38	0.51	8.25	88
3550	5.75	1.01	3.00	89
3550	5.75	1.01	13.5	92
2275	4.38	0.51	8.25	96
3550	5.75	1.01	13.5	94
4825	4.38	1.50	8.25	89
6100	5.75	1.01	13.5	80
4825	4.38	1.50	18.75	89
3550	5.75	1.01	13.5	91
2275	4.38	1.50	8.25	98
2275	7.13	0.51	8.25	93
2275	7.13	1.50	8.25	94

concentrations. Similar results were also obtained for the other yeasts (data not shown). In this way, the maximum area value was obtained when the slope of the growth curve and the upper OD asymptote were higher, but the lag phase was shorter.

Results of catechol measurement

The HPLC analysis of the culture medium with phenol showed a peak at 270 nm at 5.5 RT, which indicated that there was an intermediate of degradation of phenol compared with standard phenol, which showed a peak on 1 RT, which might indicate the formation of other intermediate compounds (Figure 8 and Table 6).

Discussion

Effect of pH

The medium pH is one of the significant factors in the success of the biological treatment process which significantly affects the biochemical reactions required for phenol degradation. Most of the microorganisms cannot tolerate pH levels above 9.5 or below 4.0. However, the optimum pH for different microorganisms is different. *S. cerevisiae* can adapt over a wide pH range, indicating that *S. cerevisiae* can be applied to different climates without the pH value changing. These results support the statement that the growth rate of most yeasts are usually maximum within the pH range of 4-5.5. Finally, the pH effects on phenol degradation were checked, because pH is a major factor controlling fungal growth. In the present work, the medium pH was considered to be 3-8.5 for further degradation studies. As illustrated in Figure 3, the rate of phenol degradation by *S. cerevisiae* did not fluctuate significantly in the range of 3-8.5. Even with a pH above 7, *S. cerevisiae* was able to degrade phenol and grew well; loss of degradation was low. Results demonstrated that the yeast efficacy values under the vast pH value of 3-8.5 were 93% and 92%, respectively. In a study by Park et al (20), phenol degradation by *Fusarium oxysporum* GJ4 was not affected by pH values under 6, and retardation of degradation was shown only in pH values above 7. Even at a pH above 7, *Fusarium*

Table 4. Optimization results of statistical analysis and confidence levels

pH	Phenol con.	Biomass con.	HRT	%Removal	Desirability
4.38	4615.20	1.50	11.86	0.8994	0.958
4.38	4615.15	1.50	11.98	0.8994	0.958
4.38	4619.10	1.50	11.79	0.8993	0.958
4.38	4614.36	1.50	11.63	0.8994	0.958
4.38	4638.81	1.50	12.23	0.9884	0.958
4.38	4617.55	1.50	12.32	0.8993	0.958

Table 5. Confirmation of experiment conditions and results

Run	Phenol concentration	Biomass concentration	HRT	pH	% Efficiency
A	4615.20	1.50	11.86	4.38	0.83
B	4615.20	1.50	11.86	4.38	0.81

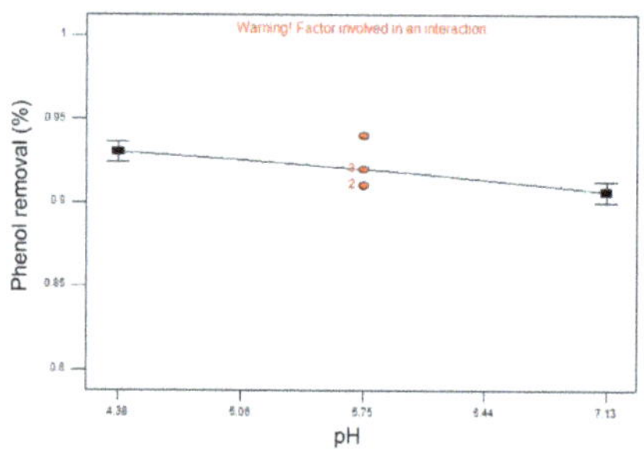

Figure 3. Effect of pH on phenol removal in ASBR reactor.

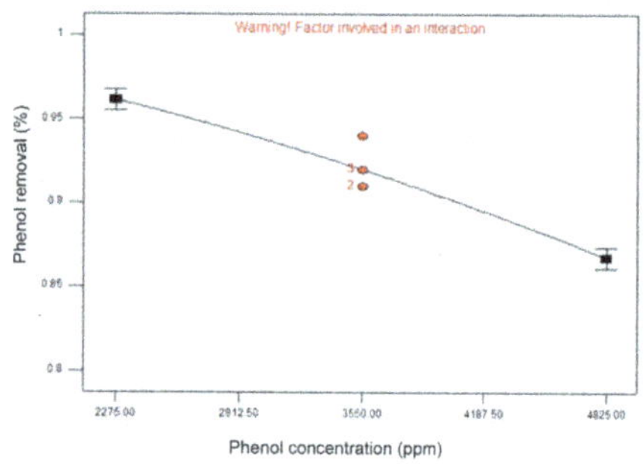

Figure 4. Effect of phenol concentration on phenol removal in ASBR reactor.

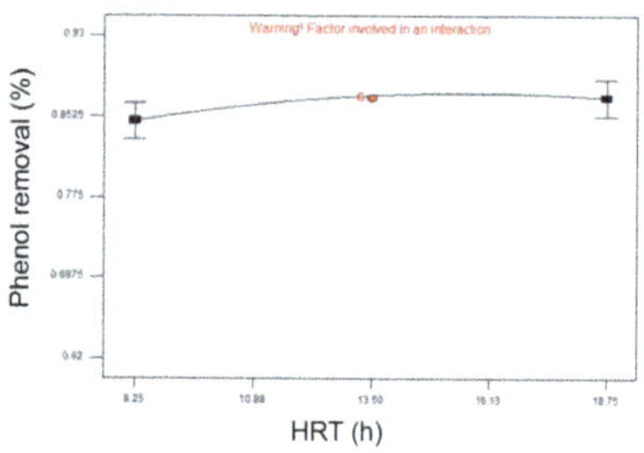

Figure 5. Effect of HRT on performance of batch system.

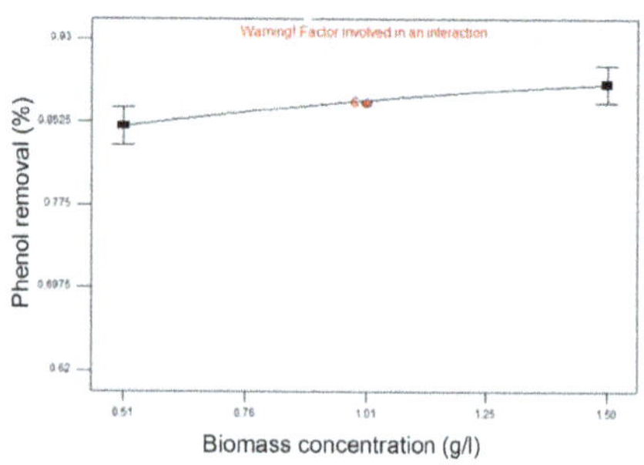

Figure 6. Effect of biomass concentration on phenol removal.

oxysporum GJ4 was still able to degrade phenol and grew well.

Effect of phenol concentration

At first, phenol degradation started once glucose concentration was significantly depleted. The degradation profile shows that the phenol degradation rate was initially high, but later it decreased until the end of the cycle, because

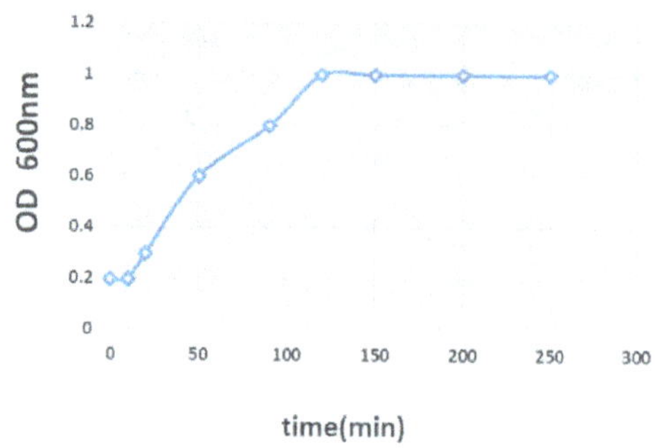

Figure 7. Optical density (OD) versus time growth curves for *S. cerevisiae* yeast

initially, the microorganism has a large amount of phenol available which is food for them, so they degrade it faster. Steady state conditions were reached after 3 days of continuous operation at 100 mg/L, with a phenol removal efficiency of 100%. Average phenol removal was close to 100% at an influent phenol concentration of 500 mg/L with each of the 3 support materials tested. The response of the degradation rate to the initial phenol concentration appeared to have 2 stages. At initial phenol concentrations between 500 to 1200 mg/L, increased phenol meant only a slight deterioration in the degradation rate, indicating insensitivity to phenol in that range. Beyond 2275 mg/mL (Figure 4), the negative effect of phenol was more marked. According to a study by Wang et al (21), the *Paecilomyces variotii* JH6 strain was able to utilize phenol as the sole source of carbon and energy at concentrations up to 1800 mg/l.

The effect of HRT

Biological wastewater treatment processes are cost-effective options, so that they not only can remove contaminants at a high efficiency with a low retention time, but also, the size and cost of the facility can be more appropriate. In an SBR system, the biggest fraction of cycle time is allocated to the aeration phase. HRT is defined as the full volume of the reactor divided by the total volume of wastewater fed into the reactor during one day. Under these operational conditions, the mean phenol removal efficiencies for a phenol concentration of 1000 mg/l were 66%, 75%, 86.5% and 99.9% in HRTs of 3, 8.25, 18.75 and 24 hours, respectively (Figure 5). Wei et al (22) reported that *Rhizobium* sp. CCNWTB701 could grow well in 900 mg/l of phenol and degrade 99.5% in 64 hours. It also degraded 78.3% in 66 hours in 1000 mg/l of phenol. In this study, the *Acinetobacter* sp. XA05 and *Sphingomonas* sp. FG03 strains could grow well in 800 mg/l of phenol and degrade 99.5% and 97.6% within 45 hours, respectively.

Effect of biomass concentration

The initial sludge has an mixed liquid suspended solids (MLSS) concentration of 0.01 g/l. After the conditioning period, MLSS increased to 2 g/l. To test the influence of inoculums volume on the rate of phenol degradation, cell

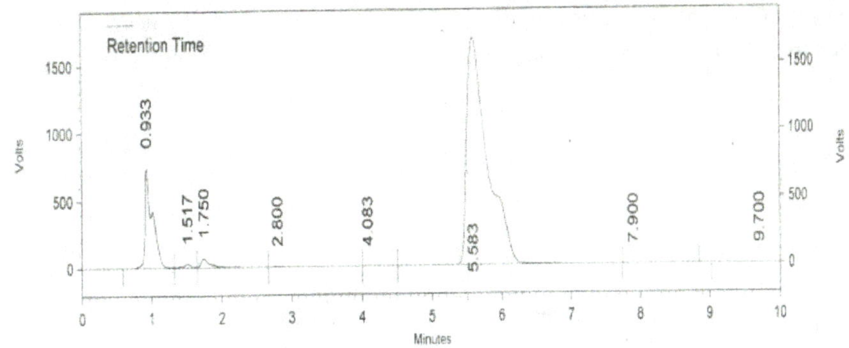

Figure 8. Chromatogram of HPLC analysis of phenol biodegradation by *S. cervisiea*

Table 6. HPLC analysis of catechol on Ascentis® RP-Amide application for HPLC

UV result name	Retention time	Area	% Area	Height	% Height
	0.933	5632782	13.5	741906	21.29
	1.517	247081	0.59	28392	1.12
	1.750	688103	1.65	72170	2.84
	2.800	85450	0.21	3068	0.12
	4.083	9030	0.02	484	0.02
	5.583	39116061	83.93	1692928	66.66
	7.900	18485	0.04	476	0.02
	9.700	7984	0.02	229	0.01
Total		41602976	100.00	2539653	100.00

suspensions with different densities (OD600 nm 0.2, 0.4, 0.5, and 0.7) were added to the phenol (1000 g/l)-containing glucose minimal medium under the same conditions. Results of this study showed a different rate of phenol degradation. An increase in the cell volumes resulted in an increased phenol degradation rate. Phenol degradation occurred after 3, 8.25, 13.5, 18.25, and 24 hours for cell densities with OD600 nm 0.2, 0.4, 0.5, 0.7 and 1, respectively (Figure 6).

When a higher amount of biomass was inoculated, tolerance to the phenol toxicity was observed at even higher initial concentrations of up to of 3550-4825 mg/L, although the growth was quite low. In this case, the degradation efficiency for phenol was also lower. Moreover, degradation was still observed for phenol in the concentration of 6100 mg/L; however, cell lyses could possibly occur and the biomass achieved was relatively low when the concentration exceeded 4825 mg/L. Therefore, it is possible to achieve efficient phenol biodegradation using S. *cerevisiae* with a low amount of sludge produced in the treatment of waste water containing phenol. In the same study by Duque et al (3), tolerance to phenol toxicity was observed at even higher initial concentrations (up to 2500 mg/L) when a higher amount of biomass was inoculated, although the growth was quite low. Moreover, degradation was still observed for phenol in the range of 3000-4000 mg/L, but it also lower.

Conclusion

Aqueous solutions of phenol are produced as a waste of industries and are discharged into the environment. The primary objective of this study was to investigate the performance of the ASBR when treating a synthetic wastewater containing high concentrations of phenol. It was revealed that pH had less of an effect on the phenol degradation rate by *S. cerevisiae* than bacteria did. Results concerning the effect of phenol concentrations revealed that these starving cells are able to promote phenol degradation efficiency slightly. Results also showed that the more HRT there is, the greater phenol removal efficiency will be. A direct relationship between phenol removal efficiency and biomass concentrations was also observed. Therefore, based on the results of the current study, this technology can be developed for the bio-decomposition of phenol.

Competing interests

The authors declare that they have no competing interests.

Acknowledgments

The authors wish to thank the Department of Environmental Health for funding this project.

Authors' contributions

AZ wrote the manuscript, and performed the calculations

and experiments; MD and AS performed a portion of the experiment and helped in the calculations; AAN contributed to the experiment design and the preparation of final manuscript. HA, BM, AH and SJ participated in drafting the article and revising it.

References

1. Stoilova I, Krastanov A, Stanchev V, Daniel D, Gerginova M, Alexieva Z. Biodegradation of high amounts of phenol, catechol, 2,4-dichlorophenol and 2,6-dimethoxyphenol by Aspergillus awamori cells. Enzyme Microb Technol 2006; 39(5): 1036-41.
2. Bergauer P, Fonteyne PA, Nolard N, Schinner F, Margesin R. Biodegradation of phenol and phenol-related compounds by psychrophilic and cold-tolerant alpine yeasts. Chemosphere. 2005; 59(7): 909-18.
3. Duque AF, Bessa VS, Carvalho MF, de Kreuk MK, van Loosdrecht MCM, Castro PML. 2-Fluorophenol degradation by aerobic granular sludge in a sequencing batch reactor. Water Res 2011; 45(20): 6745-52.
4. Liu H, Yu QJ, Wang G, Ye F, Cong Y. Biodegradation of phenol at high concentration by a novel yeast Trichosporon montevideense PHE1. Process Biochem 2011; 46(8): 1678-81.
5. Ravikumar S, Parimala PS, Gokulakrishnan R. Biodegradation of phenolic compounds by using halotolerant microbes. International Journal of Plant, Animal and Environmental Sciences 2011; 1(2): 38-45.
6. Dos Santos VL, Monteiro Ade S, Braga DT, Santoro MM. Phenol degradation by Aureobasidium pullulans FE13 isolated from industrial effluents. J Hazard Mater 2009; 161(2-3): 1413-20.
7. Rajeshwari KV, Balakrishnan M, Kansal A, Lata K, Kishore VVN. State-of-the-art of anaerobic digestion technology for industrial wastewater treatment. Renewable and Sustainable Energy Reviews 2000; 4(2): 135-56.
8. Dey S, Mukherjee S. Biodegradation kinetics of Bi-substrate solution of phenol and resorcinol in an aerobic batch reactor. KSCE J Civ Eng 2013; 17(7): 1587-95.
9. Bakhshi Z, Najafpour G, Kariminezhad E, Pishgar R, Mousavi N, Taghizade T. Growth kinetic models for phenol biodegradation in a batch culture of Pseudomonas putida. Environ Technol 2011; 33: 1835-41.
10. Firozjaee TT, Najafpour GD, Khavarpour M, Bakhshi Z, Pishgar R, Mousavi N. Phenol biodegradation kinetics in an anaerobic batch reactor. Iranian Journal of Energy and Environment 2011; 2: 68-73.
11. Moussavi G, Mahmoudi M, Barikbin B. Biological removal of phenol from strong wastewaters using a novel MSBR. Water Res 2009; 43: 1295-302.
12. Sharifian H, Kirk D. Electrochemical oxidation of phenol. J Electrochem Soc 1986; 133(5): 921-4.
13. Rosenkranz F, Cabrol L, Carballa M, Donoso-Bravo A, Cruz L, Ruiz-Filippi G, et al. Relationship between phenol degradation efficiency and microbial community structure in an anaerobic SBR. Water Res 2013; 47(17): 6739-49.
14. Li Y, Liu Z, Cui F, Xu Y, Zhao H. Application of statistical experimental design to optimize culture requirements of Aspergillus sp. Zh-26 producing xylanase for degradation of arabinoxylans in mashing. J Food Sci 2007; 72(5): E320-9.
15. Nuhoglu A, Yalcin B. Modelling of phenol removal in a batch reactor. Process Biochem 2005; 40(3-4): 1233-9.
16. Shen J, He R, Yu H, Wang L, Zhang J, Sun X, et al. Biodegradation of 2,4,6-trinitrophenol (picric acid) in a biological aerated filter (BAF). Bioresour Technol 2009; 100(6): 1922-30
17. Monteiro AA, Boaventura RA, Rodrigues AE. Phenol biodegradation by Pseudomonas putida DSM 548 in a batch reactor. Biochem Eng J 2000; 6(1): 45-9.
18. Carucci A, Milia S, Cappai G, Muntoni A. A direct comparison amongst different technologies (aerobic granular sludge, SBR and MBR) for the treatment of wastewater contaminated by 4-chlorophenol. J Hazard Mater 2010; 177(1-3): 1119-25.
19. Buitron G, Schoeb ME, Moreno-Andrade I, Moreno JA. Evaluation of two control strategies for a sequencing batch reactor degrading high concentration peaks of 4-chlorophenol. Water Res 2005; 39(6): 1015-24
20. Park JY, Hong JW, Gadd GM. Phenol degradation by Fusarium oxysporum GJ4 is affected by toxic catalytic polymerization mediated by copper oxide. Chemosphere 2009; 75(6): 765-71.
21. Wang L, Li Y, Yu P, Xie Z, Luo Y, Lin Y. Biodegradation of phenol at high concentration by a novel fungal strain Paecilomyces variotii JH6. J Hazard Mater 2010; 183(1): 366-71.
22. Wei G, Yu J, Zhu Y, Chen W, Wang L. Characterization of phenol degradation by Rhizobium sp. CCNWTB 701 isolated from Astragalus chrysopteru in mining tailing region. J Hazard Mater 2008; 151(1): 111-7.

3

Using ANN and EPR models to predict carbon monoxide concentrations in urban area of Tabriz

Mohammad Shakerkhatibi[1*], Nahideh Mohammadi[2], Khaled Zoroufchi Benis[3], Alireza Behrooz Sarand[4], Esmaeil Fatehifar[5], Ahmad Asl Hashemi[6]

[1]Assistant Professor, Department of Environmental Health Engineering, School of Health, Tabriz University of Medical Sciences, Tabriz, Iran
[2]MSc Student, Student Research Committee, Tabriz University of Medical Sciences, Tabriz, Iran
[3]Assistant Professor, Environmental Engineering Research Center, Faculty of Chemical Engineering, Sahand University of Technology, Tabriz, Iran
[4]Assistant Professor, Department of Chemical Engineering, Urmia University of Technology, Urmia, Iran
[5]Professor, Environmental Engineering Research Center, Faculty of Chemical Engineering, Sahand University of Technology, Tabriz, Iran
[6]Lecturer, Department of Environmental Health Engineering, School of Health, Tabriz University of Medical Sciences, Tabriz, Iran

Abstract
Background: Forecasting of air pollutants has become a popular topic of environmental research today. For this purpose, the artificial neural network (AAN) technique is widely used as a reliable method for forecasting air pollutants in urban areas. On the other hand, the evolutionary polynomial regression (EPR) model has recently been used as a forecasting tool in some environmental issues. In this research, we compared the ability of these models to forecast carbon monoxide (CO) concentrations in the urban area of Tabriz city.
Methods: The dataset of CO concentrations measured at the fixed stations operated by the East Azerbaijan Environmental Office along with meteorological data obtained from the East Azerbaijan Meteorological Bureau from March 2007 to March 2013, were used as input for the ANN and EPR models.
Results: Based on the results, the performance of ANN is more reliable in comparison with EPR. Using the ANN model, the correlation coefficient values at all monitoring stations were calculated above 0.85. Conversely, the R^2 values for these stations were obtained <0.41 using the EPR model.
Conclusion: The EPR model could not overcome the nonlinearities of input data. However, the ANN model displayed more accurate results compared to the EPR. Hence, the ANN models are robust tools for predicting air pollutant concentrations.
Keywords: Forecasting, ANN, EPR, Carbon monoxide, Modeling

***Correspondence to:**
Mohammad Shakerkhatibi
Email: shakerkhatibim@tbzmed.ac.ir

Introduction

Air pollution is still a serious environmental challenge in the world and is a notable environmental threat to human health (1). The problem is much more severe in urban areas of developing countries, where it affects quality of life and public health. It is usually caused by industrial activities, energy production by power plants, residential heating, fuel burning vehicles and natural disasters (1-4). Carbon monoxide (CO) is one of the most common air pollutants produced by incomplete combustion of hydrocarbons (1,5,6). Epidemiologic studies have reported short-term associations of ambient CO with daily mortality and morbidity from cardiovascular diseases (5).

For plans on how to scale down the levels of air pollutants and prevent their adverse effects, the uninterrupted assessment of air quality is required. For this purpose, measurement of air pollutants in certain points is possible by the use of fixed monitoring stations. So, in a homogeneous environment, measurements from these stations may indicate the levels of air pollutants at each station. However in most cases, dispersion of the actual pollutants remain unknown due to heavy influence by the prevailing dispersion conditions, distribution of emission sources and topography of the region (7).

Nowadays, modeling tools are widely used in many scientific fields, especially in environmental sciences such as air pollution (1). In such cases, various statistical and computational methods can be used to predict the concentrations of air pollutants using a series of reliable data captured in advance. In recent years, the artificial neural network (ANN) model is regarded as a cost effective method to obtain reliable prediction values of air pollutants (8). It is a computational model, which replicates the simple function of a biological network and is used to solve complex nonlinear functions. The neurons are located in the network layers of the model. The layers are defined as the input, the output and the hidden layers. There are many different types of neural networks. The most common structure of the neural network is the "feed forward" where the data flow from input to output units is strictly feed forward. The typical schematic of this structure is shown in Figure 1. ANNs are able to find and identify complex patterns in datasets which may not be well described by a simple mathematical formula or a set of known processes (9).

It has been used to predict hourly air pollutant concentrations in China (10) and has also been applied for forecasting daily PM_{10} and SO_2 concentrations in Taiyuan (11). In a study conducted to predict air pollution index (API), the ANN showed the smallest error in comparison to the autoregressive integrated moving average (ARIMA) and fuzzy time series (FTS) (12). In another study for forecasting PM_{10} concentrations in Turkey, the ANN presented more accurate results when compared with multi-linear regression (MLR) (13). Recently, similar studies have been conducted in Tehran (14), Düzce Province in Turkey (15), in Lisbon (16), in Algeciras (17) and in Spain (18), based on ANN models for forecasting air pollution.

On the other hand, the evolutionary polynomial regression (EPR) as a hybrid method in combination with the genetic algorithm (GA) and nonlinear regression has recently been used in some environmental studies for predicting the shear strength of municipal solid waste landfill (20), prediction of total sediment load of Malaysian rivers and some other environmental issues (21-24).

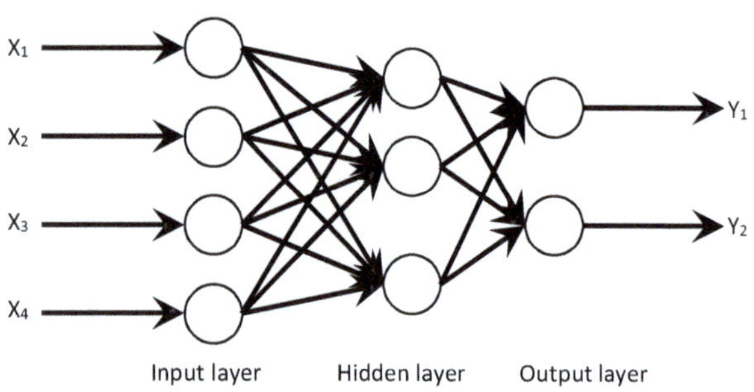

Figure 1. Typical schematic of back propagation feed forward neural network.

This research compared the ability of ANN and EPR models to forecast CO concentrations in the urban area of Tabriz. Considering the high fluctuations in the meteorological parameters of the study area (as an example: there is a temperature difference of about 50°C between the hot days of summer and the cold days of winter), an individual ANN and EPR model was constructed for each month. Having in mind that similar frameworks were used in the modeling procedures, the constructed model for March, 2013 has been explained in this study.

Methods

Study area

Tabriz, located in the northwest of Iran, the capital city of East Azerbaijan lies at 46.13 east and 38.8 north with an altitude of 1351 m above the sea level (Figure 2). According to the census conducted in 2011, it has a population exceeding 1.5 million. It has a semi-arid climate with annual precipitation around 380 mm and the mean, maximum and minimum temperatures are 13, 38 and -15°C, respectively. Table 1 presents the statistical analysis of meteorological variables.

ANN and EPR models

The hourly CO concentrations from March 2007 to March 2013 were obtained from five fixed monitoring stations designated as S1, S2, S3, S4, and S5 (Figure 3), operated by the East Azerbaijan Environmental Office and were used in the modeling procedures. Selection of model input variables with the most significant impact on model performance, is an important step in the ANN model development process. The next step is to build an input-output database required for ANN training. Since the main objective of constructing the ANN model is to forecast pollutant concentrations, the meteorological parameters which are predictable by conventional weather forecasting were used as model inputs (4). The selected meteorological variables included air temperature, relative humidity and wind speed and direction, were obtained from the East Azerbaijan Meteorological Bureau. In addition to

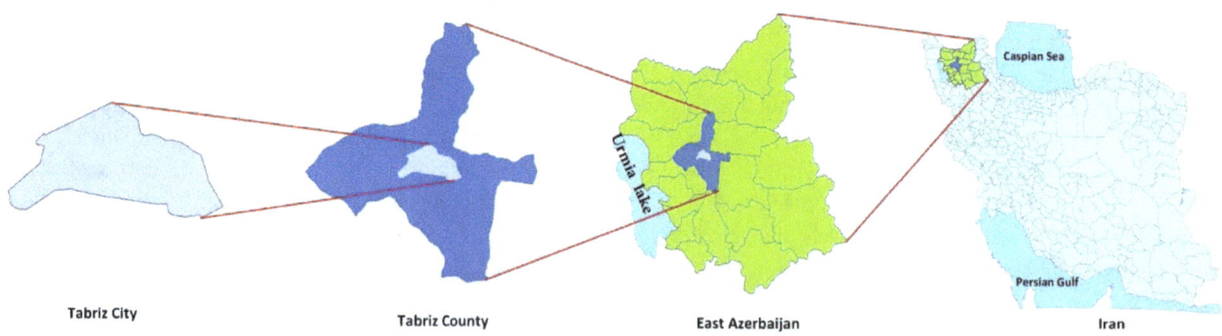

Figure 2. The location of Tabriz in the northwest of Iran.

Table 1. Statistics of meteorological variables

Parameter	Average	Median	SD	Min.	Max.
Temperature (°C)	4.7	4.4	5.7	-12.4	23
Wind speed (m/s)	3.5	3	2.5	0	14
Wind direct	156	120	121.7	0	360
Relative humidity (%)	58.4	58	19.84	18	99

Abbreviations: SD, standard deviation; Min, Minimum; Max, Maximum.

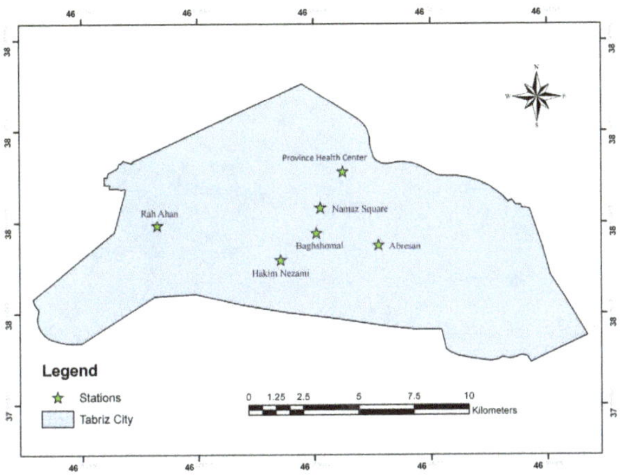

Figure 3. Locations of fixed air pollution monitoring stations in Tabriz.

meteorological variables, the hour of the day and day of the week were chosen as model inputs to cover sub-daily and sub-weekly variations in traffic pattern. For example, traffic patterns during weekends are significantly different from those on weekdays in the middle of the week, and weekdays right before and after the weekends.

A feed forward multi-layer perceptron network was used to forecast CO concentrations at the monitoring sites. The settings of ANN used in this study are presented in Table 2. The CO concentrations dataset were divided into 3 subsets, namely training (70%-80% of all), validation (10%-15% of all) and a test set (10%-15% of all) as an input for the ANN. The training set is a set of samples used to adjust or train weights in the neural network to produce the desired outcome. The validation set was used to further refine the neural network construction and find the best network configuration. The testing set was used to determine the performance of the fully trained neural network by computation of an error metric i.e., mean squared error (MSE) or maximum absolute error (MAE). The EPR model was carried out according to the procedure proposed by Giustolisi and Savic (25). To avoid network overflow, as a result of very large or very small values of input variables, all meteorological and pollutant values as model input had to be normalized (26), before entering the model. To this end, all pollutant and meteorological data were normalized ahead of prediction using Equation 1 in the range of -0.9-0.9. After prediction with Equation 2, the output data were transformed back to the real values.

$$X_{norm}=\frac{X-X_{min}}{X_{max}-X_{min}}\times(r_{max}-r_{min})+r_{min} \quad (1)$$

Table 2. The settings of the ANN

Train parameter	Value
Train function	Train lm
Divide function	Divide rand
Train ratio	0.7-0.8
Valid ratio	0.1-0.15
Test ratio	0.1-0.15
Performance function	MAE
Validation checks	300
Number of epochs	10 000
Number of layers	3-5
Number of neurons	8-25

Abbreviation: ANN, artificial neural network.

$$X=\left(\frac{(X_{norm}-r_{min})\times(X_{max}-X_{min})}{r_{max}}\right)+r_{min} \quad (2)$$

Where X_{norm} is the normalized value, X is the original value, X_{min} and X_{max} are the minimum and maximum values of X, and r_{min} and r_{max} are the values of -0.9 and 0.9, respectively.

In order to evaluate the accuracy of the constructed models to predict the CO levels, four statistical parameters were calculated. These parameters are: MSE, root mean squared error (RMSE), MAE and correlation coefficient (R^2). These parameters were calculated using Equations 3 to 6 as follows:

$$MSE=\frac{1}{N}\Sigma(Pi-Oi)^2 \quad (3)$$

$$RMSE=\left[\frac{1}{N}\Sigma_{i=1}^{N}(Pi-Oi)]^{1/2}\right] \quad (4)$$

$$MAE=\frac{1}{N}\Sigma||(Pi-Oi)| \quad (5)$$

$$R^2=\frac{\sum_{i-1}^{n}\left[P_i-\bar{O}_i\right]^2}{\sum_{i-1}^{n}\left[P_i-\bar{O}\right]^2} \quad (6)$$

Results

Table 3 presents the statistical analysis of measured CO concentrations, at 5 monitoring stations. The 8-hour average concentrations of 1.4, 2.6, 3.9, 2.8, and 3.7 ppm were measured for CO concentration at the monitoring stations of S1, S2, S3, S4 and S5, respectively.

The ANN performance and its comparison with the EPR results and real time measured values in stations S1-S5 are shown in Figures 4 to 8, respectively. The results revealed good agreement between measured and ANN predicted CO concentrations at all stations; however, the measured data were not associated with EPR outputs.

Totally, the performance of ANN and EPR models in predicting CO concentrations is shown in Figure 9. As illustrated, the levels of CO predicted using EPR, were less accurate ($R^2=0.41$) compared to the results with the ANN

Table 3. Statistical analysis of CO concentrations (ppm)

Station	Average	Median	SD	Min.	Max.
S1	1.4	1.1	0.6	0.1	14.3
S2	2.6	2.5	1.6	0.0	12.2
S3	3.9	2.9	1.9	0.0	24.1
S4	2.8	2.5	1.9	0.0	21.9
S5	3.7	3.5	2.2	0.0	19.3

Abbreviations: CO, carbon monoxide; SD, standard deviation; Min, Minimum; Max, Maximum.

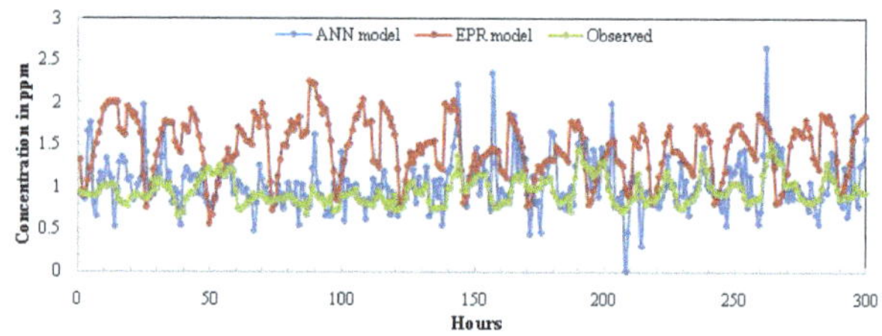

Figure 4. Hourly mean predicted and measured concentrations for CO at station S1.

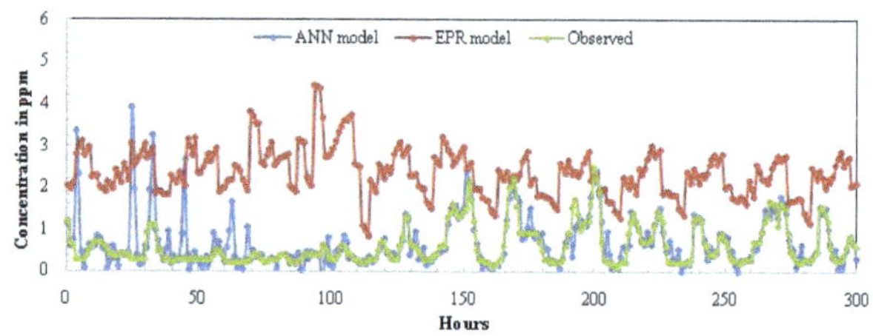

Figure 5. Hourly mean predicted and measured concentrations for CO at station S2.

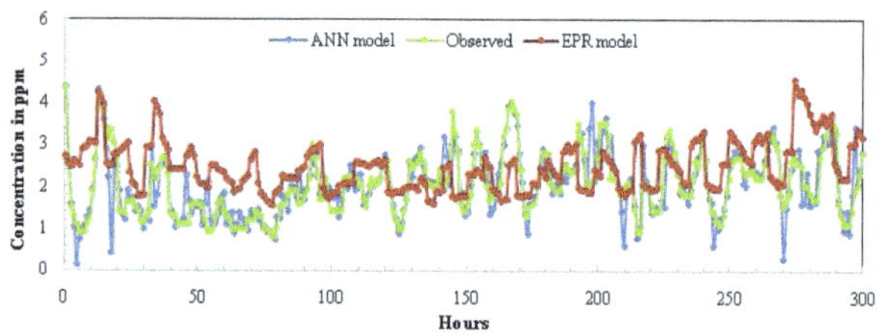

Figure 6. Hourly mean predicted and measured concentrations for CO concentration at station S3.

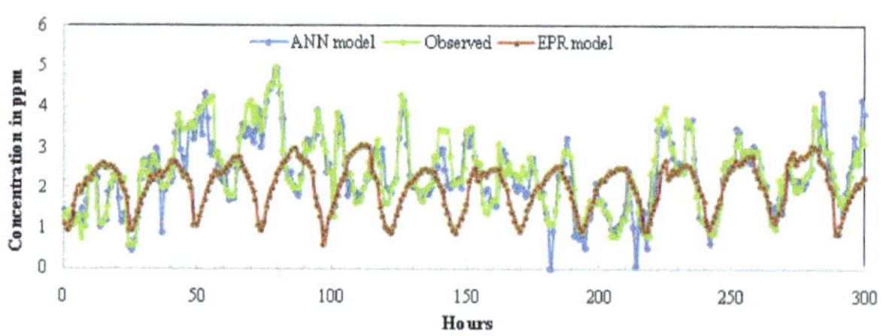

Figure 7. Hourly mean predicted and measured concentrations for CO concentration at station S4.

(R^2=0.93), which indicate that the EPR model could not overcome the nonlinearities of the variables such as meteorological parameters. The performance of constructed models were assessed by calculating MAE, MSE, RMSE and R^2 for all studied monitoring stations (Table 4).

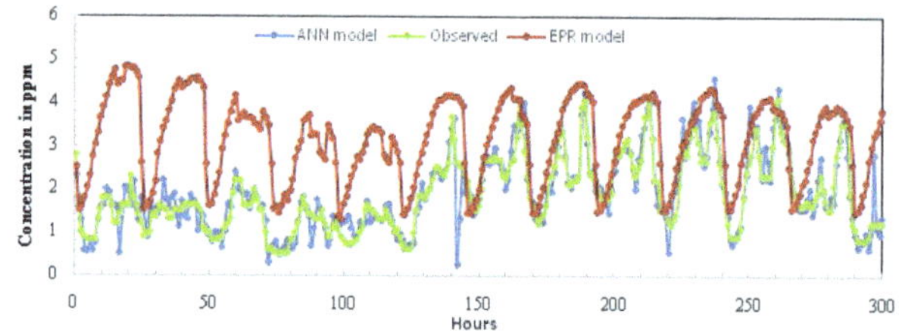

Figure 8. Hourly mean predicted and measured concentrations for CO concentration at station S5.

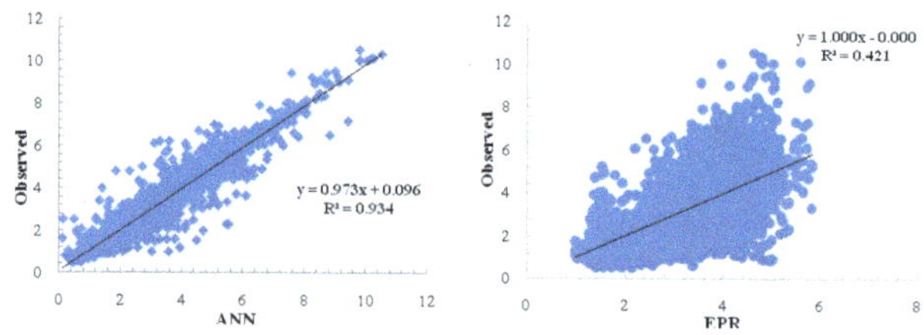

Figure 9. Predicted with ANN and EPR models vs. observed concentrations for CO concentration.

Discussion

A comparison of CO concentrations with the National Ambient Air Quality Standards (35 ppm) revealed that the CO concentration was at an acceptable level at all monitoring stations, during the study period. As previously mentioned, a separate model was built for each month of year, resulting in 60 ANN/EPR models for 5 monitoring stations at 12 months of the year. The important benefit of constructing a monthly ANN/EPR model is that it reduces the modeling errors caused by the inherent variability of the meteorological parameters. The input parameters were selected based on several previous studies which have frequently used these parameters for training ANN to predict hourly air pollutant concentrations (11,13,15,18,27,28). Also, examination of various configurations of input variables and evaluation of model performance was carried out to select the most effective input variables. The results of investigations which are consistent with those of Cai et al (10) and Arhami et al (4) showed that adding or replacing other meteorological variables did not translate to better predictions. The sensitivity analyses were done by omitting input variables one at a time and constructing a new model using the remaining input variables. The results showed that the maximum performance of the model was reached when all six parameters were used as inputs and all parameters had significant influence on the performance of the ANN model. As can be seen in Table 4, at all stations the values of calculated MAE, MSE and RMSE were lesser for ANN predicted values. In addition, at all stations the values of correlation coeficients were much more for ANN than EPR. These results reveal the fact that the ANN model is a successful tool for forecasting of not only the CO concentration, but also the concentration of other air pollutants. For primary pollutants such as CO, which have inert behavior in the

Table 4. Results of ANN and EPR models for predicting CO concentration

Monitoring station	Model	MAE (ppm)	MSE (ppm)	RMSE (ppm)	R^2 (%)
S1	ANN	0.22	0.14	0.38	0.85
	EPR	0.69	0.82	0.90	0.17
S2	ANN	0.19	0.18	0.46	0.93
	EPR	1.28	2.19	1.48	0.17
S3	ANN	0.25	0.20	0.45	0.91
	EPR	1.09	1.18	1.09	0.26
S4	ANN	0.19	0.10	0.33	0.90
	EPR	0.74	0.94	1.04	0.28
S5	ANN	0.25	0.18	0.42	0.93
	EPR	0.97	1.60	1.26	0.41

Abbreviations: CO, carbon monoxide; ANN, artificial neural network; EPR, evolutionary polynomial regression; MSE, mean squared error; MAE, maximum absolute error; RMSE, root mean squared error.

atmosphere, the input varibles considered in this study are enough to reach an acceptable performance of the model. However, it is important to take into account the other input varibles i.e., solar radiation and photochemical data, when using ANN models to forecast secondary pollutants such as O_3 (4,19,29,30).

Conclusion

This research studied the potential of applying ANN and EPR models for ambient CO prediction. The ANN model can be used as a reliable model for the prediction of hourly CO concentrations in urban areas. However, in the case of the EPR model, the results were not satisfactory at all monitoring stations. The presented ANN model can produce reliable simulations of not only CO, but also the concentration of other air pollutant levels. Although the presented model is only valid for Tabriz monitoring stations, but the ANN-based approach can be applied to other urban areas as well.

Acknowledgments

The authors would like to give special thanks to the East Azerbaijan Environmental Office and Tabriz Meteorological Organization for providing air pollutants and meteorological data, used in this study.

Competing interests

The authors declare they have no competing interests.

Authors' contributions

All authors were involved in study design, data collection, and article approval.

References

1. Najafpoor AA, Hosseinzadeh A, Allahyari S, Javid AB, Esmaily H. Modeling of CO and NO_X produced by vehicles in Mashhad, 2012. Environ Health Eng Manag J 2014; 1(1): 45-9.
2. Kurt A, Oktay AB. Forecasting air pollutant indicator levels with geographic models 3 days in advance using neural networks. Expert Syst Appl 2010; 37(12): 7986-92.
3. Lu WZ, Wang WJ. Potential assessment of the support vector machine method in forecasting ambient air pollutant trends. Chemosphere 2005; 59(5): 693-701.
4. Arhami M, Kamali N, Rajabi M. Predicting hourly air pollutant levels using artificial neural networks coupled with uncertainty analysis by Monte Carlo simulations. Environ Sci Pollut Res 2013; 20(7): 4777-89.
5. Chen R, Pan G, Zhang Y, Xu Q, Zeng G, Xu X, et al. Ambient carbon monoxide and daily mortality in three Chinese cities: the China Air Pollution and Health Effects Study (CAPES). Sci Total Environ 2011; 409(23): 4923-28.
6. Levy RJ. Carbon monoxide pollution and neurodevelopment: a public health concern. Neurotoxicol Teratol 2015; 49: 31-40.
7. Zoroufchi Benis K, Fatehifar E. Optimal design of air quality monitoring network around an oil refinery plant: a holistic approach. International J Environ Sci Technol 2015; 12(4): 1331-42.
8. Azid A, Juahir H, Toriman M, Kamarudin M, Saudi A, Hasnam C, et al. Prediction of the level of air pollution using principal component analysis and artificial neural network techniques: a case study in Malaysia. Water Air Soil Pollut 2014; 225(8): 1-14.
9. Zare Abyaneh H. Evaluation of multivariate linear regression and artificial neural networks in prediction of water quality parameters. J Environ Health Sci Eng 2014; 12: 40.
10. Cai M, Yin Y, Xie M. Prediction of hourly air pollutant concentrations near urban arterials using artificial neural network approach. Transportation Research Part D: Transport and Environment 2009; 14(1): 32-41.
11. Wang P, Liu Y, Qin Z, Zhang GA. Novel hybrid forecasting model for PM_{10} and SO_2 daily concentrations. Sci Total Environ 2015; 505: 1202-12.
12. Rahman N, Lee M, Suhartono Latif M. Artificial neural networks and fuzzy time series forecasting: an application to air quality. Qual Quant 2014.
13. Ozdemir U, Taner S. Impacts of meteorological factors on PM_{10}: Artificial Neural Networks (ANN) and Multiple Linear Regression (MLR) approaches. Environmental Forensics 2014; 15(4): 329-36.
14. Nejadkoorki F, Baroutian S. Forecasting extreme

PM_{10} concentrations using artificial neural networks. Int J Environ Res 2012; 6(1): 277-84.
15. Taspinar F. Improving artificial neural network model predictions of daily average PM_{10} concentrations by applying PCA and implementing seasonal models. J Air Waste Manag Assoc 2015; 65(7): 800-9.
16. Russo A, Lind PG, Raischel F, Trigo R, Mendes M. Neural network forecast of daily pollution concentration using optimal meteorological data at synoptic and local scales. Atmos Pollut Res 2015; 6(3): 540-9.
17. Munoz E, Martin ML, Turias IJ, Jimenez-Come MJ, Trujillo FJ. Prediction of PM_{10} and SO_2 exceedances to control air pollution in the Bay of Algeciras, Spain. Stoch Environ Res Risk Assess 2014; 28(6): 1409-20.
18. Sharma N, Chaudhry K, Rao CC. Vehicular pollution modeling using artificial neural network technique: a review. J Sci Ind Res (India) 2005; 64(9): 637-47.
19. Viotti P, Liuti G, Di Genova P. Atmospheric urban pollution: applications of an artificial neural network (ANN) to the city of Perugia. Ecol Modell 2002; 148(1): 27-46.
20. Keramati M, Reshad SK, Asgarpour S, Tutunchian MA. Predicting shear strength of municipal waste material by evolutionary polynomial regression (EPR). Electronic Journal of Geotechnical Engineering 2014; 19: 53-62.
21. Abdul Ghani NA, Shahin MA, Nikraz HR. Use of evolutionary polynomial regression (EPR) for prediction of total sediment load of Malaysian rivers. International Journal of Engineering 2012; 6(5): 265-77.
22. Baawain MS, Al-Serihi AS. Systematic approach for the prediction of ground-level air pollution (around an industrial port) using an artificial neural network. Aerosol Air Qual Res 2014; 14(1): 124-34.
23. Laucelli D, Giustolisi O. Scour depth modelling by a multi-objective evolutionary paradigm. Environ Model Softw 2011; 26(4): 498-509.
24. Giustolisi O, Doglioni A, Savic DA, Webb BW. A multi-model approach to analysis of environmental phenomena. Environ Model Softw 2007; 22(5): 674-82.
25. Giustolisi O, Savic DA. A symbolic data-driven technique based on evolutionary polynomial regression. Journal of Hydroinformatics 2006; 8(3): 207-22.
26. Gardner MW, Dorling SR. Neural network modelling and prediction of hourly NOx and NO_2 concentrations in urban air in London. Atmos Environ 1999; 33(5): 709-19.
27. Zhang H, Liu Y, Shi R, Yao Q. Evaluation of PM_{10} forecasting based on the artificial neural network model and intake fraction in an urban area: a case study in Taiyuan city, China. J Air Waste Manag Assoc 2013; 63(7): 755-63.
28. Russo A, Raischel F, Lind PG. Air quality prediction using optimal neural networks with stochastic variables. Atmos Environ 2013; 79: 822-30.
29. Biancofiore F, Verdecchia M, Di Carlo P, Tomassetti B, Aruffo E, Busilacchio M, et al. Analysis of surface ozone using a recurrent neural network. Sci Total Environ 2015; 514: 379-87.
30. Luna AS, Paredes ML, De Oliveira GC, Correa SM. Prediction of ozone concentration in tropospheric levels using artificial neural networks and support vector machine at Rio de Janeiro, Brazil. Atmos Environ 2014; 98: 98-104.

4

Prevalence of noise induced hearing loss among vehicle drivers at Bandar Abbas freight terminal, south of Iran

Leila Rezaei[1], **Vali Alipour**[2*]

[1]MSc, Bandar Abbas Health Center, Hormozgan University of Medical Sciences, Bandar Abbas, Iran
[2]Assistant Professor, Environmental Health Engineering Department, School of Health, Hormozgan University of Medical Sciences, Bandar Abbas, Iran

Abstract

Background: Traffic noise is one of the major sources of environmental pollution that can cause permanent or temporary loss of hearing in drivers. The purpose of this study was to estimate the prevalence of hearing loss among professional long-distance drivers in Bandar Abbas freight terminal.

Methods: One thousand long distance occupational drivers in Bandar Abbas freight terminal not certified by underlying medical conditions were selected for this study. The demographic background, experience, type and kind of vehicles were recorded in a check list. Audiometry test was done at 500, 1000, 2000, 3000, 4000, 6000, and 8000 Hz using Welton 1300 audiometer equipped with AD-19 supra-aural earphones. Statistical analysis was done using analysis of variance (ANOVA).

Results: The age, experience, vehicle kind and weight of drivers were 34.02 ± 13.19, 8.21 ± 7.84, and 8.73 ± 6.12 years and 68.30 ± 15.61 kg. Approximately 52% of drivers studied had a degree of hearing loss. The most common type of hearing loss was sensorineural with mild loss of 69% and 70.9% for the left and right ears, respectively.

Conclusion: Periodic medical examination with emphasis on the audiometry can be a way of diagnosing hearing loss in the drivers In addition to providing training courses for the drivers on hearing protection, the use of ear muffs equipment in the truck noise can also be considered as a solution.

Keywords: Hearing loss, Driver, Bandar Abbas freight terminal, Vehicle

***Correspondence to:**
Vali Alipour
Email: V_alip@yahoo.com

Introduction

Noise exposure at work can harm workers' health. The most well-known effect of noise at work is loss of hearing. Psychological, physiological and social effects such as feelings of disturbance, stress reactions and sleep disorders, some hormonal changes, increased blood pressure, increased risk of myocardial infarction and impairment of wellbeing and general quality of life can be caused by noise (1,2). There exist a close relationship between prolonged exposure to noise at high intensity, damage to the sensory hair cells of the inner ear and development of permanent hearing threshold shift in noise intelligibility (3,4). Noise from the work place environment can influence the development of cardiovascular diseases and hypertension in addition to hearing defect. High noise level is a causal factor for severe stress which has impacts on the health and daily life, for example through performance disorders, sleep disorders, and conversation interference (5). Sound damages the ear first at a frequency of about 4 kHz (A4 kHz notch) and one of the reasons for this is the acoustic resonance characteristics of the external ear. This hard-walled tube, closed at one end, amplifies acoustic energy in the upper frequencies by about 10 decibels. In addition, individual variation in the acoustic transfer characteristics of the tube is a factor in large variability in people's susceptibility to noise (6).

Nowadays, noise pollution is one of the major sources of environmental pollution caused by traffic. Excessive levels of noise are encountered due to traffic noise, and this situation can cause a permanent or temporary loss of hearing for the drivers. Professional drivers are the most susceptible to high noise levels for long duration (7-9). Injuries such as hearing loss caused by noise is called noise induced hearing loss (NIHL). This can be caused by several factors other than noise, but NIHL which is different in one important way can be reduced or prevented altogether (10). NIHL a type of HL is characterized by irreversible character and progressive evolution such as sensorineural hearing loss, almost always bilateral and symmetrical, not exceeding 40 dB (NA) at low frequencies and 75 dB (NA) at high frequencies, self-manifestation at 6000, 4000 and or 3000 Hz, extending up to frequencies of 8000, 2000, 1000, 500, 250 Hz, but preventable (11,12).

There is a great lack of good quality data describing the

epidemiology of acquired driver's sensorineural hearing impairment worldwide.

Age, sex and some demographic characteristics are the factors influencing the prevalence of hearing loss (13,14). Previous studies have reported a significant correlation between the worker's knowledge of hearing protection in petrochemical industry and their experience (15). The use of other countries data to estimate the prevalence of NIHL is not recommended in this study. On the other hand, few studies were done on drivers hearing loss in Iran. According to the study of Janghorbani et al (16) on the prevalence and correlates of hearing loss of drivers in Isfahan, the prevalence of bilateral NIHL was 18.1%. In another study by Karimi et al (17) on NIHL risk in truck drivers, the results showed that hearing damage of professional drivers was expected to occur sooner at 4000 and 8000 Hz than lower frequencies. An assessment of noise exposure by job and dosimeter parameter in automobile press factories revealed that the levels exceeded 85 dBA, recommended by the US National Institute for Occupational Safety and Health (NIOSH) in all leaders and forklift drivers and in 83.3%, 97.4% and 91.7% of press operators, palette men and crane operators, respectively (18). A study in India had identified noise levels in bus and cabs at 89-106 dB. They observed that 89% of the bus drivers had abnormal audiograms that is impaired hearing (19).

Hearing loss usually develops over a period of several years. Since it is painless and gradual, it may not be noticed.

Bandar Abbas, the capital of Hormozgan province is considered as one of the most important Iranian ports on the Persian Gulf and the sea of Oman. This port is connected to other parts of Iran and the world through air, land and marine routes. More than a thousand trucks arrive and depart the Bandar Abbas freight terminal daily around the country. The drivers are within the age range of 21-65 years with different types of trucks and trailers; both old and new kinds of vehicles. There is an occupational health center in the terminal, where the center's facilities were used in the study. The purpose of this study was to estimate the prevalence of hearing loss among professional long-distance drivers in the Bandar Abbas freight terminal by examining the results of drivers audiograms collected through the audiometry tests.

Methods

This cross-sectional study was carried out from March 2013 through July 2014 in Bandar Abbas, south of Iran. One thousand long-distance occupational drivers arriving at Bandar Abbas freight terminal, that are not certified to have an underlying medical condition such as hearing loss, deafness, family history, high blood pressure, blood sugar etc were randomly selected for the study. A check list was used for recording the demographic background, experience and type of vehicles.

Hearing loss was detected and quantified by pure-tone audiometric testing (20). This consists of presenting sounds at different frequencies (Hz) at various intensities (dB) to each ear independently and recording the lowest intensity at which the sound was heard; that is, the threshold of hearing for that frequency in the tested ear. A higher threshold indicates poorer hearing.

The test was conducted in a sound treated booth, using an audiometer (model of Welton 1300, made in Denmark), equipped with AD-19 supra-aural earphones. The selected frequencies used for mid-frequency hearing loss were frequencies pure tone average of hearing levels at 500, 1000, 2000, and 3000 Hz. In order to evaluate hearing impairment, high frequency range of 3000, 4000, 6000, and 8000 Hz were used. The calculation of hearing was also carried out using 0 dB (HL) as reference (9). Guideline of the American Speech-Language-Hearing Association (ASHA) (21,22) was used as audiometric testing method. The index for hearing loss was a threshold at 0.5, 1, 2, 3, 4, 6, and 8 kHz for pure-tone average and greater than 25 dB of HL in the worse ear. The severity of classification of HL was as follows: (mild: between >25 to ≤40 dB), (moderate: between >40 to ≤60 dB) and greater than 60 dB of HL was classified as severe (23). Bilateral and unilateral HL were present when pure-tone audiometry respectively were 25 dB HL in both ears, and in one ear was equal to or below 25 dB HL and above 25 dB HL in the other ear, or when there was a value over 50 dB HL in at least one frequency. The data were stored in Microsoft Excel and descriptive statistics by mean, median, minimum and maximum values were used. For more statistical analysis, SPSS version 19 software was used; where the Pearson correlation coefficient was used to assess the correlation between the ages of the individuals surveyed and NIHL. In addition, the *t* test and analysis of variance (ANOVA) test with the level of significance at $P<0.05$ were used.

Results

General characteristics of studied drivers and vehicles are shown in Table 1.

Based on the results in Table 1, the average age of drivers and vehicle were 34.02± 13.19 years and 8.73±6.12 years respectively. It means the drivers and vehicles are almost young. The population involved in audiometry test is a sample of the related result shown in Figure 1.

After the audiometry test, the drivers were classified into 2 groups, namely drivers with 1) normal and 2) abnormal hearing. Their hearing situation was classified using the right and left ear. The results of this classification is shown in Figure 2.

After these classifications, drivers who were placed in the

Table 1. General characteristics of studied drivers and vehicles

Parameters	Mean	Standard deviation
Age (y)	34.02	13.19
Duration of work (y)	8.21	7.84
Vehicle old (y)	8.73	6.12
Weight (kg)	68.30	15.61

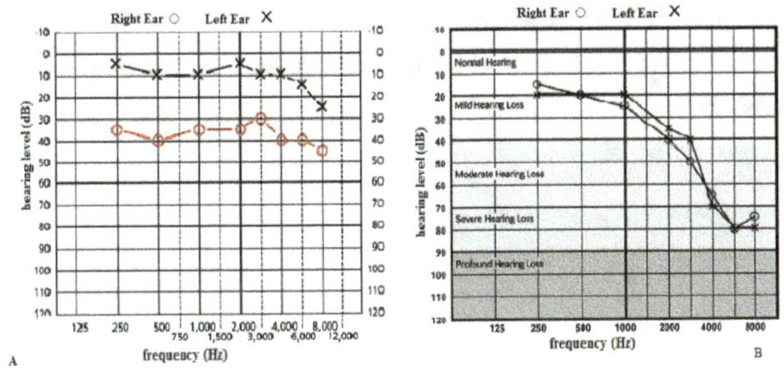

Figure 1. A sample of air-conduction thresholds audiometry result (A) a sample of audiogram classification (B) (24).

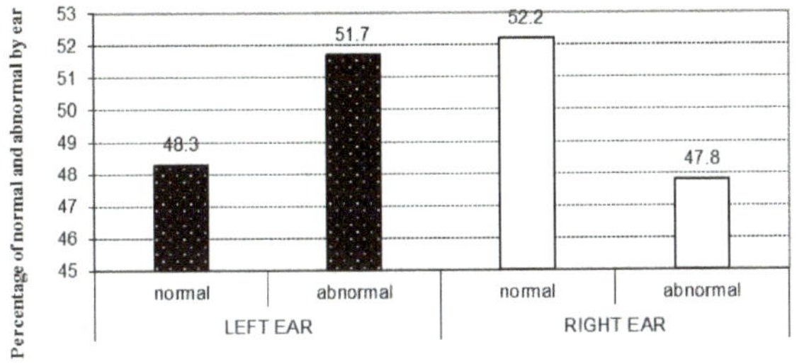

Figure 2. The drivers hearing situation classified by right and left ear.

abnormal hearing group were screened based on the severity of hearing loss by the type of hearing loss such as sensorineural hearing loss (SNHL), conductive hearing loss (CHL), and mixed hearing loss (MHL) as shown in Figure 3.

Based on the results from this study, the main type of hearing disorder was related to SNHL and mixed type had the minimum percent of HL in both ears.

In order to evaluate the effect of the related parameters, an analysis was done on data and the results (the mean and standard deviation for air-conduction thresholds of the drivers with HL are presented by ear, experience and age group in Tables 2 and 3.

According to the results from Tables 2 and 3, the mean of drivers' age with abnormal HL is more than the other

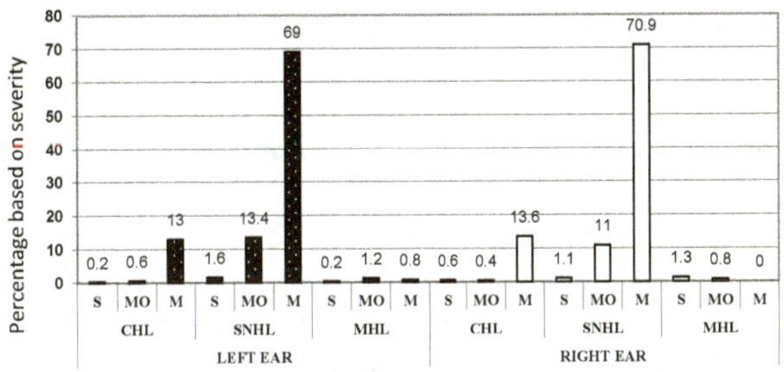

Figure 3. Abnormal hearing loss classification based on severity by left and right ear. Abbreviations: S, for Sevier; MO, for moderate; M, for mild.

group; normal HL means that a higher duration of driving significantly increased the risk of HL in both ears.

Discussion

According to the results of this study, approximately 52% of studied heavy vehicle drivers have some degree of hearing loss. The *t* test showed no statistically significant difference between the 2 averages of hearing loss in both ears ($P<0.03$). Since there was no significant difference in the rate of hearing loss for the left and right ear, one can conclude that the main source is released sound in the cabin of the truck and particularly road traffic does not interfere. The drivers with normal hearing have an average age of about 36.5 years old. However, the average age of drivers with hearing loss are about 42.5 years old. *T* test which was performed to test for statistically highly significant difference between these 2 traditions mean is shown. *T* test indicated significant differences between age and hearing loss in drivers with and without HL ($P=0.000$). Given the observed results (Table 2), the average experience of driving with and without hearing loss were 15.5 and 7.5 years respectively. It is likely that there is a relationship between experiences and hearing loss, therefore, it can be stated that road driving is a hard job and it is necessary that pension legal should be considered for this job.

Table 2. The Mean and standard deviation for air-conduction thresholds of drivers by ear, experience and age group

Right ear				Left ear			
Normal		Abnormal		Normal		Abnormal	
Mean age	SD	Mean age	SD	Mean age	SD	Mean age	SD
36.49	8.55	42.46	9.74	36.74	8.60	42.87	9.78
Experience mean	SD	Experience mean	SD	Experience mean	SD	Experience mean	SD
10.91	7.55	15.37	8.43	10.96	7.41	15.67	8.57

Table 3. Driver with hearing loss by ear, type of Hl and age

HL type	Left ear			Right ear		
Index	Average Age	Number	SD	Average Age	Number	SD
CHL	37.7	70	8.8	37.7	69	7.9
SNHL	43.3	426	9.7	43.5	392	9.9
MHL	45.1	11	10.9	45.8	10	10.3

Abbreviations: SNHL, sensorineural hearing loss; CHL, conductive hearing loss; MHL, mixed hearing loss.

More severe degrees of hearing loss are less in 11% of ears in 13.40 of the average hearing loss in the left ear and the percentage of high-grade, respectively, for 1.3 and 1.6%. One-way ANOVA was used to examine the relationship between age and driving record of the hearing loss, which was found to be between moderate to severe. This analysis revealed a highly significant relationship between the variables of age and hearing loss there. Thus, it can be stated that the risk of NIHL is high in vehicle drivers.
The regulated standard for occupational exposure by NIOSH and OSHA to noise specifies a maximum exposure limit of 85 dB for a duration of 8 h/day. But in many cases, the duration of work in a day will be more than 8 h. Noise protection is not an easy matter for drivers; due to the sensitive nature of driving and the importance of visual and auditory senses, it may not be able to isolate the source and the recipient. Because drivers need to be in aural contact with the outside environment they on the other hand need to be protected from the health damaging consequences of noise. So the use of personal protective equipment (ear plug and ear muff) will not be a suitable solution too. Typically options for the drivers include audiometer test, reduction of drivers work time by implementation of regulations, and standardizing the amount of noise generated in the vehicles engines. The use of silencers between driver cabin and engine is also recommended. By abiding to the mentioned instructions, not only will professional drivers reduce the degree of hearing loss, there will also be a significant improvement in noise pollution.

Conclusion

A truck driver can encounter engine and road traffic noise during professional experience; hence the problem of NIHL has been reported in truck drivers. Among the 1000 vehicle drivers studied, approximately 52% have some degree of hearing loss. The rate of HL among studied drivers needs actions to be taken to reduce the problem. As vehicle noise cannot be totally eliminated, but can be reduced to some degrees, it is therefore necessary to take up intermediation to reduce the risk factors of noisy situations for the occupationally exposed truck drivers. Periodic medical examination with emphasis on the audiometry can be a way of diagnosis of hearing loss in the drivers. In addition providing training courses for drivers on the hearing protection and use of equipment in the truck noise reduction can be considered as a solution.

Acknowledgements

The authors appreciate the department of occupational health of the Bandar Abbas health center, Hormozgan University of Medical Sciences.

Competing interests

The authors are committed to declare that they have no competing interests.

Authors' contributions

All authors contributed equally and were involved in study design, data collection, and article approval.

References

1. Paunović K, Jakovljević B, Belojević G. Predictors of noise annoyance in noisy and quiet urban streets. Sci Total Environ 2009; 407(12): 3707-11.
2. Lin FR, Thorpe R, Gordon-Salant S, Ferrucci L. Hearing Loss Prevalence and Risk Factors among Older Adults in the United States. J Gerontol A Biol Sci Med Sci 2011; 66(5): 582-90.
3. Henderson D, Bielefeld EC, Lobarinas E, Tanaka C. Noise-induced hearing loss: Implication for tinnitus. In: Møller AR, ed. Text book of Tinnitus. Berlin: Springer; 2011. p. 301-9.
4. Vipperman JS, Bauer ER, Babich DR. Survey of noise in coal preparation plants. J Acoust Soc Am 2007; 121(1): 197-205.
5. Kim KS. Occupational hearing loss in Korea. J Korean Med Sci 2010; 25 (Suppl):S62-9.
6. Azizi MH. Occupational noise-induced hearing loss. Int J Occup Environ Med 2010; 1(3): 51-68.
7. Sensogut C, Cinar I. An empirical model for the noise propagation in open cast mines – a case study. Applied Acoustics 2007; 68(9): 1026-35.
8. Kraus KS, Ding D, Jiang H, Lobarinas E, Sun W, Salvi RJ. Relationship between noise-induced hearing-loss, persistent tinnitus and growth-associated protein-43 expression in the rat cochlear nucleus: does synaptic plasticity in ventral cochlear nucleus suppress tinnitus? Neuroscience 2011; 194(27): 309-25.
9. Majumder J, Mehta CR, Sen D. Excess risk estimates of hearing impairment of Indian professional drivers. Int J Ind Ergon 2009; 39(1): 234-8.
10. Abreu-Silva RS, Rincon D, Horimoto AR, Sguillar AP, Ricardo LA, Kimura L. The search of a genetic basis for noise-induced hearing loss (NIHL). Ann Hum Biol 2011; 38(2): 210-8.
11. Hanger MR, Barbosa-Branco A. Auditory effects resulting from occupational noise exposure in workers at quarries in the Federal District. Rev Brazilian Med Assoc 2004; 50(4): 396-9.
12. Thurston FE. The worker's ear: a history of noise-induced hearing loss. Am J Ind Med 2013; 56(3): 367-77.
13. Masterson EA, Tak S, Themann CL, Wall DK, Groenewold MR, Deddens JA, et al. Prevalence of hearing loss in the United States by industry. Am J Ind Med 2013; 56(6): 670-81.
14. Pawlaczyk-Luszczynska M, Dudarewicz A, Zaborowski K, Zamojska M, Sliwinska-Kowalska

M. Noise induced hearing loss: research in Central, Eastern and South-Eastern Europe and Newly Independent States. Noise Health 2013; 15(62): 55-66.
15. Miri M, Fallahzadeh RA, Ehrampoush MH, Salmani MH. Knowledge, attitude and performance of wood painter about harmful effects of solvents and dyes on human health. Environ Health Eng Manag J 2014; 1(1): 25-8.
16. Janghorbani M, Sheikhi A, Pourabdian S. The Prevalence and Correlates of Hearing Loss in Drivers in Isfahan, Iran. Arch Iranian Med 2009; 12(2): 128-34.
17. Karimi A, Nasiri S, Kazerooni FK, Oliaei M. Noise induced hearing loss risk assessment in truck drivers. Noise Health 2010; 12(46): 49-55.
18. Jeong JY, Park S, Yi GY, Lee N, You KH, Park J, et al. An assessment of noise exposure by job and dosimeter parameters setting in automobile press factory. J Korean Soc Occup Environ Hyg 2001; 11: 190-7.
19. Patwardhan MS, Kolate MM, More TA. To assess effect of noise on hearing ability of bus drivers by audiometry. Indian J Physiol Pharmacol 1991; 35(1): 35-8.
20. Yueh B, Shapiro N, MacLean CH, Shekelle PG. Screening and management of adult hearing loss in primary care: Scientific review. JAMA 2003; 289(15): 1976-85.
21. American Speech-Language-Hearing Association (ASHA) Guideline for manual pure-tone. Threshold audiometry. ASHA 1978; 20: 297-301.
22. American National Standards Institute, Specification for Audiometers, American National Standards of the Acoustical Society of America. ANSI; 1996. p. 38.
23. World Health Organization (WHO). World Health Organization International Classification of Impairments, Disabilities, and Handicap. Geneva: WHO; 1980.
24. American Speech-Language-Hearing Association (ASLHA). Guidelines for manual pure-tone threshold audiometry. http://www.asha.org/policy. Published 2005.

5

Antimicrobial activity, toxicity and stability of phytol as a novel surface disinfectant

Mohammad Taghi Ghaneian[1], **Mohammad Hassan Ehrampoush**[2], **Ali Jebali**[3], **Seyedhossein Hekmatimoghaddam**[3], **Mohammad Mahmoudi**[4*]

[1]Associate Professor, Department of Environmental Health, Faculty of Public Health, Shahid Sadoughi University of Medical Sciences, Yazd, Iran

[2]Professor, Department of Environmental Health, Faculty of Public Health, Shahid Sadoughi University of Medical Sciences, Yazd, Iran

[3]Assistant Professor, Department of Laboratory Sciences, School of Paramedicine, Shahid Sadoughi University of Medical Sciences, Yazd, Iran

[4]MSc Student, Department of Environmental Health, Faculty of Public Health, Shahid Sadoughi University of Medical Sciences, Yazd, Iran

Abstract

Background: Although various surface disinfectants have been introduced, most of them are toxic. The use of natural antimicrobial agent e.g. phytol, extracted from *Leptadenia pyrotechnica* is a new strategy. The aim of this study was to evaluate the antimicrobial activity, toxicity, and stability of phytol.

Methods: The serial concentrations of phytol were prepared, and separately incubated with four microbial isolates. Then, its Minimum Inhibitory Concentration (MIC) was measured for each microorganism. For toxicity test, serial concentrations (62.5, 125, 250, 500 and 1000 µg/mL) of phytol were incubated with mouse skin cells, and then cell viability was calculated by MTT assay. For stability test, three common surfaces (stone, steel, and MDF) were considered. Then, 100 µL of phytol was separately spread over their surface, and they have been kept at lab panel for 12, 24 and 36 hours. After incubation, two samples were obtained from each surface and inoculated on nutrient agar plates. Finally, colony count was read for each surface. T-test was used to evaluate the significant differences between groups, and $P>0.05$ considered as level of significant difference.

Results: The MIC50 of phytol against *E.coli, C.albicans*, and *A.niger* was 62.5 µg/mL, and against *S.aureus* was >1000 µg/mL. MTT assay showed that the toxicity of phytol was dose and time dependent. The stability test demonstrated that phytol was stable on the stone, MDF, and steel surfaces until 36 hours.

Conclusion: It can be concluded that phytol has high antimicrobial activity, high stability, and low toxicity. This substance must be evaluated at actual conditions.

Keywords: Antimicrobial activity, Phytol, Toxicity, Stability

***Correspondence to:**
Mohammad Mahmoudi
Email: mahmoodi170@yahoo.com

Introduction

Elimination of pathogenic microorganisms such as bacteria, molds, yeasts and viruses is one of the main concerns of human. Historically, so many natural and synthetic materials have been used for this purpose. Also, various disinfectants including Deconex, Microten, Cidex, and Alprocide have been introduced to remove pathogens from surfaces. Isopropyl alcohol and ethanol were applied to reduce pollution and to minimize nosocomial infections in medical centers. Moreover, to eliminate pathogenic fungi on work surfaces, different materials such as Betadine, Detol, and Savlon have been applied (1-3).

Following the failure of antibiotics and the emergence of new resistant strains, nowadays, scientists are interested to work on plant antimicrobial agents. Several researchers have studied the antimicrobial effects of essential oils, and it has been established that certain essential oils have antiseptic and antimicrobial effects (4,5).

Leptadenia pyrotechnica is a desert plant, and grows in tropical regions of Pakistan, India, Iran, Saudi Arabia, Egypt, Sudan, Somalia, Chad, Libya, and Algeria. The plant has been used as an anti-seizure, anti-inflammatory, anti-allergic, and anti-bacterial material. Also, new studies have proven that this plant is analgesic, anabolic, astringent, and laxative (6-8). Studies have shown that *L. Pyrotechnica* has some bioactive compounds such as phytols, steroidal glycosides, cardenoids, alkaloids, flavonoids, and terpenes. Phytol (3,7,11,15-tetramethylhexadec-2-EN-1-OL) is an important member of branched chain unsaturated terpene, and is a product of chlorophyll metabolism in plants. Interestingly, phytol can inhibit microbes (6-8).

The aim of this study was: 1) to evaluate the antimicrobial activity of phytol, 2) to evaluate its toxicity on mouse skin cells, and 3) to evaluate its stability on different surfaces.

Methods

Preparation of microbial strains

The standard strain of *Escherichia coli* and *Staphylococcus aureus* was obtained from Iranian Research Organization for Science and Technology (IROST). These strains were cultured on nutrient agar (Invitrogen, UK) at 37 °C (Table 1). Also, standard strain of *Candida albicans* and *Aspergillus niger* provided from IROST were cultured on Sabouraud dextrose agar (Invitrogen, UK) at 25 °C. For each strain, a single colony was added to Mueller Hinton broth (Invitrogen, UK) to reach ½ McFarland.

Antimicrobial test

At this stage, 100 µL serial concentrations (62.5, 125, 250, 500 and 1000 µg/mL) of phytol (Sigma-Aldrich, USA) were prepared in 96-well plates. In each well, 100 µL of fungal and bacterial suspension was separately added. Then, bacterial and fungal strains were incubated at 37 °C and 25 °C for 24 hours, respectively. After incubation, the optical density of each well was determined by ELISA reader (Novin Gostar, Iran) at 405 nm. In the control group, 100 µL of distilled water was separately added to bacterial and fungal strains, and incubated in the same way as test wells (9).

Toxicity test

To evaluate the toxicity of phytol,3-(4,5-dimethylthiazol-2-yl)-2, 5-diphenyl-tetrazolium bromide (MTT) assay was used. First, serial concentrations (62.5, 125, 250, 500, 1000 µg/mL) of phytol were prepared. Then, 100 µL of each concentration was added to 100 µL of mouse skin suspension, and incubated for 12, 24, and 36 hours at 37 °C. Mouse skin suspension was prepared according to standard protocol (10), and adjusted at 10,000 cells/mL. After incubation, 25 µL of 5- mg/mL MTT (Sigma-Aldrich, USA) was added to each well and then was incubated at 37 °C for 3 hours. Finally, the optical density of each well was read by ELISA reader at 492 nm. Such as antimicrobial test, in control well, 100 µL of distilled water was added to 100 µL of mouse skin suspension. Finally, the percentage of cell viability was calculated (10).

Stability test

In the first step, three surface models including stone, steel, and MDF were purchased from different shops of Yazd. All surfaces were washed by 70% ethanol. Then, 100 µL of phytol at 1000 µg/mL was separately added to all surfaces, spread using a sterile swab, and dried at room temperature. All surfaces were maintained at lab panel for 12, 24, and 36 hours at room temperature. After incubation, two samples were obtained from each surface using a sterile swab, and inoculated on nutrient agar plates under sterile conditions. Then, the cultures were incubated for 48 hours at 37 °C, and finally the number of colonies grown on each plate was counted (11).

Table 1. Standard microbial strains which used in this study

Species	ATCC
E.coli	25922
S.aureus	25923
C.albicans	10231
A.niger	16888

ATCC= American Type Culture Collection

Statistical analysis

All experiments were done three times, and the results were shown as mean ± standard deviation. Here, T-test was used to evaluate significant differences between groups at P>0.05.

Results

The MIC50 and MIC90 of phytol against two bacterial and fungal strains are shown in Table 2. As seen, MIC50 of phytol against *E.coli*, *C.albicans*, and *A.niger* was 62.5 µg/mL, and against *S.aureus* was >1000 µg/mL (P<0.05). It means that *S. aureus* is resistant to phytol. The MIC90 of phytol against all strains was more than 1000 µg/mL, i.e. none of concentrations could inhibit 90% of microbial strains.

The results of MTT assay were shown in Figure 1. The results revealed the toxicity of phytol was dose-dependent, i.e. the minimum concentration (31.2 µg/mL) caused maximum cell viability (97%) and vice versa. Such a

Table 2. The MIC50 and MIC90 of phytol against microbial strains.

	MIC_{50} (µg/mL)	MIC_{50} (µg/mL)
Aspergillus Niger	62.5	>1000
Candida albicans	62.5	>1000
Escherichia coli	62.5	>1000
Staphylococcus aureus	>1000	>1000

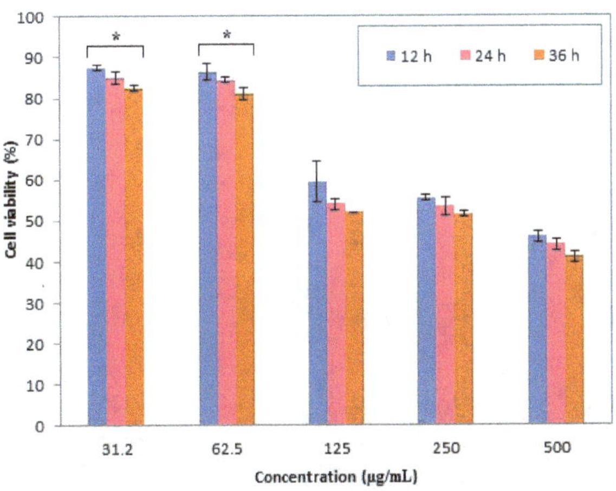

Figure 1. The results of MTT assay. *P<0.05 compared with 125, 250, and 500 µg/mL.

pattern was observed for all incubation times. Statistically, significant difference (P<0.05) was observed between the cell viability of phytol at concentration of 31.2 µg/mL and 62.5 µg/mL versus the cell viability of phytol at concentration of 125, 250, and 500 µg/mL. Another finding showed that the toxicity of phytol was time-dependent. Thus, the decrease of incubation time led to an increase of cell viability. Note that, the lowest cell viability (near 40%) which can be seen in this figure corresponds to concentration of 1000 µg/mL with incubation time of 36 hours (P<0.05) compared with 125, 250, and 500 µg/mL.
The results of stability test are shown in Table 3. As seen, the stone surfaces pre-treated with phytol and incubated for 12 and 24 hours at lab panel had the same colony count, but colony count was increased after 36 hours in both control and test surfaces. There were significant differences between colony count of pre-treated stone surfaces and that of control surfaces (P<0.05). Also, the MDF surfaces pre-treated with phytol had approximately the same colony count at three incubation times. Significant differences were also observed between the colony count of pre-treated MDF surfaces and that of control surfaces (P<0.05). As shown, the colony count of steel surfaces pre-treated with phytol and incubated for 12 hours was 2±2, but the colony count at other times was zero. Here, the significant differences were observed between pre-treated MDF surfaces and control (P<0.05). It can be revealed that phytol can maintain its stability on the stone, MDF, and steel surfaces over the 36-hour period.

Discussion

Although various disinfectants, e.g. Deconex, Microten, Cidex, and Alprocide have been introduced in the two last decades, most of them are toxic and unstable (1-3). In this study, we used phytol, extracted from *L. Pyrotechnica* as a new disinfectant. According to previous studies, this material is anti-inflammatory, anti-allergic, and anti-bacterial (6-8). Phytol (3,7,11,15-tetramethylhexadec-2-EN-1-OL) is an important member of the branched chain unsaturated terpene, and is a product of chlorophyll metabolism in the plant. The mechanism of its antimicrobial activity is not fully described. It is suggested that protein and enzyme inactivation is one of the important mechanisms for inactivation of microbes (6-8). In this study, antimicrobial activity of phytol, its toxicity on mouse skin cells, and its stability on different surfaces were investigated. We found that phytol is an approximately good antimicrobial agent. Moreover, it had no remarkable toxicity and had high stability.
Compared with other studies, the antimicrobial efficacy of phytol is comparable with other traditional disinfectants (12,13). In this section, some related articles have been reported to be compared with this study. Pejin *et al* considered on antiradical and antimicrobial activities of phytol. Its antiradical activity was evaluated by electron paramagnetic resonance. Also, its antimicrobial activity was evaluated by the microdilution method against eight bacterial and eight fungal strains. Its MIC was 0.003–0.038 mg/mL and 0.008–0.016 mg/mL against bacteria and fungi, respectively (14). Kumar *et al* studied the anthelminthic activity of *L. pyrotechnica*. Two concentrations (50 and 100 mg/ml) of methanolic extract were studied in this research. They declared that methanolic extract of this plant exhibited significant anthelmintic activity at highest concentration of 100 mg/ml (15).

Table 3. The results of stability test at 3 incubation times

	Control (cfu/cm^2)	Phytol(cfu/cm^2)
Stone		
12 h	63±5	2±2*
24 h	92±2	2±0*
36 h	183±3	7±7*
MDF		
12 h	65±2	1±1*
24 h	70±3	1±1
36 h	76±2	0*
Steel		
12 h	42±2	2±2*
24 h	105±2	0*
36 h	227±1	0*

*shows significant difference when compared with its control (P<0.05)

Conclusion

Based on the results, it can be concluded that phytol is a good choice for disinfection of surfaces, because: 1) it had antimicrobial activity against *E.coli*, *C.albicans*, and *A.niger* 2) it had no remarkable toxicity, and 3) it was stable on all three surfaces (stone, MDF, and steel) until 36 hours. This material must be evaluated at actual conditions in future studies.

Acknowledgments

The authors thank the laboratory staff of Yazd Pajoohesh Medical lab. This study was financially supported by Shahid Sadoughi University of Medical Sciences, Yazd, Iran.

Competing interests

The authors declare that they have no competing interests.

Authors' contributions

In this study, MTG and MHE were supervisors of MM, as MSc student. Also, AJ and SHHM were advisors.

Reference

1. Rios MP, Morgano SM, Stein RS, Rose L. Effects of chemical disinfectant solutions on the stability and accuracy of the dental impression complex. J Prosthet Dent 1996; 76(4): 356-62.
2. Martin H. Chemical disinfectant and sterilant composition comprising acidic glutaraldehyde. Google Patents; 1984.
3. Mbithi JN, Springthorpe VS, Sattar SA. Chemical disinfection of hepatitis A virus on environmental surfaces. Appl Environ Microbiol 1990; 56(11): 3601-4.
4. Knobloch K, Pauli A, Iberl B, Weigand H, Weis N. Antibacterial and antifungal properties of essential oil components. Journal of Essential Oil Research 1989; 1(3): 119-28.
5. Lv F, Liang H, Yuan Q, Li C. In vitro antimicrobial effects and mechanism of action of selected plant essential oil combinations against four food-related microorganisms. Food Res Int 2011; 44(9): 3057-64.
6. Alqasoumi SI, Soliman G, Awaad AS, Donia A. Anti-inflammatory activity, safety and protective effects of Leptadenia pyrotechnica, Haloxylon salicornicum and Ochradenus baccatus in ulcerative colitis. Phytopharmacology 2012; 2(1): 58-71.
7. Khasawneh MA, Elwy HM, Hamza AA, Fawzi NM, Hassan AH. Antioxidant, anti-lipoxygenase and cytotoxic activity of Leptadenia pyrotechnica (Forssk.) decne polyphenolic constituents. Molecules 2011; 16(9): 7510-21.
8. Dagla HR, Paliwal A, Rathore MS, Shekhawat NS. Micropropagation of Leptadenia pyrotechnica (Forsk.) decne: a multipurpose plant of an arid environment. Journal of Sustainable Forestry 2012; 31(3): 283-93.
9. Pfaller MA, Castanheira M, Diekema DJ, Messer SA, Moet GJ, Jones RN. Comparison of European Committee on Antimicrobial Susceptibility Testing (EUCAST) and Etest methods with the CLSI broth microdilution method for echinocandin susceptibility testing of Candida species. J Clin Microbiol 2010; 48(5): 1592-9.
10. Jebali A, Kazemi B. Triglyceride-coated nanoparticles: skin toxicity and effect of UV/IR irradiation on them. Toxicol in Vitro 2013; 27(6): 1847-54.
11. Chan LY, Zhang VM, Huang Yh, Waters NC, Bansal PS, Craik DJ, *et al.* Cyclization of the antimicrobial peptide gomesin with native chemical ligation: influences on stability and bioactivity. Chem Bio Chem 2013; 14(5): 617-24.
12. Munazir M, Qureshi R, Arshad M, Gulfraz M. Antibacterial activity of root and fruit extracts of Leptadenia pyrotechnica (asclepiadaceae) from Pakistan. Pak J Bot 2012; 44(4): 1209-13.
13. Khan ME, Hanatu I. Anti-nutritional/nutritional analysis and anti-microbial investigation of the ethanol extract of the stem bark of Leptadenia hastata (Asclepiadaceae). Journal of Environmental Treatment Techniques 2013; 1(3): 208-12.
14. Pejin B, Savic A, Sokovic M, Glamoclija J, Ciric A, Nikolic M, *et al.* Further in vitro evaluation of antiradical and antimicrobial activities of phytol. Nat Prod Res 2014; 28(6): 372-6.
15. Kumar S, Chaudhary S, Jha KK. Anthelminthic activity on the Leptadenia pyrotechnica (forsk.) decne. J Nat Prod Plant Resour 2011; 1(4): 56-9.

6

Performance evaluation of non-incineration treatment facilities for disinfection of medical infectious and sharps wastes in educational hospitals of Shahid Beheshti University of Medical Sciences in 2013

Anooshiravan Mohseni Band-pay[1], Monireh Majlesi[1], Mona Tabrizi Azad[2*]

Associate Professor, Department of Environmental Health Engineering, School of Public Health, Shahid Beheshti University of Medical Science, Tehran, Iran

[2]MSc in Environmental Health, Department of Environmental Health, Shahid Beheshti University of Medical Sciences, Tehran, Iran

Abstract

Background: In 2007, a rule prohibiting the use of incinerators was ratified by the Iranian Islamic Parliament. Based on this rule, the Ministry of Health emphasized the sterilization of infectious waste at its production source by means of non-incineration equipment and methods. This research examined the performance of non-incineration technologies in treating medical infectious and sharps wastes at educational hospitals affiliated with Shahid Beheshti University of Medical Sciences.

Methods: This cross-sectional descriptive study was conducted in 12 educational hospitals of Shahid Beheshti University of Medical Sciences. First, a questionnaire was designed and its validity approved. Then the required data was gathered during visits to participating hospitals. Finally, the collected data were analyzed using Microsoft Excel and SPSS version 16.

Results: Findings showed that the daily production of infectious and sharps wastes in the studied hospitals generally equaled 3387 kg. All hospitals were equipped with non-incineration systems; however, only 83.3% of them were active. Some infectious waste was disposed of along with urban wastes without being sterilized. Monthly biological assessments of treatment equipment were implemented for only 41.7% of the equipment.

Conclusion: The failures of the non-incineration systems demand that appropriate investigations be conducted prior to the purchase of these devices. Monthly biological assessments are essential to ensure the accuracy of the systems' performance in hospitals.

Keywords: Waste treatment, Non-incineration technologies, Infectious waste, Sharps waste, Hospital

***Correspondence to:**
Mona Tabrizi Azad
Email: m.tabrizizad2011@gmail.com

Introduction

Over the last several decades, huge amounts of different kinds of waste have been produced by human activities and alterations in man's lifestyle and consumption patterns (1). Medical sciences are among the world's top advanced professional sections. While providing medical services, hospitals and healthcare facilities produce wastes, including body parts and tissue, sharp items, and other types of infectious waste, which are hazardous to the environment and to health (2). Hospital wastes can be divided into 2 categories based on their potential hazards and risks: non-hazardous wastes (quasi-municipal wastes), which include about 75% to 90%, and hazardous wastes which make up the remaining 10% to 25% of total clinical solid wastes (3). Based on World Health Organization (WHO) investigations, 80% of clinical solid wastes in developing countries can be identified as non-hazardous wastes and can be treated just like other municipal wastes. The rest of these clinical wastes are comprised of infectious and pathological waste (15%), sharps waste (1%), chemical and pharmaceutical waste (3%), and other kinds of hazardous waste (up to 1%), like radioactive and cytotoxic wastes, broken thermometers, etc. However, a World Bank report stated that the current proportions of hospital wastes produced in Iran are contrary with those of other developing countries; in the other words, about 75% of hospital waste in Iran should be identified as hazardous and only 25% as non-hazardous (4).

Even though contemporary waste classification differs from that of 5 or 10 years ago, it still goes hand in hand with the advancement of treatment methods. Therefore, meeting the medicinal solid waste manual's requirements is essential to ensuring occupational safety and public and environmental health. Environmental and public health specialists recognized the importance of infectious waste management long ago (5).

Disregard for standards in the collection, storage, conveyance, and disposal of hospital wastes can challenge the country with serious teething troubles in their public health and environmental programs (6,7). One estimate shows that approximately 5.2 million people globally (including 4 million children) die each year from waste-related diseases (8). Furthermore, according to WHO estimates in 2002, 23 million people in the world have acquired infectious diseases such as Hepatitis B (20 million people), hepatitis C (2 million), and AIDS (260000 people) from contact with hospital waste (9). Epidemiological studies have also identified the risk of acquiring infectious diseases like hepatitis B (30%), hepatitis C (1.8%), and AIDS (0.3%) for people who have contact with sharp needles (10). Hospitals, as one of the most prodigious clinical waste producers in Iran, produce 400 tons of clinical wastes a day. However, according to official statistics from the Ministry of Health, 236 hospitals from a total of 875 hospitals in the country are not equipped with clinical waste treatment facilities (11). Falahzadeh et al (12) reported in 2012 that 31% of non-incineration treatment facilities in Yazd hospitals were used in source production. Bioudaghi et al (13) reported in 2011 that 31% of non-incineration treatment facilities in Mazandaran hospitals were used in source production. In 2010, Babai et al (14) studied 5 hospitals of Shahid Beheshti University of Medical Sciences. They reported 80% of them performed the disinfection, cleaning, and elimination of hazardous waste in accordance with the regulations. In their 2004 study in Korea, Jang et al (15) showed that 10% of wastes were treated with incinerators and autoclaves.

Any imperfection in management and disposal of clinical waste can lead to severe health and environmental problems; the best standard methods for managing hospital waste should be used (11). This study examined the performance of non-incineration technology for the management of waste in educational hospitals affiliated with Shahid Beheshti University of Medical Sciences.

Methods

The population of this cross-sectional descriptive study comprised educational hospitals of Shahid Beheshti University of Medical Sciences. Sampling was performed using a complete census. Data were gathered from field investigations, observations, and interviews using an integrated questionnaire designed and validated for data collection. This questionnaire contained 198 questions in 4 categories of common information: disinfection related personnel status, disinfection, and the position of disinfection, treatment and disposal apparatus. This study proposes some appropriate applicable strategies based on the results. Trends for assessing the performance of non-incineration disinfection apparatus used to treat infectious and sharps wastes in the studied hospitals were investigated. Data were analyzed using Microsoft Excel and SPSS version 16.

Results

This study was implemented in 2013 in 12 hospitals affiliated with Shahid Beheshti University of Medical Sciences in Tehran composed of general hospitals (25%), specialty hospitals (8.3%), advanced specialty hospitals (41.7%), and specialty-advanced specialty hospitals (25%). Investigations showed that 25% of the hospitals achieved a first grade of excellence score and 75% of them acquired a first grade score. In the 12 studied hospitals, in only 66.7% of situations were produced wastes weighed accurately; the weight of the remaining 33.3% of the wastes were inferred from container volume. Average daily production of solid wastes equaled 9516 kg of non-hazardous waste, 3090 kg of infectious waste, and 297 kg of sharps waste. These hospitals had 3048 available beds, and the average amount of waste produced for each bed was 4.2 kg per day. The average amount of infectious waste produced was estimated to be around 1.11 kg per bed per day (Figure 1).

It is essential to segregate infectious waste from non-hazardous waste to prevent contamination of the latter. Findings showed that infectious waste was segregated from non-hazardous wastes in 100% of the studied hospitals, but not completely. Sometimes mixing and contamination occurred. The quality of segregation varied from excellent to very poor among hospitals. Two hospitals had a frequency percentage of 16.7%, so segregation was rated as excellent. Segregation at 3 hospitals was rated good with a frequency percentage of 25%, intermediate at three hospitals with a frequency percentage of 25%, and poor at one hospital with a frequency percentage of 8.3%. Three other hospitals received ratings of very poor with a frequency percentage of 25% (Figure 2). Safety boxes were used to collect sharps waste; however, non-hazardous and infectious wastes were also observed in some of these safety boxes. The quality of segregation of sharps waste in the studied hospitals varied from excellent to very poor. It received a rating of excellent with a frequency percentage of 33.3% in four hospitals, a rating of good in 6 hospitals with a frequency percentage of 50%, a rating of poor in one hospital with a frequency percentage of 8.3%, and a

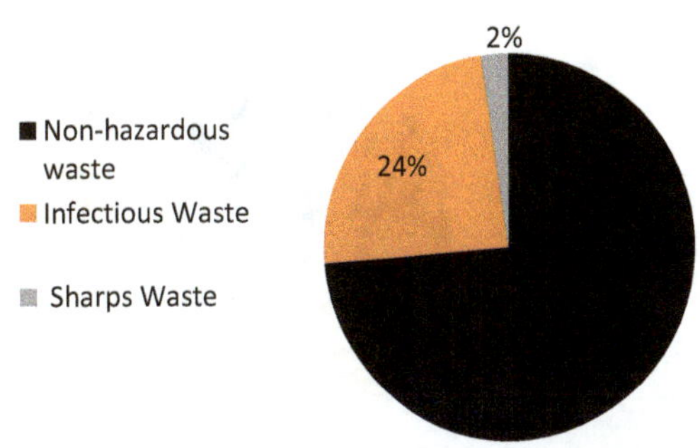

Figure 1. Frequency distribution of hospital waste.

rating of very poor in one hospital with a frequency percentage of 8.3% (Figure 3).

Findings showed that all studied hospitals were equipped with non-incineration disinfection facilities. In 11 (91.7%) of the 12 studied hospitals, the apparatuses were installed. The remaining hospital (8.3%) used a non-incineration disinfection apparatus which belonged to a private company. Eleven hospitals (91.7%) used thermal disinfection methods, and one hospital used a chemical disinfection method. Among the first 11 hospitals, 7 (63.6%) used autoclaves, 3 (27.3%) used hydroclaves, and 1 (9.1%) used the dry-heat sterilization method.

As shown in Table 1, among the 15 apparatuses installed in 12 hospitals, 12 devices (80%) were active and 3 others (20%) were not. In other words, 9 autoclaves (60%), 3 hydroclaves (20%), 2 dry-heat sterilization apparatuses were installed, and 1 hospital (6.7%) was using a chemical disinfection method. Among the 9 autoclaves, 6 (66.7%) were active and 3 others (33.3%) were not.

An investigation of each facility's failure rate in 2013 revealed that 21.4% had more than 5 instances of failure per year, 7.1% had 4 failures per year, 21.4% had 3 failures per year, 21.4% had just 1 instance of failure per year, and 28.6% of the apparatuses had no failures (Figure 4).

To examine the performance of disinfection operations, the hospital waste management manual states it is necessary for hospitals to perform chemical tests in every cycle for autoclave apparatuses and biological tests by means of *Bacillus stearothermophilus* or *Bacillus subtilis* vials for thermal and chemical methods every month. Among the 6 active autoclaves, 1 apparatus (16.7%) had never had chemical assessments, 3 (50%) had some chemical assessments, but not for every cycle, and 2 apparatuses (33.3%) were chemically assessed every cycle (Figure 5). Two apparatuses (16.7%) had no biological assessment, 5 (41.7%) had some biological assessments, but not every month, and 5 (41.7%) were biologically tested every month (Figure 6).

Discussion

The importance of environmental conservation and urban population health requires that infectious wastes from hospitals and other healthcare sectors be disposed of separately from municipal wastes. Furthermore, it is essential

Table 1. Activity status of the disinfection apparatuses in studied hospitals

Hospital name	No. of installed apparatus	No. of active apparatus	No. of inert apparatus
Taleghani	1	1	-
Shahid Modares	1	1	-
Shohada e Tajrish	1		1
Koodakan e Mofid	1	1	-
Imam Housein	2	1	1
Akhtar	1	1	-
Panzdah e Khordad	1	1	-
Labafai Nejad	2	2	-
Mahdieh	1		1
Loghman e Hakim	1	1	-
Tarfeh	1	1	-
Masih e Daneshvari	2	2	-

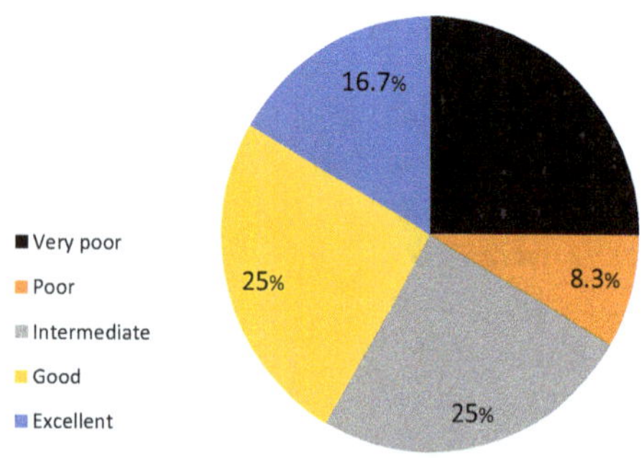

Figure 2. Infectious waste quality of segregation ratings.

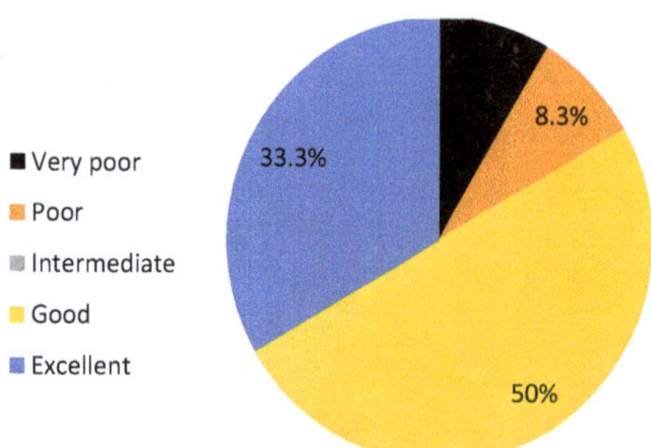

Figure 3. Sharps waste quality of segregation ratings.

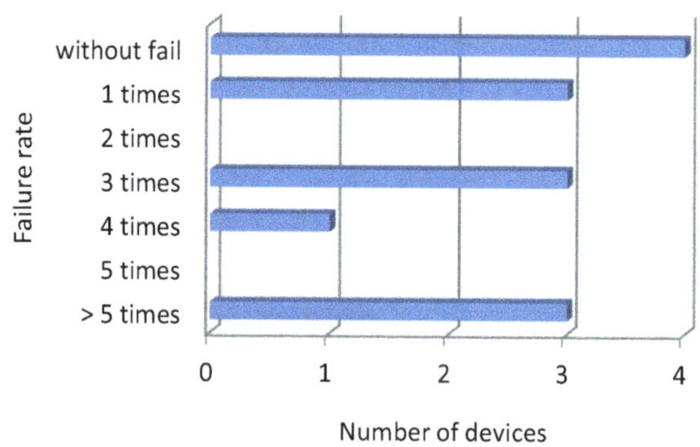

Figure 4. Failure rate of disinfection facilities in studied hospitals.

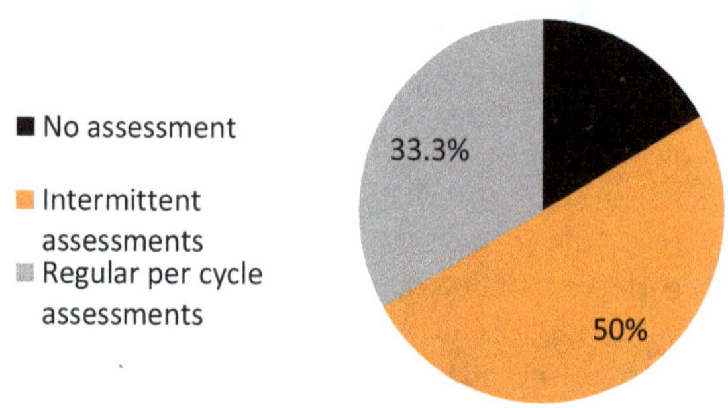

Figure 5. Status of chemical assessments of active autoclaves.

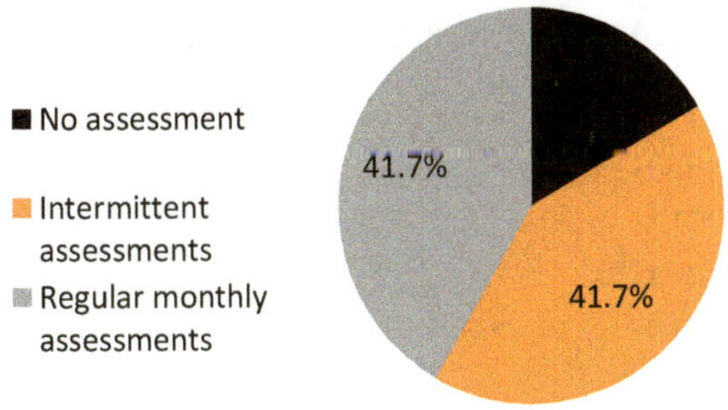

Figure 1. Status of biological testing for all active disinfection facilities

that these wastes be disinfected prior to being discharged in to the environment. If these wastes find their way into municipal waste disposal or recycle areas, they can cause serious problems.

The amount of infectious and sharps wastes in the studied hospitals equaled about 35.6% of total produced waste, which is much more than that predicted by WHO. Segregation of these wastes at the point of production should be controlled wisely. Non-hazardous wastes, like syringes and paper, and chemical wastes, like serum bottles, were observed in an infectious waste container, and blood-stained gauzes were found in safety boxes. Farzadkia et al (16) reported 51.4% of 5 hospitals in Tehran produced waste, and Falahzadeh et al (12) reported this 46.7% of 20 hospitals in Yazd. In Pakistan in the years 2004-2006, the amount of waste generated was determined to be 2 kg per bed per day, and 0.5 kg of that was hazardous waste (17).

Only 83.3% of the disinfection sets were active; 16.7% of them were inactive because of the high costs of repair and part replacement in addition to inappropriate application and interference by untrained personnel. The report conducted by Health Care Without Harm (HCWH) in 2010 on the successful implementation of waste disinfecting in a hospital in Tanzania showed that from October 2008 to reduce the risks of autoclaves and crushers waste before disposal is used (18). The findings of Majlesi (19) showed that, at that time, none of the hospitals had been equipped with disinfection facilities. The current study found that hospitals affiliated with Shahid Beheshti University of Medical Sciences have made marked advancements since 2005; however, the inactivity of disinfection sets can lead to aggravated health problems, since infectious waste is being disposed of in municipal waste landfills without being disinfected and in combination with non-hazardous waste (quasi-municipal waste). Furthermore, the cost of conveying the infectious waste is being paid to the municipality, which is not economical. A serious problem exists because of the inactivity of these devices. The most adverse limitations of such apparatuses include a high annual failure rate and high repair and part replacement costs. The best way to assess the performance of disinfection is through monthly biological tests. Results from this study showed that monthly biological tests were implemented regularly for 41.7% of the apparatuses, while for another 41.7% of them, testing occurred intermittently. The remaining 16.7% had no biological testing done. The findings of Aghapour et al (20) in their study of 39 Tehran hospitals showed that biological tests were implemented in 45.45% of the sets, but the other 54.55% of the apparatuses had no biological testing performed (20). If all steps of waste management are executed wisely and different stages of the set operation observed but no biological testing is done, assessing device performance is impossible. Moreover, if the operation is not performed perfectly, the release of infectious waste into the environment will lead to serious environmental and health problems.

Conclusion

According to results of the current study, some suggestions and guidelines are proposed: (*a*) Employees involved in the disinfection process should be informed about special wastes; (*b*) Medical waste management training should be implemented for healthcare managers, nurses, and physicians to inform them about different kinds of wastes and how to segregate them at the point of production; (*c*) Monthly biological assessments of the disinfection sets should be performed; (*d*) Regular assessments of the sets should be scheduled and their failure prevented by the hospitals; (*e*) The producers or importers of the apparatuses should be obliged to execute periodic technical inspections and provide technical information about the devices application, installation, and biological assessment.

Acknowledgments

The authors would like to thank the cooperating hospitals' executives, environmental health specialists, and set operators.

Competing interests

The authors declare they have no competing interests.

Authors' contributions

All authors were involved in study design, data collection, and article approval.

References

1. LaGrega MD, Buckinham P, Evans JC. Hazardous Waste Management. 2nd ed. New York: McGraw-Hill; 2001.
2. Patil GV, Pokhrel K. Biomedical solid waste management in an Indian hospital: a case study. Waste Manag 2005; 25(6): 592-9.

3. Katoch S. Biomedical waste classification and prevailing management strategies. International Conference on Sustainable Waste Management; 5-7 September 2007; Chennai, India. p. 196-75.
4. Shojaei S, Tehrani H. Textbook of Preventive and Social Medicine. Tehran: Samat; 2004. [In Persian]
5. Beiglu MA. A report of survey on Qazvin hospital wastes. Qazvin: Qazvin Municipality; 2002. p. 67-74. [In Persian].
6. Dehghani MH, Azam K, Changani F, Dehghani Fard E. Assessment of medical waste management in educational hospitals of Tehran university medical sciences. Iran J Environ Health Sci Eng 2008; 5(2): 131-6.
7. Bazrafshan E, Kord Mostafapoor F. Survey of quantity and quality of hazardous wastes produced in Sistan and Baluchestan in 2007. Tabib-e-shargh, Zahedan Journal of Research in Medical Sciences 2008; 10(4): 305-14.
8. Abd El-Salam MM. Hospital waste management in El-Beheira Governorate, Egypt. J Environmental Manage 2010; 91(3): 618-29.
9. World Health Organization (WHO). Health-care waste management, policy paper. WHO; 2004. http://www.who.int/entity/water_sanitation_health/medicalwaste/en/hcwmpolicye.pdf.
10. Environment Protection Training & Research Institute. Bio-medical waste management self-learning document for doctors, superintendents and administrators; 2010.
11. Nadafi K. Comprehensive plan operations program of waste management. 2nd International conference and Exhibition of Waste Management, Recycling, Biomass; 2012 Nov14-17; Tehran, Iran. p. 48-57. [In Persian].
12. Falahzadeh A, Dashti MM, Farahzadi MH, Ghadirian D. The survey of management of hazardous wastes in hospitals of Yazd. 14th National Conference on Environmental Health; 2010 Nov; Yazd, Iran. p.175-192. [In Persian].
13. Bioudaghi H, Panahi Roudsari R, Abadi MH, Mojdeh R. A survey of the medical waste management situation hospitals in Mazandaran province in 2011. 15th National Conference on Environmental Health; 2012 Oct- Nov 30-1; Gillan, Iran. p. 66-7. [In Persian]
14. Babai M, Balvayeh M , Abbasi Moghadam H, Mostafie D. A survay Fulfillmen to fcriteria and special waste management procedures in Shahid Beheshti University of Medical Sciences Hospitals in 2011. 6th National and International Conferences on Waste Management; 2012 May; Mashhad, Iran. p.142-52. [In Persian].
15. Jang YC, Lee C, Yoon OS, Kim H. Medical waste management in Korea. J Environ Manage 2006; 80(2): 107-15.
16. Farzadkia M, Gholamy H, Emam Jomeah MM, Kermany M. Study of the hospital solid waste management in 5 hospitals in Tehran city and presentation of improvement approaches. 14th National Conference on Environmental Health; 2010 Nov; Yazd, Iran. p. 179-91. [In Persian].
17. Jawed A. Hospital waste management issues and steps taken by the government of Pakistan. Ministry of Environment 2006; 22(4): 101-6.
18. Successful implementation of medical waste treatment in Tanzania, 2010. Health Care without Harm press Release. https://noharm-global.org/articles/news/global/successful-implementation-medical-waste-treatment-tanzania. Updated September 22, 2010.
19. Majlesi M, Kashitarash Esfahani Z, Alizadeh S, Forutani F, Gachkar L. Evaluating the solid waste management of hospitals affiliated with shaheed beheshti medical university. Pajoohandeh Journal 2007; 12(4):299-311. [In Persian].
20. Aghapour P, Nabizadeh R, Monavari M,Yaghmaeian K, Nouri J. The analysis of health and environmental statues of using sterilizers in hospital waste -case stady: hospitals of Tehran. 14th National Conference on Environmental Health; 2010 Nov; Yazd, Iran. p. 162-74. [In Persian].

7

Knowledge, attitude and performance of wood painter about harmful effects of solvents and dyes on human health

Mohammad Miri[1], Reza Ali Fallahzadeh[2], Mohammad Hassan Ehrampoush[3], Mohammad Hossien Salmani[4*]

[1]Ph.D Student of Environmental Health, Department of Environmental Health Engineering, School of Health, Shahid Sadoughi University of Medical Sciences, Yazd, Iran
[2]MSc of Environmental Health, Department of Environmental Health Engineering, School of Health, Shahid Sadoughi University of Medical Sciences, Yazd, Iran
[3]Professor of Environmental Health, Department of Environmental Health Engineering, School of Health, Shahid Sadoughi University of Medical Sciences, Yazd, Iran
[4]Ph.D Student of Analytical Chemistry, Department of Environmental Health Engineering, School of Health, Shahid Sadoughi University of Medical Sciences, Yazd, Iran

Abstract
Background: Solvents, which are widely used in industry, are able to dissolve another substance for creating a solution. Solvents have various effects on human health based on their type and chemical composition.
Methods: This was a cross-sectional study to investigate the harmful effects of solvents on wood painters in Yazd city. To achieve information, a census questionnaire was prepared and distributed among wood painters. The studied parameters include the mean score of knowledge, attitude, and practice of wood painters about harmful effects of dyes and solvents on body according to age, work experience, education, hours worked per day, and smoking. The data of survey were analyzed by Chi-square test and T-test in SPSS.
Results: The average age and work experience of wood painters were 29 and 7.5 years, and the age of 25 years and work experience of 5 years had the highest frequency among them. Analysis of data indicated that 71.8% of people had middle school and lower education level, 68.3% was married, 31.7% was single, and 37.5% was smoking. Average working hours were 8 hours in day.
Conclusion: Results show that attitudes had significant correlation with education level and different age groups. None of the studied parameters were not significant correlation with performance. Also, there was significant correlation between knowledge with experience.
Keywords: Solvent effects, Knowledge, Attitude, Practice, Wood painter

***Correspondence to:**
Mohammad Hossien Salmani
Email: : mhsn06@yahoo.com

Introduction

Solvent refers to a substance that dissolves another substance to create a homogenous solution. Liquid solvents are classified into two groups: organic and inorganic solvents. The main groups of organic solvents are saturated hydrocarbons, unsaturated hydrocarbons, aromatic hydrocarbons, halogenated ethers, alcohols, amines, and carbonyl (1). Solvents are extensively used in construction works and chemical industries, so the workers are exposed to solvents in coloring and painting industry, refineries, and many other jobs (2).

Solvents have a variety of health effects, depending on their type and chemical composition. Some of solvents have short-term effects, such as eyes irritation, effects on lungs and skin, nausea, dizziness, and headache (3). Also solvents and dyes have long-term effects, such as skin diseases and cancers. They can cause loss of consciousness and death at high concentrations or long-term contact (4). On the other hand, we have more traumatic effects when we are dealing with chemical solvents. All organic solvents are irritants to skin and cause dermatitis that occurs by degreasing or fat-dissolving properties of skin, also due to their effect on the nervous system and reduction in performance, they can cause problems, such as headache, nausea, dizziness, and drowsiness (5). Organic solvents have the potential to cause injuries and diseases in many organs, including the nervous system, heart, kidneys, skin, and liver (2,6). People were exposed to a mixture of solvents in this job (7). Solvents are used for ductility of the color and are components of dye. One of the solvents is thinner that has plenty of use to dilute colors in painting industry and contains a mixture of toxic organic solvents (2).

Most ingredients of dyes are somewhat toxic and contaminated. All dyes are flammable than water-based dyes. Some solvents are quite toxic and others have some damage to organisms. However, all these problems can be solved with precising control and safety compliances (8). In this study, we analyzed some information of wood painters about the solvents, harmful effects.

Methods

This was a cross-sectional study that was done on wood painters in Yazd city. The information was taken through distributing the census questionnaire among 120 wood painters (wood painter selected by census method). Validity and reliability have also been approved by experts and Cronbach's alpha test.

Twenty questionnaires were distributed among the target population to obtain Cronbach's alpha. Cronbach's alpha was achieved 72.68% after completing questionnaires. The scoring method of questionnaires was one score for each correct answer and zero score for the wrong option. In attitude questionnaires we have the best possible choice of 5 score, and it gets lower on the next level to one. The performance questions were contractually scored from 1 to 4.

The studied parameters include the mean score of knowledge, attitude and practice of wood painters about dyes and solvents effects on body according to age, work experience, education, hours worked per day, and smoking. The data from the survey were analyzed with SPSS statistical software by Chi-square test and T-test. In this study, questionnaire were completed by satisfaction of individuals so there was no ethical limitation.

Results

The average age was 29 years and work experience was 7.5 years. Having 25 years age and 5 years work experiencehad the highest frequency among the participants. In terms of education, more than 71.8% of people have middle school and lower education levels. The results are shown in Table 1.

Also, data showed that 68.3% were married, 31.7% were single, and 37.5% of people were smoking. Average working hours were 8 hours per day.

According to the obtained scores by wood painters from questionnaires and use of T-test (P=0.05), the mean scores of attitude, knowledge, and performance were correlated based on their age group, experience, education, and smoking. The correlation coefficients are listed in Table 2.

Also, wood painters were classified into categories in terms of work experience (below and above 10 years) and smoking (smokers and non-smokers). There was no significant correlation in the attitude scores in different age groups based on their work experience (P= 0.059). There was no significant correlation between/with knowledge scores in different age groups based on their work experience (P= 0.852). The relation of performance scores in different age groups based on their work experience is dubious (P= 0.05), and it can make a significant correlation if the number of samples is increased. There was no significant correlation between/with the mean attitude score in both groups of smokers and non-smokers (P= 0.686). There was significant correlation between/with the mean knowledge score in both groups of smokers and non-smokers (P= 0.001), and there was a significant correlation between/with the mean performance scores in both groups of smokers and non-smokers (P= 0.003).

Table 1. Distribution of educational status of Yazd wood painters

Education	Number	Percent
Illiterate	16	13.3
Elementary school	36	30
Middle school	23	27.5
High school	32	18.3
Associate and Bachelor degree	8	6.7
Master›s degree or higher	5	4.2
Sum	120	100

Table 2. The correlation coefficients of studied parameters

Variables	Age	Experience	Education	Smoking
Knowledge	0.103	0.020	0.058	0.723
Attitude	0.000	0.523	0.000	0.825
Performance	0.162	0.438	0.059	0.050

Discussion

To achieve a comprehensive view of behavior about the health effects of solvents and dyes on the painters, we conduct a study on comparison of individual characteristics including work experience, education level, and individual age on people with an average age of 29 years and the average work experience of 7.5 years; this is consistent with the study done by Ghasemi and Karami; They conducted a study on the attitudes and behaviors of Fars greenhouse owners with the median age of 31 years and 1-3 years of experience about using chemical pesticides in greenhouses (8).

The effect of age

According to study's findings we can say that there was a difference between individual attitudes with various work experience and there was no significant correlation, but, there was a significant correlation between individual attitudes with their education and different age groups. In Ghasemi and Karami study (8), younger workers with less education and work experience had a poor attitude in using pesticides. Dadgari *et al* (9) studied the nurses' attitudes regarding sex, age, education and work experience. In this study, none of the variables had significant correlation with attitude that confirms the relationship between experience and attitude in our research, but it is unlike in other parameters that was obtained in the present study. These differences may be resulted from differences in the studied population (9). This result can be seen in Fung's study as well (10).

The effect of performance

Additionally, we studied wood painters' performance that work with dyes and solvents in terms of parameters such as age, education, and work experience.

The results show that there was no significant correlation between/with the individual performance with work experience, age, and education that confirms the results of Dadgari *et al* study (9). In another study conducted in India, this conclusion was obtained that education alone does not affect performance (11).

The effect of knowledge

Knowledge about the effects of solvents and dyes on body among wood painters has been studied with different education levels, age groups, and experience. The results show that painters' knowledge has no relation with age and level of education, but there was a significant correlation between individual knowledge and work experience that confirms Jahangiri *et al*'s result of study (12). In addition, they reported a significant correlation between worker's knowledge of hearing protection in petrochemical industry and their experience (12).

The results of Hosseini *et al* (13) showed that there was a significant correlation between farmers, who works with pesticides, knowledge of safety precautions and protective equipments and their age and experience. Whereas, the results of our study are not correlated with age, but are correlated with work experience. In a study conducted among Qom farmers, no correlation has been reported between farmers' knowledge and experience and their age (14). The knowledge and experience of older workers increased when workers received specialized training in their workplace.

The effect of smoking

The correlation between the attitudes of two groups of smokers and non-smokers was not significant, so the attitude in two groups did not differ, while knowledge and performance had a significant correlation in both groups. This result is similar to Abedzadeh *et al*'s conclusion about knowledge, attitude, and performance of women referring to health care centers in Kashan for breast cancer (15).

Conclusion

Results showed that painter's attitude had significant correlation with education level. It is evident, all of the solvents that are used to dilute the dyes are harmful to human health and exposure of solvents and dyes increase the health risk. Tacking to account all the above, give information and awareness of solvents harmful, it can help to reduce its effects. It is recommended that it will be important to survey the concentration of these compounds in various tissues of painting body and his workplace air.

Acknowledgements

This project was financially supported by the Faculty of Public Health, Shahid Sadoughi University of Medical Sciences. The authors are grateful to the head of Environmental Chemistry Laboratory for his help.

Competing interests

The authors declare that they have no competing interests.

Authors' contributions

MHS and MM participated in the design of the study and draft the manuscript. MHE helped to design and draft the manuscript. MM and MHF carried out the studies and performed statistical analysis of the collected data. All authors read and approved the final manuscript.

References

1. Hajighasemkhan A. Industrial toxicology. Tehran: Tomorrow publications; 2007. [In Persian]
2. Ladou J. Occupational and environmental medicine. 3rd edition. Philadelphia: McGraw-Hill; 2004.
3. Baker EL, Fine LJ. Solvent neurotoxicity: the current evidence. J Occup Med 1986; 28(2): 126-9.
4. Lindbohm ML. Effects of parental exposure to solvents on pregnancy outcome. J Occup Environ Med 1995; 37(8): 87-93.
5. Ghasemkhani M. Detect chemical agents at work (gases and steams). 3rd Edition. Tehran: Cultural development of palm publications; 1995. [In Persian]
6. Rom WN. Occupational and environmental medicine. 3rd edition. New York: US Lippington-Raven; 1998.
7. Rosenstock L, Cullen MR, Brodkin CA, Redlich CA. Clinical occupational and environmental medicine. 2nd edition. Edinburgh: WB Saunders; 2005.
8. Ghasemi S, Karami EA. Attitudes and behaviors about pesticides use among greenhouse workers in Fars province. Journal of Economics and Agricultural Development 2009; 23(1): 28-40. [In Persian]
9. Dadgari A, Yaghmaie F, Shahnazarian J, Dadvar L. Nurses knowledge, attitude and practice in prevention of ICU syndrome. Knowlede and Health Journal 2007; 2(3): 29-35. [In Persian]
10. Fung L, Yuan Y. Performance enhancement drugs: knowledge, attitude, and intended behavior among community coaches in Hong Kong. The Sport Journal 2006; 9(3): 103-8.

11. Shah VN, Verma PB, Tripathi CB. Knowledge, attitude and practice regarding tobacco consumption among the college students of Bhavnagar city (Gujarat). Indian J Community Med 2005; 30(1): 1-4.
12. Jahangiri M, Mirzaei R, Ansari H. Risk perception, knowledge and safety attitude and hearing protector use in petrochemical industry workers. Audiol 2008; 17(1): 11-8. [In Persian]
13. Hosseini MH, Ramazani A, Hanafie Bojd M, Hamidi H, Samimi K, Mohsenzadeh MA, *et al.* Farmers' knowledge of occupational poisonings in South Khorasan. Journal of Birjand University of Medical Sciences 2011; 18(1): 47-54. [In Persian]
14. Heydari A, Razavi Asl SM. Agricultural occupational health knowledge and practice of farmers in 2007 in Qom province. Qom University of Medical Sciences Journal 2007; 1(3): 51-7. [Persian]
15. Abedzadeh M, Sadat Z, Saberi F. Knowledge, attitude, and performance of women referring health care centers in Kashan towards breast cancer and its screening tests. Feyz Journal of Kashan University of Medical Sciences 2003; 7(2): 85-92.

8

Determination of the level of parasitic infection (Cryptosporidium and Giardia) of the vegetables marketed in Ilam city

Moyad Avazpoor[1*], Mohammad Taqi Yousefipoor[2], Majid Dusty[3], Mohsen Mehdipour[4], Fariba Seifipour[5], Zeinab Gholami[6]

[1]Faculty instructor, Department of Environmental Health Engineering , Ilam University of Medical Science, Ilam Iran

[2]BS of Environmental Health Engineering, Ilam University of Medical Science, Ilam, Iran

[3]MSc, Department of Parasitology, Ilam University of Medical Science, Ilam, Iran

[4]PhD Student of Environmental Health in SBMU, Member of Environmental Health Engineering Research Center, Kerman University of Medical Sciences, Kerman, Iran

[5]MSc Department of Environmental Health Engineering, Ilam University of Medical Science, Ilam, Iran

[6]MSc Student of Environmental Health, Tehran University of Medical Science, Tehran, Iran

Abstract

Background: Infected with intestinal parasites is one of the most important health and economical problems, which could have different effects, such as diarrheal diseases or death associated. The purpose of this study was to determine the level of prevalence of Cryptosporidium and Giardia parasites in the vegetable marketed in Ilam city.

Methods: This study was performed on 280 samples of fresh vegetables and lettuce in Ilam. The samples were taken at the level of 500 grams from the places where vegetables and lettuce are sold. Micro liters of each sample was placed on the slide using automatic micropipette, and Logel and Zyl-Nelson stainings were performed in order to identify Cryptosporidium and Giardia.

Results: From 200 samples, 54 samples were contaminated to Cryptosporidium oocyte and 13 samples to Giardia cysts. From 80 lettuce samples also 32 samples were contaminated to Cryptosporidium oocyte, and 6 samples contaminated to Giardia cysts. The results showed that the overall infection was 37%. Infection with Giardia cysts was 6.8% and infection with Cryptosporidium oocyte was 30.7%, and Cryptosporidium infection rates in vegetables and lettuce were different. This difference was statistically significant ($P<0.05$).

Conclusion: As a result of this research it is determined that the prevalence of Giardia and Cryptosporidium in Ilam vegetables is significantly higher, and the contamination of lettuce is far greater. Therefore, authorities should be more attentive to the field of education and the control of parasitic diseases.

Keywords: Cryptosporidium, Oocyte, Giardia lamblia, Vegetables

***Correspondence to:**
Moyad Avazpoor
Email: m_f_1859@yahoo.com

Introduction

Parasitic diseases are among the diseases that are closely related to personal and public health. Our country is not free from various parasitic infections and requires efforts to identify more pathogens and little known or unknown factors. Vegetable consumption, especially those that are eaten raw have a major role in the transmission of parasites (1). Vegetables can transmit oocytes and protozoan-cysts and eggs and larvae of worms, that can cause diseases in humans (2). Cryptosporidiosis and giardiasis are protozoan infections that can cause digestive disorders and chronic diarrhea in recent years in healthy and unhealthy individuals who have impaired immune systems. This disease is more common in patients who have normal immune deficiencies from birth to middle age. In cases the disease leads to severe weight loss in children and patients with immune deficiency and jeopardizes their lives assecondary infectious agent. Several studies have been conducted indifferent parts of the world to investigate vegetable parasites. In the studies that have been conducted in Turkey, Saudi Arabia, Vietnam, Nigeria, and India the rate of parasite infection in consumption of vegetables are respectively 6%, 16%, 26%, 36% and 44%, and maximum contamination have been reported in vegetables, cabbage, chives and watercress (3-6). Iran is one of the areas in which the prevalence of parasitic infections is noteworthy

(7). In most parts of Iran also, eating raw vegetables with meals is a current nutritional habit, that provide a significant parentage of essential vitamins and nutrients of the body and always expose people to parasites (8,9). In Iran also, during the past years, studies have been conducted in various cities and the results indicate that there is always the risk of parasitic infections for the consumption of raw, unwashed, and not disinfected vegetables. In Ardabil contamination was higher in vegetables, spinach and basil so that the cysts of Entamoeba coli, Giardia, eggs Tinia, Dicrocoelium, and Ascaris have the highest reported rate (10). In Tehran the highest rate of infection was in leek and parsley, and Giardia cysts, eggs Trichostrongylus and Ascaris were reported as the most parasitic (11). Due to the lack of accurate epidemiological study in Ilam, there is no complete information about the release of parasitic diseases. Vegetables which are supplied as nonstandard by the vendors in the city, downtown, and along the street play a major role in the pathogenesis of people. This study examines parasitic vegetables. There is the possibility of vegetables being contaminated in the fields due to using the wastewater and well water in irrigated vegetables and access of animals to farms due to lack offences around the fields. In this study parasitic infected vegetables are considered in Ilam city. Thus, identification of cryptosporidium and giardia infected vegetables marketed in Ilam can assist health authorities with thee exercise of control and finally promotion of public health.

Methods

This study was performed in the winter of 2013 on 280 samples of edible vegetables and lettuce in Ilam. First vegetable supplies of shops in the city were identified and then 500 g of samples were randomly taken from each of them. First the leaves of each sample was completely separated using disposable and clean gloves. Each sample was kept in a separate container, which contains three liters of water with 6 ml dish washing liquid for 8 hours. During this period, it was stirred regularly every half hour to facilitate these parathion of oocysts from the plant. After that, the dish was left for 1 hour until the isolated oocysts were deposited. Then the vegetable was removed gently and the dishwashing water content was fixed in place for 16 hours, to ensure the complete precipitation of oocysts (12,13).
In the next step, about 2 liters of water in the container were slowly discharged using an electric pump. The precipitate and the remaining water were passed from sieve No. 100 (one hundred pores per inch, every pore diameter 150 microns) which is buffered on two layers, to remove coarse particles. After integration the suspensions were centrifuged twice for five minutes at 1000 rpm, and the contents of each tube were enriched by adding physiology serum to a final volume of two cubic centimeters and the number of samples were inserted, and kept in the fridge until testing. In the next step, the samples were placed on a lam and add 10 microliters of each sample using an automatic micropipette and we added a drop of logel solution and then put a lamella on it. Now the lam is ready to identify and recognize giardia cysts (14).
In the next step, 10 µl of each sample were placed on the slide using an automatic micropipette. Expansion obtained after drying for 3 minutes in methanol fixation. And it was placed in cold carbol fuchsin dye and then was had with running water. The bleaching stage was done using a solution of acid methanol for 10 to 15 seconds. After being washed with running water, slides were placed at 0.4% malachite color for 30 seconds, and after washing, dried and examined under a microscope with lens No. 100. If there is contamination (see oocyst and Giardia cysts), the mean number of oocysts and Giardia cysts in at least 50 microscopic fields were counted and their total numbers calculated based on the initial volume of the suspension.

Results

In this study, according to Table 1, 280 samples of vegetables and lettuce were tested in laboratory. From the total samples, 105 samples were polluted, and 175 samples were not contaminated. The results showed that infection in all samples was 33.6%. Infection with Giardia was 6.8%. Infection with Cryptosporidium was 30.7%, with Giardia on lettuce 7.5%, and in vegetables 5.6%. Infection with Cryptosporidium on lettuce was 40% and on vegetables was 27%. According to Table 2, the overall infection in the form of vegetables and lettuce was different, and these differences were meaningful in terms of statistics. (chi-square test: df=1, $P<0.05$) (prevalence of infection is higher in lettuce). In terms of infection with Giardia, the difference between the two types of vegetables and lettuce was not significant (chi-square test: df=1, $P>0.05$). Infection with Cryptosporidium on lettuce and vegetables was different and this difference was statistically significant, (chi-square test: df =1, $P<0.05$) (lettuce is more infected).

Discussion

In this research the total 200 samples of vegetables were taken, each of which is included (parsley, basil, leeks,

Table 1. General information, Cryptosporidium and Giardia contamination levels in vegetables consumed in the city of Ilam

	No. of samples infected with Cryptosporidium	No. of samples infected with Giardia	No. of samples of non-infected	Total
Vegetable samples	54	13	133	200
Lettuce samples	32	6	42	80
Total	86	19	175	280

Table 2. The overall infection rate in terms of types of vegetables (for both species)

Descriptions	Infection		Total
	Positive	Negative	
Number	59	101	200
%, According to lettuce/vegetable	29.5%	27.5%	100%
Number	35	45	80
%, According to lettuce/vegetable	43.8%	56.2%	100%
Number	94	186	280
%, According to lettuce/vegetable	36.6%	66.4%	100%

thorp, oregano, mint, watercress). Fifty-four samples were infected with Cryptosporidium oocyst, and 13 samples were contaminated with Giardia cysts. From 80 samples of lettuce, 32 samples were infected with Cryptosporidium oocyst, and 6 samples were infected with Giardia cysts. Totally, 86 samples contained Cryptosporidium oocyst, and 19 samples were contaminated with Giardia cysts.

The total numbers of samples infected with Giardia were 19 samples. As a result, the number of samples infected with Giardia cysts was 6.8% of the whole samples (the overall prevalence of Giardia). Based on the results of research done by Malakoutian et al in 2009 in the city of Kerman, contamination of different vegetables with Giardia cysts was reported 0.74%. In this study, scallion had the highest rate of infection, and basil and radishes had the lowest rate (15). But in the research conducted in Norway from 1999 to 2001 it was observed that 6% of infections were with Giardia cysts (16). The survey conducted in Ramhormuz by Arab and Rahdar, showed that the rate of prevalence of Giardia was detected about 4.6% in vegetables (17). In a study conducted in Isfahan city, 480 samples were collected from different fields in this city. Seven types of Giardia were observed in the edible vegetables (11). Depending on the type of used fertilizer (organic or chemical), drinking water, and transportation of animals on the farm, the type and the percentage of infection is different in different regions.

Cryptosporidium oocyst infection percentage of the whole samples was 30.7%, and the total number of infected samples were 86. Of these 86 samples, 54 samples were vegetables and 32 samples were lettuce. Accordingly the number of lettuce samples taken is much lower than those of vegetables, percentage of Cryptosporidium oocyst infection of lettuce is more than those of vegetables. In the study on Cryptosporidium infection of lettuce marketed indifferent areas of Shiraz city, in two seasons of spring and summer, the number of 47 samples from 200 samples of lettuce (23.5%) with Cryptosporidium infection were found positive (18). Overgaauw et al, analyzing 475 samples of various vegetables such as lettuce and beans, reported the rate of Cryptosporidium infection 6% in Norway. There searchers reported that the infection rate of beans, is higher than the lettuce infection rate. Separating the parasites from farms, they concluded that contamination of vegetables and decontamination were linked to the use of contaminated water (19). In another study Paula et al, by studying 60 samples of a self-service foodstuff in Nitro in Brazil, they proved that 16 cases (26%) were infected with Cryptosporidium, which was proved to be more contaminated than the previous study (20). In the present study, Giardia infection in lettuce is 7.5% and in vegetables is 6.5%. Cryptosporidium infection in lettuce is 40% and in vegetables is 27%. Cryptosporidium has a wide host range and infects not only humans but also infects other animals such as poultry, sheep, goats, cattle, otter, carnivorous and fish (21). Inpatients with impaired immune systems, 3.6% of patients with diarrhea, were reported to be infected with Cryptosporidium (22). Wastes of birds, animals, or humans are infected with Cryptosporidium on farmlands, if used, the infection is transmitted through fertilizer, and infected agricultural products such as vegetables. In addition to soil contamination, there is the possibility of transmitted contamination of water. There are many reports of outbreaks caused by Cryptosporidium and Giardia with the source of water pollution, that has been originated from leaking sewage or direct infection with the feces of human or animals.

Conclusion

In this study the levels of Giardia infection were less than Cryptosporidium. It might have different reasons, but because there is no completely effective treatment for Cryptosporidium, a wide range of hosting and asymptomatic carriers, resistan of oocysts to disinfectant agents, and increasing incidence of the disease involved. Also, the over all infection and Cryptosporidium infection is higher in lettuce. Bivalves such as lettuce, due to the large surface of the leaves, and the special form where the leaves are attached to each end, causes Cryptosporidium oocyst maintain their level and are more contaminated than other vegetables. The differences in terms of infection to Giardia in two types of vegetables and lettuce are not significant. According to this research findings and the role of vegetables in diets and the risk of transmitting infections to human, it is necessary to take substantial action in planting, harvesting, storage, transport, distribution, and consumption of vegetables and raising public awareness. According to the research, consumed vegetable of Ilam in the winter was supplied from Khuzestan. This issue justified further research in this area. Educating the health tips when washing vegetables, with the aim of reducing the number of oocysts and not destroying them is an important step in prevention of Cryptosporidium infection in human. Due to the importance of vegetables in our diet and the possibility of transmission of parasitic infections to human by vegetables, it is necessary to consider a plan that prevents the movement of domestic and wild animals in the farm land, because in addition to damage to agricultural lands, they may increase the probability of transmission of zoonotic parasitic diseases. The accumulated fertilizer for farms, which is uninfected (accumulated long as compost) can play a role in reducing contamination. According to the results of this research, based on the high overall infection and also high levels of cryptosporidial contamination of lettuce than vegetables, when washing, lettuce must have been separated from leaves and washed well with anionic detergent and then bed is infected.

Acknowledgements
The authors highly appreciate the sponsorship of the Vice Chancellor for Research and Technology of Ilam University of Medical Science.

Competing interests
The authors declare that they have no competing interests.

Authors' contributions
MA conceived and designed the study. MTY, MD, MM, FS and ZG performed the literature search and wrote the manuscript. All authors participated in the data acquisition, analysis, and interpretation. All authors critically reviewed, refined and approved the manuscript.

Reference
1. Robertson LJ, Gjerde B. Isolation and enumeration of Giardia cysts,Cryptosporidium oocysts and Ascaris eggs from fruits and vegetables. J Food Prot 2000; 63(6): 775-8.
2. Slifko TR, Smith HV, Rose JB. Emerging parasite zoonoses associated with water and food. Int J Parasitol 2000; 30(12-13): 1379-93.
3. Hayes EB, Matte TD, O'Brien TR, McKinley TW, Logsdon GS, Rose JB, et al. Large community outbreak of cryptosporidiosis due to contamination of a filtered public water supply.N Engl J Med 1989; 320(21): 1372-6.
4. Kozan E, Gonenc B, Sarimehmetoglu O, Aycicek H. Prevalence of helminth eggs on raw vegetables used for salads. Food Control 2005; 16(3): 239-42.
5. Damen JG, Banwat EB, Egah DZ, Allanana JA. Parasitic contamination of vegetables in Jos, Nigeria. Ann Afr Med 2007; 6(3): 115-8.
6. Uga S, Hoa NT, Noda S, Moji K, Cong L, Aoki Y, et al. Parasite egg contamination of vegetables from a suburban market in Hanoi, Vietnam. Nepal Med Coll J 2009; 11(2): 75-8.
7. Al-Megrin WA. Prevalence intestinal parasites in leafy vegetables in Riyadh, Saudi Arabia. International Journal of Tropical Medicine 2010; 5(2): 20-3.
8. Gupta N, Khan DK, Santra SC. Prevalence of intestinal helminth eggs on vegetables grown in wastewater-irrigated areas of Titagarh, West Bengal, India. Food Cotrol 2009; 20(10): 942-5.
9. Bundy DA, Cooper ES, Thompson DE, Didier JM, Simmons I. Epidemiology and population dynamics of Ascaris lumbricoides and Trichuris trichiura infection in the same community. Trans R Soc Trop Med Hyg 1987; 81(6): 987-93.
10. Arfaa F. Medical helminthology. Tehran: Daneshpajoh publication; 2007. [In Persian]
11. Izadi S, Abedi S, Ahmadian S, Mahmoodi M. Study of the current parasitic contamination of the edible in Isfahan in order to identify preventive measures. Journal of Kurdistan University of Medical Sciences 2006; 11(2): 51-8. [In Persian]
12. Daryani A, Ettehad GH, Sharif M, Ghorbani L, Ziaei H. Prevalence of intestinal parasites in vegetables consumed in Ardabil, Iran. Food Control 2008; 19(8): 790-4.
13. Robertson LJ, Gjerde B. Occurrence of parasites on fruits and vegetables in Norway. J Food Prot 2001; 64(11): 1793-8.
14. Henriksen SA, Pohlenz JF. Staining of cryptosporidia by a modified Ziehl-Neelsen technique. Accra Vet Scand 1981; 22(3-4): 594-6.
15. Malakoutian M, Hoseini M, Bahrami H. Study of parasitic contamination ofvegetablesin Kerman. Journal of Medicine of Hormozgan 2009; 13(1): 55-62. [In Persian]
16. Robertson LJ, Greig JD, Gjerde B, Fazil A. The potential for acquiring cryptosporidiosis or giardiosis from consumption of mung bean sprouts in Norway: a preliminary step-wise risk assessment. Int J Food Microbiol 2005; 98(3): 291-300.
17. Arab L, Rahdar M. Parasitic contamination of consumed vegetables from farms in Ramhormoz. Jundishapur Scientific Medical Journal 2006; 11(4): 375-82. [In Persian]
18. Razavi S, Nasirinasab-Rafsanjani M, Bahrami S. A study on cryptosporidium contamination in lettuce collected from different areas in Shiraz. Journal of Shahrekord University of Medical Sciences 2009; 12(2): 44-50. [In Persian]
19. Overgaauw PA, van Zutphen L, Hoek D, Yaya FO, Pinelli E, et al. Zoonotic parasites in fecal samples and fur from dogs and cats in The Netherlands. Veterinary Parasitology 2009; 163 (1): 115-22.
20. Paula P, Rodrigues PS, Tortora JC, Uchoa CM, Farage S. [Microbiological and parasitological contamination of lettuce (Lactuca sativa) from self service restaurants of Niterói city, RJ]. Rev Soc Brasil Med Trop 2003; 36(4): 535-7. [In Portuguese]
21. Davood J. Akbarin H. Review to cryptosporidiom, cryptosporidiosis. Jahane Andishe Publishing house; 2005.
22. Nahrevanian H, Assmar M. Cryptosporidiosis in immunocompromised patients in the Islamic Republic of Iran.J Microbiol Immunol Infect 2008; 41(1): 74-7.

9

Sulfur dioxide AQI modeling by artificial neural network in Tehran between 2007 and 2013

Saeed Motesaddi[1], Parviz Nowrouz[2*], Behrouz Alizadeh[3], Fariba Khalili[4], Reza Nemati[2]

[1]Associate Professor, Department of Environmental Health Engineering, School of Public Health, Shahid Beheshti University of Medical Sciences, Tehran, Iran
[2]Ph.D Student of Environmental Health Engineering, Department of Environmental Health Engineering, School of Public Health, Shahid Beheshti University of Medical Sciences, Tehran, Iran
[3]PhD Student of Medical Informatics, Department of Medical Informatics, School of Allied Medical Sciences, Shahid Beheshti University of Medical Sciences, Tehran, Iran
[4]Ph.D Student of Environmental Health Engineering, Department of Environmental Health Engineering, School of Public Health, Tehran University of Medical Sciences, Tehran, Iran

Abstract
Background: Air pollution and concerns about health impacts have been raised in metropolitan cities like Tehran. Trend and prediction of air pollutants can show the effectiveness of strategies for the management and control of air pollution. Artificial neural network (ANN) technique is widely used as a reliable method for modeling of air pollutants in urban areas. Therefore, the aim of current study was to evaluate the trend of sulfur dioxide (SO_2) air quality index (AQI) in Tehran using ANN.
Methods: The dataset of SO_2 concentration and AQI in Tehran between 2007 and 2013 for 2550 days were obtained from air quality monitoring fix stations belonging to the Department of Environment (DOE). These data were used as input for the ANN and nonlinear autoregressive (NAR) model using Matlab (R2014a) software.
Results: Daily and annual mean concentration of SO_2 except 2008 (0.037 ppm) was less than the EPA standard (0.14 and 0.03 ppm, respectively). Trend of SO_2 AQI showed the variation of SO_2 during different days, but the study declined overtime and the predicted trend is higher than the actual trend.
Conclusion: The trend of SO_2 AQI in this study, despite daily fluctuations in ambient air of Tehran over the period of the study have decreased and the difference between the predicted and actual trends can be related to various factors, such as change in management and control of SO_2 emissions strategy and lack of effective parameters in SO_2 emissions in predicting model.
Keywords: Sulfur dioxide, Neural networks, Air quality index, Tehran.

***Correspondence to:**
Parviz Nowrouz
Email: Nowrouzp@gmail.com

Introduction

Air pollution is a serious challenge for human health and annually millions of tons toxic pollutants due to human activities are released into the atmosphere (1). Therefore, many of the metropolitan cities of the world are exposed with the challenge of air pollution that causes citizens exposure to air pollution and has created health problems. With increase in population growth and industries, the possibility of air pollution gradually increased, such that the most likely outcome is threat of human health and environmental damage (2). Tehran is one of the most polluted metropolitan cities of the world. Much of this pollution in other countries is due to over population, the use of fossil fuels, heavy traffic, a lot of old vehicles, poor development of industry and other pollution related to the geographical location of Tehran to the southern slopes of the Alborz mountains and surrounded by mountains at the north and east. In addition, the impact of climate conditions, such as calm winds and stable weather and lack of rainfall are highly effective in Tehran, thus intensifying air pollution (3). Several pollutants are involved in creating and intensifying air pollution; sulfur dioxide (SO_2) is one of the most important air pollutants and one of the criteria of pollutants of air quality index (AQI). Large amounts of SO_2 are emitted from diesel vehicles (all commercial vehicles and buses), especially in congested downtown areas (4,5). Generally, SO_2 emissions in a region is related to various factors, such as economic growth, pollution control laws, fossil fuel consumption and etc (6). The importance of SO_2 is found in the wide range of consequences of air pollution and climate changes. Generally, three major environmental consequences of SO_2 pollution will be considered: photochemical smog, acid rain, and global climate change (7). Results of a study in China showed that SO_2 emissions have increased to 53% in the period between 2000 and 2006, which is approximately 3.7% annual increase (4). In Klang Valley of Malaysia, the trend of SO_2 concentration showed significant increase in high traffic stations (8). The trend of SO_2 in seven major cities of Korea between 1989 and 2010 showed that much higher concentrations of SO_2 occurred in winter (9). Considering the importance of air pollution, the use of preventive strategies and predicting is very important. Air pollution predicting can be used through models and available tools. Nowadays, modeling tools are widely used in many scientific fields, especially in environmental sciences, such as air pollution (10). Artificial neural networks (ANN) developed in recent years, have been used to model pollutant concentrations with promising results (11-13). This is regarded as an intelligent, cost-effective approach and has received much attention in environmental engineering. ANN is an information processing paradigm that is inspired by the biological nervous systems, such as the brain processing formation. It is composed of a large number of highly inter connected processing elements (neurons) working in unison to solve specific problems. The goal of this network is to create a model that can correctly map the input to the output using historical data, so that the model can then be used to produce the output when the desired output is unknown. An ANN has a parallel distributed structure and consists of a set of processing elements called neurons. The ANN structure consists of input layer which receives data, output layer to send computed information and one or several hidden layers lying the input and output layers. According to the architecture, all or a part of the neurons in a layer are connected with all or a part of the neurons of the previous and next layer. The number of hidden layers and neurons of each layer depends on the specific model, convergence speed generalization capability, physical process, and the training data that the network will simulate (14). Concentration variation in predicting air pollutants using neural network was used in the early 1990s and for the first time by Boznar et al who used it to predict the concentration of SO_2 in industrial areas of Slovenia (11). The ability and power of neural networks to learn the complexity of communications of air pollution systems, has led to the use of neural network model to examine environmental issues increase. Sahin et al (15) carried out a study using neural networks and nonlinear regression model for the concentration of SO_2 in Istanbul. The results of this study showed that neural network was better than nonlinear regression. Mok and Tam used ANN to predict the daily SO_2 concentration. The promising results showed that ANN could be used to develop efficient air-quality analysis and prediction models in the future (16). An autoregressive moving average model (ARMA) and time series forecasting of SO_2 in Tehran were used for the period of 2000 to 2005. The results proved that ARMA model can provide reliable, satisfactory predictions for time series and SO_2 emission was significantly high for stationary sources as compared to other pollutants (17).

Trend of air pollutant can show that strategy of air pollutant emission control has been useful or not. Considering the above and the proper performance of the neural network, the aim of this study was to investigate SO_2 AQI trend between 2007 and 2013 and forecasting model in Tehran using neural network.

Methods

Study area

The present study was carried out in Tehran. Tehran is located at the foot of the Alborz mountains, south of the Caspian Sea and is the largest urban area of Iran that has the highest population (8 700 000 in 2011). The city is also ranked as one of the largest cities in Western Asia and 19th in the whole world. As in other large cities, Tehran is faced with serious air quality problems. In general, 20% of the total energy of the country is consumed in Tehran. Compounding Tehran's air pollution problem is its geographical location. With the location of 35° 41' N - 51° 25' E and altitude of 1000 to 1800 m above mean sea level, Tehran is located in valleys and is surrounded on the north, northwest, east and southeast by high to medium high (3800 to 1000 m) mountain ranges (18).

SO_2 data

The daily SO_2 AQI and concentration between 2007 and 2013 were obtained from 16 air quality monitoring stations that belonged to the Department of Environment (DOE). In monitoring stations of the DOE, UV fluorescence analyzers (model AF22M of Environment SA, France) were used to measure SO_2. Complete datasets would have contained 2550 days measured values.

Methodology for ANN implementation

The nonlinear autoregressive (NAR) neural network through Matlab software (R2014a) was used for the SO_2 trend and forecasting. As previously mentioned, the implementation of ANN consists of several phases. Our conducted procedure is described as follows:

Data normalizing

For data normalizing, data convolution with Gaussian function was used to move a window while maintaining the nature of the data, and largely eliminates unwanted noise in the data. Averaging window techniques was used and 31 windows were chosen for noise removal.

Network structure

Considering the existing number of hidden layers and number of neurons in each layer, the number of choices available for network design increase, therefore the design and testing of all cases is actually not feasible. Cybenco proved that a hidden layer if having sufficient number of neurons could provide all the certain conditions (19). Depending on the appropriate inputs, the use of simpler structure is more favorable and network with one or two hidden layers can actually be able to solve a variety of issues. However, a program of data processing with the aim of finding the best neural network architecture by trial and error according to the number of layers was designed with the number of architectures (20,21). Therefore, the network consists of two hidden layers obtained with 50 neurons in the first hidden layer and 50 neurons in the second hidden layer and Bayesian regularization algorithm is used as shown in Figure 1.

Transfer functions

Tansig transfer functions were used each time separately to obtain the best combination of transfer and linear function for realizing a good approximation of every type of functions.

Training/Test set

The maximum number of training generations of 500 was considered when there was no significant change after the fifth generation of network training. During training of network, 70% of data was considered as the training and 30% as the test.

The error diagram and validation for different repeats to simulate SO_2 based on mean-square error is as shown in Figure 2. It is clear that the selected network has very high accuracy. Figure 3 shows the correlation between actual output and estimated output through network and R = 0.999 represents high correlation between actual data and estimated data.

The results for network training are as shown in Figure 4. Test data (green) completely overlap the actual data (blue) and the used model shows that error (orange) is also very low. Therefore, the results show a high power of network to predict the time series trend of SO_2.

Data input

For simulation and forecasting of SO_2 AQI, 810 days were used as input data and the next 90 days was predicted.

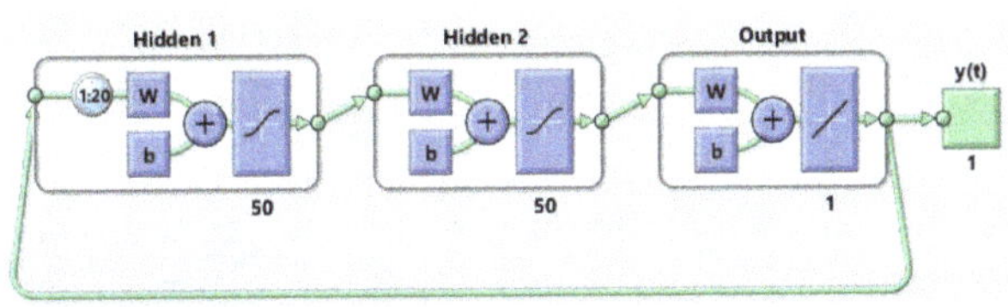

Figure 1. Artificial neural network.

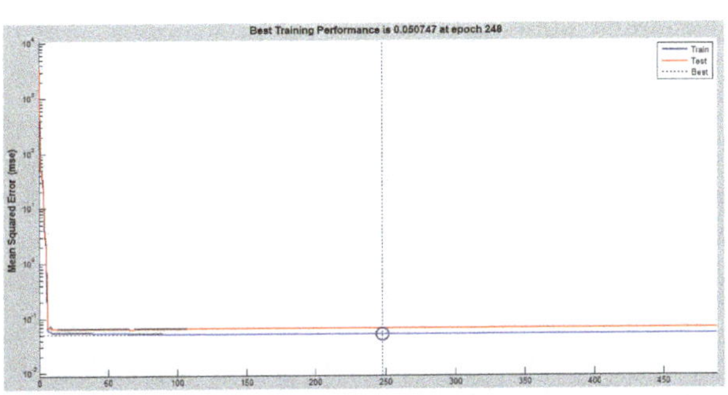

Figure 2. The training error rate and validation for SO_2 simulation based on mean-square error.

Results

So_2 pollution data

The seasonal and annual mean concentration (standard deviation) of SO_2 in Tehran is shown in Table 1. The lowest annual mean concentration of SO_2 was 0.018 ppm in 2013 and maximum was 0.037 ppm in 2008. Winter of 2007 had the highest mean concentration of SO_2 (0.049 ppm) among the seasons.

Trend of SO_2 AQI

AQI trend of SO_2 in Tehran for the period of 7 years (2007 to 2013) is as shown in Figure 5. Trend of SO_2 in several days did not have a constant pattern over the time that has been studied, especially between 2007 and 2010 (1400 days), there were a lot of fluctuations, but in the last three years (2010 to 2013), trend and fluctuations regularly declined.

For forecasting of SO_2 AQI, 810 days were used as input data and the result of 90 days forecasting is as shown in Figure 6. It can be observed that the predicted trend is

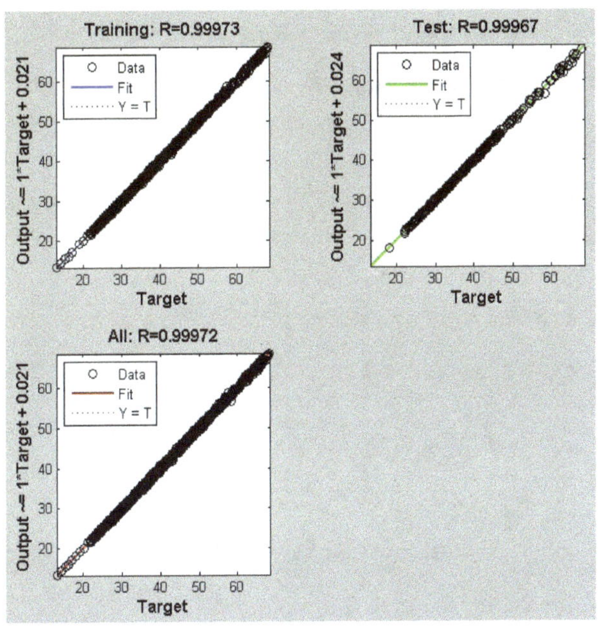

Figure 3. Correlation between actual output and estimated output by network.

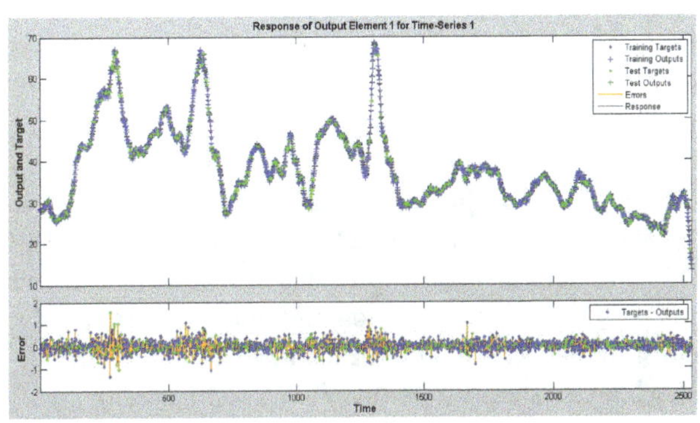

Figure 4. Comparison simulation of trend with actual trend of sulfur dioxide AQI in Tehran.

Table 1. Seasonal and annual mean concentration of SO_2 (unit: ppm ± SD)

Year	Season				Annual
	Spring	Summer	Autumn	Winter	
2007	0.019± 0.003	0.022± 0.006	0.034± 0.006	0.049± 0.009	0.033± 0.02
2008	0.029± 0.003	0.033± 0.004	0.033± 0.009	0.034± 0.01	0.037± 0.01
2009	0.021± 0.003	0.028± 0.003	0.027± 0.005	0.029± 0.003	0.025± 0.005
2010	0.033± 0.004	0.030± 0.003	0.035± 0.012	0.023± 0.006	0.033± 0.018
2011	0.021± 0.002	0.023± 0.002	0.026± 0.004	0.025± 0.004	0.024± 0.004
2012	0.020± 0.002	0.023± 0.003	0.021± 0.003	0.023± 0.004	0.022± 0.003
2013	0.020± 0.002	0.018± 0.002	0.016± 0.003	0.020± 0.004	0.018± 0.003

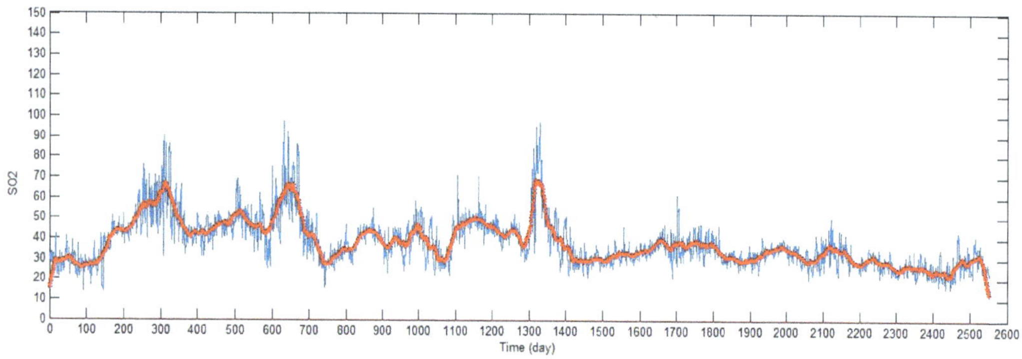

Figure 5. Trend of SO_2 AQI between 2007 and 2013 in Tehran.

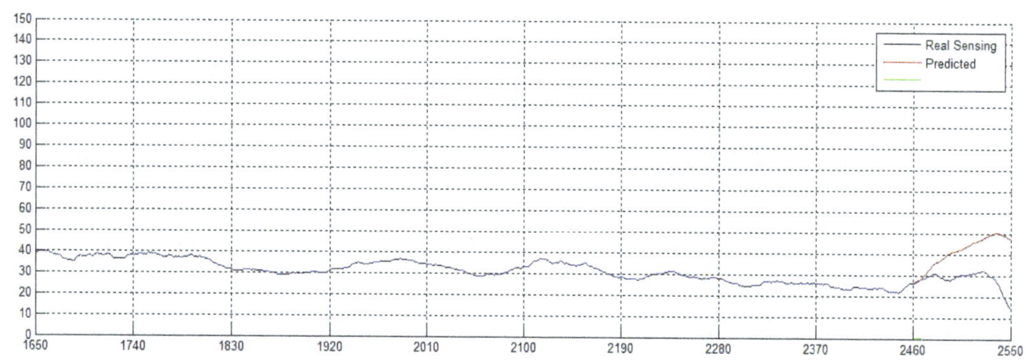

Figure 6. Forecasting of sulfur dioxide AQI trend using neural network.

higher than the actual trend and the predicted trend shows that SO_2 in air of Tehran can be increased in the future.

Discussion

Distributions of daily and annual mean concentrations for SO_2 for the period of 2007 to 2013 show that almost the annual average concentrations of SO_2 in ambient air of Tehran except 2008 were less than the standard (ppm 0.03). Also, in all the days studied, the concentration of SO_2 was not higher than the 24-hour standard (ppm 0.14). SO_2 emissions in a region is related to various factors and can vary in different situation and unlike this study, SO_2 emission between 2000 and 2005 in Tehran was considerably high for stationary sources as compared to other pollutants (17). The seasonal variation of SO_2 concentration was found from the daily means and presented in Table 1. The differences between the various seasons can be observed. The winter of 2007 had the highest SO_2 mean concentration (0.049 ± 0.009 ppm) among the other seasons. The high SO_2 emission is due to anthropogenic activities, such as domestic heating and industry and high concentration in winter could be the result of inversion.

There are several estimating and forecasting techniques. ANN was chosen for finding trend and forecasting of SO_2 in Tehran. Trend of SO_2 AQI over a period of 7 years is as shown in Figure 5 and can be observed despite daily fluctuations in the ambient air of Tehran, over the years studied, especially after 1700 days trend of SO_2 has decreased. Asrari et al (22) between 1995 and 2002 studied SO_2 trend in Tehran; this study showed high fluctuations and in most days they were much higher than the standard. This could depend on many factors, such as fluctuations in economic growth, better control of SO_2 sources, such as power plants near the city or refining diesel fuel quality and good management strategy in emissions control. The same study between 2005 and 2012 in relation with trend of SO_2 in Yangtze of China had been conducted and results showed a significant decline in SO_2 trend, especially after 2008 due to effectiveness of control and reduction of SO_2 emissions occurred at this area (23).

Predicted trend of SO_2 AQI using NAR model is as shown in Figure 6. It can be observed that predicted 90 days trend is higher than the actual trend. Therefore, we cannot predict the future trend of SO_2 in Tehran by this method. It could be the result of changes in management strategy in emission control or lack of effective parameters in SO_2 emissions in predicting model.

Conclusion

In this study, all the peaks of AQI were less than 100 showing good and moderate category. Trend of SO_2 AQI over the years studied in the ambient air of Tehran, has decreased. Difference between actual trend of SO_2 and predicted trend shows that the actual trend is well and unlike the predicted trend which declined and this can be related to various factors, such as good management and control of SO_2 emissions in Tehran.

Acknowledgements

The authors appreciate the Iran's Environmental Protection Organization for their cooperation in gathering data.

Competing interests

The authors have declared that no competing interests exist.

Authors' contributions

All authors contributed equally, and all authors participated in the data acquisition, analysis, and interpretation. All authors critically reviewed, refined, and approved the manuscript.

References

1. Piraino F, Aina R, Palin L, Prato N, Sgorbati S, Santagostino A, et al. Air quality biomonitoring: assessment of air pollution genotoxicity in the province of Novara (North Italy) by using Trifolium repens L. and molecular markers. Sci Total Environ 2006; 372(1): 350-9.
2. Mohan M, Kandya A. An analysis of the annual and seasonal trends of air quality index of Delhi. Environ Monit Assess 2007; 131(1-3): 267-77.
3. Keykhosrowi G, Lashkari H. Analysis of the relationship between the thickness and height of the inversion and the severity of air pollution in Tehran. Journal of Geography and Planning 2014; 18(49): 231-57. [In Persian].
4. Lu Z, Streets DG, Zhang Q, Wang S, Carmichael GR, Cheng YF, et al. Sulfur dioxide emissions in China and sulfur trends in East Asia since 2000. Atmos Chem Phys 2010; 10(13): 6311-31.
5. Lu WZ, Wang WJ, Wang XK, Yan SH, Lam JC. Potential assessment of a neural network model with PCA/RBF approach for forecasting pollutant trends in Mong Kok urban air, Hong Kong. Environ Res 2004; 96(1): 79-87.
6. Carmichael GR, Streets DG, Calori G, Amann M, Jacobson MZ, Hansen J, et al. Changing trends in sulfur emissions in Asia: implications for acid deposition, air pollution, and climate. Environ Sci Technol 2002; 36(22): 4707-13.
7. Stern DI. Reversal of the trend in global anthropogenic sulfur emissions. Glob Environ Change 2006; 16(2): 207-20.
8. Azmi SZ, Latif MT, Ismail AS, Juneng L, Jemain AZ. Trend and status of air quality at three different monitoring stations in the Klang Valley, Malaysia. Air Quality, Atmosphere & Health 2010; 3(1): 53-64.
9. Ray S, Kim KH. The pollution status of sulfur dioxide in major urban areas of Korea between 1989 and 2010. Atmos Res 2014; 147-148: 101-10.
10. Khatibi MS, Mohammadi N, Zoroufchi K, Sarand AB, Fatehifar E, Hashemi A. Using ANN and EPR models to predict carbon monoxide concentrations in urban area of Tabriz. Environmental Health Engineering and Management Journal 2015; 2(3): 117-22.
11. Boznar M, Lesjak M, Mlakar P. A neural network-based method for short-term predictions of ambient SO2 concentrations in highly polluted industrial areas of complex terrain. Atmos Environ 1993; 27B(2): 221-30.
12. Broomhead D, Lowe D. Multivariable functional interpolation and adaptive networks. Complex Syst 1988; 2(3): 321-55.
13. Hadjiiski L, Hopke PK. Application of artificial neural networks to the modeling and prediction of ambient ozone concentrations. J Air Waste Manage Assoc 2000; 50(5): 894-901.
14. Shaddel M, Seyed Javan D, Baghernia P. Estimation of hourly global solar irradiation on tilted absorbers from horizontal one using artificial neural network for case study of Mashhad. Renewable and Sustainable Energy Reviews 2016; 53: 59-67.
15. Sahin U, Ucan ON, Bayat C, Oztorun N. Modeling of SO2 distribution in Istanbul using artificial neural networks. Environmental Modeling & Assessment 2005; 10(2): 135-42.
16. Mok KM, Tam SC. Short-term prediction of S02

concentration in Macau with artificial neural networks. Energy Build 1998; 28: 279-286

17. Hassanzadeh S, Hosseinibalam F, Alizadeh R. Statistical models and time series forecasting of sulfur dioxide: a case study Tehran. Environ Monit Assess 2009; 155(1-4): 149-55.
18. Amini H, Taghavi SM, Henderson SB, Naddafi K, Nabizadeh R, Yunesian M. Land use regression models to estimate the annual and seasonal spatial variability of sulfur dioxide and particulate matter in Tehran, Iran. Sci Total Environ 2014; 488-489: 343-53.
19. Cybenco G. Approximation by super positions of a sigmoidal function. Mathematics of Control, Signals and Systems 1989; 2(4): 303-14.
20. Berry Michael J, Linoff G. Data mining techniques: for marketing, sales, and customer support. John Wiley & Sons, Inc; 1997
21. Boger Z, Guterman H. Knowledge extraction from artificial neural network models. Systems, Systems, Man, and Cybernetics, 1997. Computational Cybernetics and Simulation, 1997 IEEE International Conference on (volume 4); Orlando, FL. IEEE; 1997.
22. Asrari E, Ghole V, Sen P. Study on the Status of SO2 in the Tehran- Iran. J Appl Sci Environ Mgt 2006; 10(2): 75-82.
23. Qi HX, Lin W, Xu XB, Yu XM, Ma QL. Significant downward trend of SO2 observed from 2005 to 2010 at a background station in the Yangtze Delta region, China. Sci China Chem 2012; 55(7): 1451-8.

10

Evaluation of quality of urban life with emphasis on health

Khalilullah Kazemi Khabiri[1], Mohammad Ajza Shokouhi[2*], Omid Ali Kharazmi[2], Mohammad Reza Bemanian[3]

[1]Department of Geography, School of Urban Planning, International Campus, Ferdowsi University, Mashhad, Iran
[2]Department of Geography, School of Urban Planning, Ferdowsi University, Mashhad, Iran
[3]Department of Architecture, School of Art and Architecture, Tarbiat Modares University, Tehran, Iran

Abstract
Background: The quality of life of the citizens is one of the most important issues studied in different countries and used in the planning and monitoring of public policies. The present study measured and evaluated the indicators of quality of urban life among citizens of Mashhad city.
Methods: This analytical study was conducted on 375 citizens of various regions in Mashhad city. The random sampling method using population distribution and short-form questionnaires for data collection were applied. The validity of the questionnaires was verified by experts and the points given each question based on a 5-point Likert scale, and the Cronbach αcoefficient was used to measure the reliability of the questionnaire; the questionnaire rated 0.853%. To analyze the variables under study, SPSS and other statistical methods such as average answers and *t* test for independent variables were used.
Results: Findings of this research showed that the average health-sanitation dimension and environmental quality dimension are lower than 50% in Mashhad city. Sanitation and health, with a standard deviation of 5.838, are situated below the median level. The most common weakness is related to the dietary intake of protein. Environmental quality with a standard deviation of 5.857 is lower than the median level which is related to garbage separation and landfill sites. This result indicates that the quality of health and the environment in Mashhad is undesirable.
Conclusion: Citizens' satisfaction with quality of life index is lower than average in Mashhad city. Plans for improving the quality of life and developing services are highly necessary for increasing the quality of life.
Keywords: Sanitation, Personal satisfaction, Quality of life, Urban healt

***Correspondence to:**
Mohammad Ajza Shokouhi
Email: shokouhim.um.ac.ir

Introduction

A healthy city develops a combination of a healthy and dynamic community. Urbanization is considered one of the most important factors influencing citizens' individual and social health; therefore, the people's health is greatly affected by the social, economic, and environmental conditions of their city. Raising the quality of life in urban areas depends on the promotion of health (1,2). Quality of life is a vital issue in healthcare in the present era and one of the biggest sanitation goals in an individual's health improvement (3). Accepted as an axis of the development of a society, the promotion of health is the ultimate goal of all governments, in accordance with the objectives of the Ottawa Charter (4). Quality of life is one of the accepted frameworks for studying living conditions in different societies (5,6). The Netherlands National Institute for Public Health and the Environment claims that quality of life means the objective issues associated with non-material means of life and is determined by a person's perceptions of health, environment, job, family, etc (7). In fact, quality of life is the overall level of a person's satisfaction with life, which includes both mental and environmental dimensions (8). Quality of life is broadly conceptualized as an indicator for general welfare, social welfare, satisfaction, etc (9). A sustainable city provides for the development, prosperity, and promotion of environmental, economic and social quality for all; it also seeks an integrated development in the economic, social, and environmental aspects (10,11). In the first Health Promotion Conference, the Ottawa resolution was set up for health improvement and emphasized that having a healthier community is a responsibility not just for the health sector (12). The second conference on the environment and health, held in Helsinki, focused for the first time on the importance of urban health and its priority over other issues (13). Finally, the idea of a healthy city comes with the aim of promoting health and the move towards decentralization (14).

Human population growth has led to uncontrolled and unplanned environmental changes and urbanization that has an influential effect on the quality of life (15). Hence, cities are faced with environmental effects such as water and air pollution, health services, wastes, and so on which exacerbate the environmental health risks for urban residents (16). Population density in cities and urban areas and disproportion between the growth of services and the urban infrastructure, particularly in developing countries, have converted urban areas to unhealthy and polluted places that have other various problems including sewage and waste disposal, water supply, etc (17). As a religious-metropolis in Iran (Imam Reza's Holy Shrine), Mashhad is located on the main highway of eastern Iran. Being the second largest metropolis and the main religious city of Iran, Mashhad has recently experienced high population growth. The population of Mashhad city was 3 300 000 people in 2016, and appealing tourist attractions in Mashhad city attract nearly 30 million pilgrims annually (18). Therefore, this city is dealing with population growth and its subsequent results, such as increased air pollution (92 unhealthy days in year 2016); increased noise pollution (up to 75 dB) (19); the excessive development of industries in Mashhad city; failure to complete the sewage disposal system, the implementation of 60% of the Ego project in downtown Mashhad; explosive pollution of the Kashaf Rood river due to urban wastewater flowing from treatment plants; and the existence of household waste in streams which causes environmental pollution and diseases (20). Evaluating the quality of life may accelerate the evaluation of policies, ranking places, and prioritizing social issues for urban managers in order to promote the quality of life for the citizens. The present paper has been devoted to this topic.

Methods

The descriptive-analytic research method was used in this study. A questionnaire and field surveys were used for data collection. The statistical population of the research was 375 citizens from various regions of Mashhad who were randomly chosen. The questionnaire's indices were designed based on a 5-point Likert scale (five choices) and in the two dimensions of health and hygiene (six items) and environmental quality index (seven items). To analyze the variables under study, SPSS (version 22) and other statistical methods such as average answers and t test for independent variables were used.

Results

While Mashhad city has been well-known since ancient times and is home to various historical places, it is also located in a strategic regional position; minor integrated planning has been done to revitalize and enhance the quality of urban spaces. So, the point comes to mind that the historic-cultural capabilities of Mashhad city have led to the sustainable development of Mashhad city.

To assess and evaluate the quality of life in Mashhad city, an environmental index and the relevant indices were applied. Out of 375 citizens who completed the questionnaires, 245 persons (65.3%) were male and 130 persons (34.6%) were female.

The quality of life is related to the city environment and its infrastructures. An essential part of the broad concept of quality of life is one's environmental quality, which contains fundamental concepts such as health and safety combined with aspects like attractiveness. As main elements of the environmental index, the 2 indexes of "Health and Hygiene" and "Environmental Quality" were reviewed in the present research.

Health and Hygiene Index

Hygiene is considered an important index for assessing quality of life. To investigate the index of health and hygiene in Mashhad city, the variables (Table 1) that were used included: hygiene in the living environment of citizens, insurance services, health and treatment centers (health home, clinic, and bathroom), food consumption, closeness to infected centers to drugs, etc.

Environmental Quality Index

In recent decades, the issue of environmental quality has become a specialized and public debate in communities. Moreover, the attention of the people has been attracted to the nature of life in the inefficient urban collections instead of material objectives. The obvious point is that all urban problems have an environmental quality component; in other words, most environmental problems will quickly become urban problems. This is why that to have sustainable environmental dimensions, quality of life, and healthy communities, more attention has been paid in recent years to the quality dimensions in urban and residential settings. As shown in Table 2, seven variables were used to review the status of the environmental quality index.

Discussion

The findings of the current research (Table 1) indicate that every effort to improve the quality of life in Mashhad city should initially focus on areas such as health and hygiene which have the highest impacts on quality of life. Also, the percentage of the results range from "medium" to "low" for the quality of health and hygiene. The responses of most of the citizens to the variables of "Overall satisfaction with health status," "Weekly intake of protein substances," and "Weekly consumption of vegetables and fruits," indicate an inappropriate status for these variables. The

Table 1. Percentage of responses related to health and hygiene

Row	Environmental quality index	Extremely high	High	Medium	Low	Extremely low
1	Weekly intake of protein substances in the diet	0	0	51.7	31.3	17
2	Weekly consumption of vegetables and fruits in the diet	6	17.8	46	28.2	2
3	health and treatment centers	10	25	35	20	10
4	closeness to infected centers to drugs	25	15	45	15	0
5	insurance services	12	33	43	10	2
6	Overall satisfaction of health status	2	22.2	56	17.8	2
7	Garbage separation	4	10.1	8	77.9	0

Table 2. Likert scale scores for questions about the environmental quality index

Row	Environmental quality index	Extremely high	High	Medium	Low	Extremely low
1	Sound pollution	7.7	30.2	46	14.1	2
2	Air pollution	7	15	45	33	0
3	Status of construction waste and unnecessary items	2	16.1	24.2	49.7	8
4	No placement of residential units in the vicinity of floods and rivers	2	20.1	57.7	20.2	0
5	Waste and pollution of water resources	8	15	35	25	17
6	Possessing a landfill site	2	8	24	51	15
7	Garbage separation	4	10.1	8	77.9	0

Table 3. *T* test results to understand the impact of variables related to health, hygiene, and environmental quality

Variable	Mean	SD	*df*	*P* value	*T* value
Health and hygiene	26.500	5.838	99	0.000	-5.944
Environmental quality	27.500	5.857	99	0.000	-5.963

results (Table 2) indicate a relatively inappropriate status for environmental quality variables from the citizens' points of view. As shown in Table 2, most percentages are in the range of medium to low. The responses to the variables of this index indicates not much change in these variables which arise from the citizens' opinions of the city. The responses of most citizens to a low range in the variables "landfill site" and "garbage separation" illustrate their inappropriate status. Moreover, hygienic methods are not used in collecting and disposing of sewage; in fact, outdated methods are still used.

The current study yielded results similar with those of previous studies. The results of one study about planning for the enhancement of quality of life in the Sarab neighborhood of Mashhad indicated that quality of life regarding sanitation and health at 72% was the most problematic index among others. The main issues raised were solving the problem of wastewater wells and collecting surface water and building a sewage network for the neighborhood (21).

Conclusion

The most appropriate way to measure the quality of urban life is to employ the simultaneous use of objective and subjective indicators. Ignoring any of these indicators will create problems for the city and its citizens in future planning. Therefore, the present study investigated the quality of life in Mashhad city based on these dimensions and social environment components (health and hygiene index, environmental quality index). Statistical methods such as average responses and parametric statistical *t* test (Table 3) were used for independent variables. The health and hygiene index was lower than average with a standard deviation of 5.838. Most of the weakness associated with this component was related to the weekly intake of protein substances in the diet, weekly consumption of vegetables and fruits in the diet, and the low level of services and health centers. The environmental quality index, with a standard deviation of 5.857, was below the median level. The greatest weakness associated with this component was related to waste separation and landfill site, which requires fundamental planning.

Regarding the inadequate status of indicators of quality of the social environment in Mashhad city, the following suggestions are offered according to each indicator to improve the quality of life in Mashhad metropolis:

1. Prioritize the elimination of health problems in areas where the quality of life is inappropriate.
2. Increase the environmental health of the city by constructing a sewage collection network on the margins of Mashhad city.
3. Prevent the entry of any disturbing or polluting industries based on environmental laws and the optimal use of healthcare services to promote urban environmental health.
4. Plan and set goals to create specialist clinics for better service to local citizens.
5. Improve the collection, separation, and disposal of urban waste in the region.
6. Provide public health and hygiene training to promote

the level of public culture and identification of the inhabitants of the region.

Acknowledgements

This research is derived from a PhD thesis. The authors express their appreciation to the Municipality of Mashhad for its cooperation in facilitating visits to the suburbs of Mashhad.

Competing interests

The authors declare that they have no competing interests.

Authors' contributions

All authors participated in data acquisition, analysis, and interpretation. All authors critically reviewed, refined, and approved the manuscript.

References

1. Ghadami M, Motamed S. Investigate the quality of life in small cities, with an emphasis on the personal and social health dimension (case study: Nour city, Mazandran province). Geography and Environmental Planning Journal 2013; 24(1): 33-50. [In Persian].
2. Karkehabadi Z. Comparative comparison of urbanism quality according to enviromental index (case study: Semnan worn out and new urban textures). Quarterly of Geography 2017; 25(1): 33-48. [In Persian].
3. Salari Sardari F, Heudari Moghadam M, Sobhani N, Arefi A. Examination of the quality of life in urban areas (Case Study: Lamerd City). Journal of Urban Landscape Research 2015; 1(2): 53-91. [In Persian].
4. Shah Hosseini P, Tavakkoli H. The analysis of urban life quality indices case: Vardavard locality, in the 21st district of Tehran city. Environmental Based Territorial Planning (Amayesh) 2014; 7(24): 127-44. [In Persian].
5. Sheykh Islami A, Khoshbin N. Evaluation of quality of life, case study: first district of Behshahr City. J Geography and Urban Planning of the Zagros Landscape 2012; 4(14): 99 - 114. [In Persian].
6. Zangane Shahraki S, Galin Sharifdini J, Hassanzadeh D, Salary Moghadam Z. Evaluation of the quality of life in informal settlements, Tehran metropolitan (case study: Islamabad Salehabad). Human Geography Research Quarterly 2015; 67(1):177-96. doi: 10.22059/jhgr.2014.50599. [In Persian].
7. Epley DR, Menon M. A Method of Assembling Cross-sectional Indicators into a Community Quality of Life. Soc Indic Res 2008; 88(2): 281-96. doi: 10.1007/s11205-007-9190-7.
8. Rastegar M, Hatami H, Mirjafari R. Role of social capital in improving the quality of life and social justice in Mashhad, Iran. Sustainable Cities and Society 2017; 34: 109-13. doi: 10.1016/j.scs.2017.05.024.
9. Fayers PM, Machin D. Quality of Life: The Assessment, Analysis and Reporting of Patient-Reported Outcomes. 3rd ed. Wiley-Blackwell; 2016. p. 325-42. doi: 10.1002/9781118758991.
10. Saeedi Mofard S, Gordfaramarzi M. Study of Healthy City Indices with Sustainable Urban Development Approach. 8th Symposium on Advances in Science & Tecknology Commission-III: from Vernacular Architecture to Sustainable City (VASCITY); 2013 Dec 26; Khavaran Institute of Higher-education, Mashhad; 2013.
11. Yigitcanlar T, Kamruzzaman M. Planning, development and management of sustainable cities: a commentary from the guest editors. Sustainability 2015; 7(11): 14677-88. doi: 10.3390/su71114677.
12. Barton H, Grant M. Urban planning for healthy cities. A review of the progress of the European Healthy Cities Programme. J Urban Health 2013; 90(suppl 1): 129-41. doi: 10.1007/s11524-011-9649-3.
13. Lawrence RJ, Fudge C. Healthy Cities in a global and regional context. Health Promot Int 2009; 24 Suppl 1: i11-i8. doi: 10.1093/heapro/dap051.
14. Nieuwenhuijsen MJ, Khreis H. Car free cities: Pathway to healthy urban living. Environ Int 2016; 94: 251-62. doi: 10.1016/j.envint.2016.05.032.
15. Li F, Liu H, Huisingh D, Wang Y, Wang R. Shifting to healthier cities with improved urban ecological infrastructure: From the perspectives of planning, implementation, governance and engineering. J Clean Prod 2017; 163: S1-S11. doi: 10.1016/j.jclepro.2016.11.151.
16. Joseph Sirgy M, Phillips R, Rahtz D. Community Quality-of-Life Indicators: Best Cases VI. New York: Springer; 2013. doi: 10.1007/978-94-007-6501-6.
17. Saberifar R. The effect of satisfaction of the citizens of municipalities in urban environmental sustainability, case study: District 9 Mashhad. Biannual Journal of Urban Ecology Researches 2016; 7(14): 11-24. [In Persian].
18. Statistical yearbook of Organization of Transport and Traffic Deputy of Transportation and Traffic, Mashhad Municipality; 2016. p14.
19. Annual Report of Mashhad Environmental Monitoring Center. Department of Urban Services and Environment, Mashhad Municipality; 2016. p 53.
20. Statistical yearbook of Municipality of Mashhad. Mashhad: Deputy of Planning and Development, Mashhad Municipality; 2015. p. 42.
21. Ahmadian MA, Zafrenia S. Planning to improve the quality of city life in the Sarab neighborhood of Mashhad. Geographic Sciences Journal 2016; 12(24): 1-20. [In Persian].

11

Evaluation of microbial contamination of ready-to-eat foods (pizza, frankfurters, sausages) in the city of Ilam

Akbar Eslami[1], Zeinab Gholami[2], Shokofeh Nargesi[3], Bahareh Rostami[3], Moayed Avazpour[4,5*]

[1]Associate Professor of Environmental Health Engineering, Environmental and Occupational Hazards Control Research Center, Shahid Beheshti University of Medical Sciences, Tehran, Iran
[2]MSc of Environmental Health Engineering, Student Research Committee, School of Public Health, Tehran University of Medical Sciences, Tehran, Iran
[3]BSc in Environmental Health, Ilam University of Medical Sciences, Ilam, Iran
[4]PhD Student Research Office of Environmental Health, Department of Environmental Health Engineering, School of Public Health, Shahid Beheshti University of Medical Sciences, Tehran, Iran
[5]Instructor of Environmental Health, Department of Environmental Health Engineering, Ilam University of Medical Science, Ilam, Iran

Abstract
Background: Today in the world, disease resulting from food is considered one of the most important problems in public health. This study aimed to determine the bacterial contamination of ready-to-eat foods, i.e. fast food, in Ilam city.
Methods: In this cross-sectional, analytical study, 270 samples of ready-to-eat food, including pizza, frankfurters, and sausages, were randomly collected and tested for contamination with *Staphylococcus aureus, Escherichia coli, Shigella sonnei, Salmonella arizonae*, and *Enterococcus faecalis*. After examination, the collected data was analyzed using SPSS 20 software and logistic regression.
Results: From a total of 270 samples of ready-to-eat food, 27.77% was contaminated with E. coli, 21.48% with *S. aureus*, 13.33% with *S. sonnei*, 14.44% with *S. arizonae*, and 5.9% with *E. faecalis*. The results showed higher rates of *E. coli* and *S. aureus* contamination in pizza, frankfurters, and sausages. Also, a higher percentage of frankfurters were contaminated with microbial species than pizza or sausages. There were significant differences in microbial contamination rates ($P < 0.05$) among the three groups of food. In addition, factors such as indicators (health, sanitation, and lack of hygiene), age, gender, and education level of the operating staff had no effect on the results.
Conclusion: Based on the results, it can be concluded that bacterial contamination of ready-to-eat foods is significantly high in the city of Ilam; therefore, it is suggested that the examination of food in various stages of production and distribution can help reduce bacterial contamination, and training for the operators of shopping centers' ready-to-eat food shops and controlling pathogens are essential.
Keywords: Microbial contamination, Food, Pizza, Frankfurters, Sausages

***Correspondence to:**
Moayed Avazpour
Email: m_f_1859@yahoo.com

Introduction

Foodborne diseases are a major problem affecting people in poor societies (1). Microbial food contamination affects the life of people in developing countries and has a high mortality rate (2). A large variety of micro-organisms or their toxins with different mechanisms are involved in causing foodborne illness (3,4). It is estimated that 30% of people in industrialized countries suffer from diseases caused by food at least once a year (5).National health agencies have reported that the average prevalence of foodborne diseases in the EU and third world countries is 3.38 and 8.915 cases per 100 000 people respectively (6-8). The annual cost of foodborne diseases, including direct medical costs and reduced efficiency, is $5-6 billion (9). Most cases of disease are caused by bacteria, viruses, or parasites (10). The main foodborne pathogens that can contaminate food are *Salmonella* spp., *S. aureus*, *Clostridium botulinum*, *Bacillus* spp., *Acinetobacter* spp., *Escherichia coli*, *Pseudomonas* spp., and the hepatitis A virus. Intestinal parasites include *Giardia lamblia*, *Entamoeba hystolytica*, *Ascaris lumbricoides*, and *Hookworm* (11,12). From 1990 to date, several major groups of foodborne bacteria (*E. coli*, *S. aureus*, *S. arizonae*, and *E. faecalis*), have been considered in a lot of research and have attracted the attention of the food industry (13). The incidence of food-based diseases in developed countries has had a growing trend. In developing countries such as Iran, although there are no statistics on the incidence of infections and food poisoning, infection and food poisoning occurs far more often than in developed countries because of poor conditions of production, storage, and distribution and due to the low level of health education (14). In a microbiological study, Christison et al examined 4 food distribution centers in South Africa for contamination and reported that 16% and 4% were contaminated with *Salmonella* spp. and *Listeria,* respectively (15). In a 2006 study of bacterial contamination in foods conducted in centers affiliated with Baqiyatallah University, contamination rates of *E. coli* and *Staph* were reported as 12.5% and 13.8%, respectively (16). In a 2000 study of contamination in vegetables, dairy products, and ice cream conducted in Kashan, *E. coli* infection was reported in 15% of samples (17). In a survey conducted on the bacterial contamination of raw milk in Shahre Kord, 70% of samples were contaminated with *E. coli* and 80% with coliform (18). Generally, various studies have been conducted in the field of bacterial contamination of food. In most of these studies, a specific type of bacteria in a food group was studied; therefore, a lot of information on a range of food is not available. The results of studies conducted in Iran show that the quality of ready-to-eat foods is not desirable, and the microbial contamination of these foods is higher than the standard (19,20). A lack of attention to health issues at all stages of pizza and sandwich production decreases the quality of food products. Therefore, to protect the health of consumers, this study aimed to determine the microbial quality of pizza, frankfurters, and sausages in the distribution centers of these products in the city of Ilam.

Materials and Methods

Field study

In this cross-sectional study, a wide range of bacteria (*S. aureus, S. sonnei, S. arizonae, E. coli* and *E. faecalis*) was evaluated in three groups of foods, pizza (90 samples), frankfurters (90 samples), and sausages (90 samples), in the city of Ilam. Different diagnostic tests were done on each sample. A total of 270 food samples were randomly collected by health experts from fast food within 3 months during 2015 in the city of Ilam. Under sterile conditions, the samples were sent to the microbiology laboratory of the Environmental Health Department where they were refrigerated. Experiments were performed less than 24 hours later. The experiments, designed to determine contamination in food products and identify and confirm the presence of bacteria, were performed according to the Iranian national standard 2461-1 method (21).

Bacterial identification

To identify and enumerate *S. aureus,* the surface culture method for *Staphylococcus* in a specific medium of Baird Parker agar was used. Black colonies that were colorless and encircled with a clear halo were counted using the coagulase test (22). To identify *E. coli,* the Iranian national standard 2946 method was used. In this technique, after preparation, the sample was cultured in brilliant green broth and peptone water. After 24 hours of incubation, a few drops of Kovacs indole reagent were added to the tube with a peptone water medium. If a red circle formed on the top of the tube, the sample was considered positive for contamination with *E. coli.* Each diagnosis was confirmed by IMVIC tests (23). To detect *Salmonella,* after enrichment in non-selective and selective media such as lactose broth and Tetrathionate broth, the samples were cultured linearly in a selective solid medium of Brilliant Green agar (24). Then, the suspect colonies were transferred to a Triple Sugar Iron agar (TSI) differential medium and investigated for the presence or absence of Salmonella (24). To detect and isolate *Shigella,* after enrichment, the samples in the enrichment medium were used for Xylose lysine deoxycholate agar (XLD) differential culture media (2627) (25). To isolate the bacteria *Enterococcus* the selective medium of Kanamycin aesculin azide (KAA) Agar (Merck, Germany) was used. In this medium kanamycin was the selective agent. *Enterococcus* was determined using esculin hydrolyze, the fermentation of glucose and hydrolysis of esculin, which, in the presence of ferric citrate creates a brown color. Then, from the colonies grown, a few colonies were selected and cultured again on the same specific medium (26). To evaluate the contamination of the three studied groups of food, other factors such as indicators (health, sanitation, lack of hygiene), age, gender, and education level of operators in food supply centers were evaluated using a questionnaire.

Statistical analyses

The results of tests on various food groups were analyzed using statistical software SPSS 20 and regression test, and a level of 5% ($P<0.05$) was considered significant. To comply with ethical issues in research, the names of the food supply centers sampled in this study have been withheld.

Results

In this study, contamination with *E. coli* and *S. aureus* was greater in the three studied food groups (pizza, frankfurters, sausages) than other microbial species. From the 270 food samples tested, 75 samples (27.77%), were contaminated with *E. coli,* 58 samples (21.48%) with *S. aureus,* 39 samples (14.44%) with *S. arizonae,* 36 samples (13.33%) with *S. sonnei,* and 16 samples (5.9%) with *E. faecalis.* From total samples of pizza, 12.22% were infected with *S. aureus,* 5.55% to *S. sonnei* 8.88% to *S. arizonae* 23.33% to *E. coli* and 1.11% to *E. faecalis* (Table1).

The number and percentage of frankfurters contaminated with the microbial species are shown in Table 2.

From all frankfurter samples, 27.77% were contaminated with *S. aureus,* 17.77% with *S. sonnei,* 24.44% with *S. arizonae,* 31.11% with *E. coli,* and 8.88% with *E. faecalis.* The number and percentage of sausages contaminated

Table 1. The frequency of bacteria contamination in pizza

Bacteria	Positive cases		Negative cases	
	Number	Percent	Number	Percent
S. aureus	11	12.22	79	87.78
S. sonnei	5	5.55	85	94.45
S. arizonae	8	8.88	82	91.12
E. coli	21	23.33	69	76.67
E. faecalis	1	1.11	89	98.89

Table 2. The frequency of bacteria contamination in frankfurter

Bacteria	Positive cases		Negative cases	
	Number	Percent	Number	Percent
S. aureus	25	27.77	65	72.23
S. sonnei	16	17.77	74	82.23
S. arizonae	22	24.44	68	75.56
E. coli	28	31.11	62	68.89
E. faecalis	8	8.88	82	91.12

Table 3. The frequency of bacteria contamination in sausages

Bacteria	Positive cases		Negative cases	
	Number	Percent	Number	Percent
S. aureus	22	24.44	68	75.56
S. sonnei	15	16.66	75	83.34
S. arizonae	19	21.11	71	78.89
E. coli	26	28.88	64	71.12
E. faecalis	7	7.77	83	92.23

with the microbial species are shown in Table 3.
From the total samples of sausage, 24.44% was contaminated with *S. aureus*, 16.66% to *S. sonnei*, 21.11% to *S. arizonae*, 28.88% to *E. coli* and 7.77% to *E. faecalis*. The results showed that the percentage of contamination with microbial species was higher in frankfurters than in pizza or sausages. The high contamination of frankfurters (greater than pizza or sausages) is reasonable. In relation to the contamination in the three groups of food with *S. sonnei*, and *S. arizonae*, there is a significant difference; however, the *E. coli* and E. *faecalis* contamination rates were not significant ($P>0.05$). The chance of becoming contaminated with *S. aureus*, *S. sonnei*, *S. arizonae*, *E. coli*, and *E. faecalis* was higher for frankfurters and sausages than for pizza (Table 4).
Also, the chances of contamination in three types of ready-for-consumption food were adjusted for the impact of factors such as location, age, gender, and education level, and it was found that these factors did not influence the outcome (Table 5).

Table 4. Univariate logistic regression analysis of Fast food contamination by a variety of bacteria in Ilam

Bacteria	Univariable			
	Fast food	*P*	Odd ratio	95% CI for OR
S. aureus	Pizza	0.033	-	-
	Frankfurter	0.011	2.762	1.264–6.024
	Sausages	0.037	2.325	1.051–5.128
S. sonnei	Pizza	0.041	-	-
	Frankfurter	0.015	3.676	1.283–10.526
	Sausages	0.023	3.40	1.179–9.803
S. arizonae	Pizza	0.023	-	-
	Frankfurter	0.007	3.311	1.388–7.936
	Sausages	0.025	2.739	1.200–6.666
E. coli	Pizza	0.487	-	-
	Frankfurter	0.272	1.483	0.765–2.873
	Sausages	0.397	1.333	0.684–2.604
E. faecalis	Pizza	0.128	-	-
	Frankfurter	0.044	8.695	1.062–71.428
	Sausages	0.062	7.518	0.904–62.5

Table 5. Multivariable logistic regression analysis of Fast food contamination by a variety of bacteria in Ilam

Bacteria	Multivariable			
	Fast food	*P*	Odd ratio	95% CI for OR
S. aureus	Pizza	0.029	-	-
	Frankfurter	0.009	2.873	1.295–6.369
	Sausages	0.034	2.398	0.186–1.069
S. sonnei	Pizza	0.037	-	-
	Frankfurter	0.014	3.787	1.310–10.989
	Sausages	0.022	3.496	1.200–10.204
S. arizonae	Pizza	0.021	-	-
	Frankfurter	0.007	3.378	1.406–8.130
	Sausages	0.024	2.785	1.141–6.802
E. coli	Pizza	0.464	-	-
	Frankfurter	0.226	1.526	0.769–3.030
	Sausages	0.381	1.362	0.682–2.659
E. faecalis	Pizza	0.114	-	-
	Frankfurter	0.038	9.433	1.127–76.923
	Sausages	0.056	8.064	0.948–66.666

Discussion

The food industry and available technologies and the preparation, distribution, and sale of food (including raw materials or ready-to-eat foods) in health centers are both important issues and require special attention (18). Because of people's interest in using ready-to-eat foods and fast food such as pizza and meat products (sausages, frankfurters) to resolve a lack of protein and since such meat products are cheaper than pure meat, their use in different countries has increased several times in the past decade (14). Due to the importance of contamination of ready-to-eat foods and fast food, pathogenic microbes, and their role in causing human infection, this study examined 270 samples from 3 groups of food (pizza, frankfurters, and sausages). The results showed that among the three groups of foods tested, frankfurters and pizza, respectively, have the highest and lowest bacterial contamination. Contamination was greater with *E. coli* and *S. aureus* in the three food studied groups than with the other microbial species. Also, the percentages of contamination with *E. faecalis* in pizza, frankfurters, and sausages are low. It is noteworthy that among the three groups of foods a significant difference was observed in contamination with the microbial species. In addition, as shown in Table 4, the contamination of frankfurters and sausages by the microbial species is greater than that of pizza. It is noteworthy that factors such as indicators (health, sanitation, lack of hygiene), age, gender, and education level did not impact the outcome. In studies conducted in Iran and other countries, hygiene and food contamination by pathogenic bacteria has been evaluated. In a study conducted by Mirzabeygi et al in 2006 in western Tehran, the levels of contamination with *S. aureus* in dairy products and sweetmeats were reported as 16% (27). In a study by Sultan Dallal et al in 2007 surveying the microbiological quality of chicken and red meat, 47.8% of chicken samples and 28.8% of meat samples were contaminated with *Salmonella,* which is less than *S. arizonae* contamination in the present study (28). A study by Tavakoli et al was carried out in 4 restaurants affiliated with a military facility in Tehran. A total of 288 samples of ready-to-eat food and salad were examined. In 5 samples (1.73%), *E. coli* was found. The samples did not confirm *Salmonella* contamination. Also, the mean number of coliforms and *S. aureus* in some foods was found to be more than the standard. However, in this study, the rates of contamination with *E. coli* and *S. arizonae* were higher (29). In a study by Faramarzi et al, 642 food samples (58.33% salads and 9.84% dairy products) were found to be contaminated with *E. coli,* and 4.8% of sweetmeats were contaminated with *S. aureus,* which is consistent with the current study (30). Aycicek et al examined the rate of *S. aureus* contamination of ready-to-eat salads and foods in restaurants at military centers in Ankara, Turkey. They tested 512 samples of salads, pizzas, and a variety of meat foods. Their results indicated that 48 samples were contaminated with *S. aureus*, and in meat foods and salads, *S. aureus* contamination was significantly higher than in the other samples, which is consistent with the current study (31). In a study performed by Meldrum et al conducted in the United Kingdom on 1213 salad and 1208 sauce samples, results showed that 4.7% of salad samples and 5% of sauce samples were of lower than acceptable quality, and the presence of microbial *E. coli* and *S. aureus* were confirmed in them (32). In the current study, 27.77% of food samples were contaminated with *E. coli.* In the study of Sagoo et al, 3% of salad samples had confirmed contamination with *E. coli* (33). The presence of bacterial species (*S. aureus, S. sonnei, S. arizonae, E. coli, and E. faecalis*) in the three food groups studied indicates the lack of sufficient attention paid to food hygiene standards in their procurement centers. This may be due to the staff's lack of personal hygiene, contamination of raw materials, or secondary contamination. *E. coli* and *S aureus* contamination in the studied samples is a serious warning to health officials. *S aureus* in raw food is not a good competitor for other bacteria, but in cooked foods in which other microorganisms are destroyed, it is easily grown and creates contamination (34). The tendency of a lot of people to use ready-to-eat foods, the lack of proper observance of environmental health and food processing equipment, the improper washing of hands and the long-term contact of these hands with food are the most important causes of food contamination and disease. The results of this study can be used for operators of fast food centers and also for healthcare providers in health centers. Making the staff of fast food centers aware of the dangers of these bacteria can allow them to act to reduce the bacterial contamination of ready-to-eat foods. The implementation of an HACCP system, another standard certification, and the training of operators at fast food centers can be very effective in preventing or reducing bacterial contamination. Also, a complementary study of bacterial contamination in food preparation, dining room, utensils and equipment used in processing and cooking and personal hygiene operators can be useful.

Conclusion

Based on the results of the current study, the prevalence of bacterial contamination of ready-to-eat foods can have an important role in infection and food poisoning. The spread of foodborne diseases, problems in the field of food hygiene and its importance in health and economics, a lack of awareness, and a lack of respect for the basic principles of health could be the main reasons for contamination and could endanger public health. A lot of people tend to consume fast food, and the bacterial contamination of these foods is a serious problem that needs further investigation. Training for personnel working in fast food preparation centers on the proper observance of health issues, and the overseeing of the preparation, transportation, storage, and supply of ready-to-eat foods seems necessary to prevent the transmission of microbial contamination. The amount of contamination in food must be reduced by taking appropriate actions to ensure the health of the community.

Acknowledgments

This article is the result of the research project number 22/52/93/1409, contract dated 29/11/93, approved by the Ilam University of Medical Sciences and Health Services. The authors are grateful for the financial support provided by the Deputy of Research and Technology of Ilam University of Medical Sciences.

Competing interests

The authors declare that they have no competing interests.

Authors' contributions

MA conceived and designed the study. MTY, MD, MM, FS, and ZG performed the literature search and wrote the manuscript. All authors participated in data acquisition, analysis, and interpretation. All authors critically reviewed, refined, and approved the manuscript.

References

1. Razavilar V. Pathogenic Microorganisms in Foods and Epidemiology of Food Borne Intoxications. 3rd ed. Tehran Tehran University Publications; 2010. [In Persian].
2. Isara AR, Isah EC, Lofor PV, Ojide CK. Food contamination in fast food restaurants in Benin City, Edo State, Nigeria: Implications for food hygiene and safety. Public Health 2010; 124(8): 467-71. doi: 10.1016/j.puhe.2010.03.028.
3. World Health Organization (WH). Food Safety and Food Borne Illness. Geneva: WHO; 2007.
4. Newell DG, Koopmans M, Verhoef L, Duizer E, Aidara-Kane A, Sprong H, et al. Food-borne diseases-the challenges of 20 years ago still persist while new ones continue to emerge. Int J Food Microbiol 2010; 139 Suppl 1: S3-15. doi: 10.1016/j.ijfoodmicro.2010.01
5. Abdollahzadeh E, Rezaei M, Hosseini H, Safari R. Effects of Nisin and thyme essential oil, individually and in combination, on inoculated populations of Listeria monocytogenes in minced silver carp. Iran J Nutr Sci Food Technol 2012; 6(4): 13-20. [In Persian].
6. Kilic B. Current trends in traditional Turkish meat products and cuisine. LWT- Food Science and Technology 2009; 42(10): 1581-9. doi: 10.1016/j.lwt.2009.05.016.
7. Teymori R, Ghazanfarirad N, Dehghan K, Asadzadeh J, Hajigholizadeh G, Bahmani M. A survey of bacteria and mold contamination of imported rice into West Azerbaijan Province, northwest of Iran. Asian Pac J Trop Dis 2014; 4 (Suppl 2): S833-5. doi: 10.1016/S2222-1808(14)60737-4.
8. Kagkli DM, Vancanneyt M, Hill C, Vandamme P, Cogan TM. *Entrococcus* and *Lactobacillus* contamination of raw milk in a farm dairy environment. Int J Food Microbiol 2007; 114(2): 243-51. doi: 10.1016/j.ijfoodmicro.2006.09.016.
9. Mosaferi M, Hajizadeh Y, Ostadrahimi AR, AslHashemi A. Importance of water quality control in food safety, case study: drinking, dairy and canning industries of eastern Azerbaijan. Med J Tabriz Univ Med Sci Health Serv 2007; 29(1): 93-97. [In Persian].
10. Nascimento MS, Reolon EM, Santos ARB, Moreira VE, Silva N. *Enterobcteriaceae* contamination in chocolate processing. Food Control 2015; 47: 291-297.
11. Garayoa R, Vitas AI, Díez-Leturia M, García-Jalón I. Food safety and the contract catering companies: food handlers, facilities and HACCP evaluation. J Food Control 2011; 22(12): 2006-12. doi: 10.1016/j.foodcont.2011.05.021.
12. Vanderzant C, Splittstoesser DF. Compendium of methods for the microbiological examination of foods. 3rd ed. Washington, DC: American Public Health Association; 1992.
13. Bolton DJ, Meally A, Blair IS, McDowellb DA, Cowana C. Food safety knowledge of head chefs and catering managers in Ireland. J Food Control 2008; 19(3): 291-300. doi: 10.1016/j.foodcont.2007.04.006.
14. Chapman B, Eversley T, Fillion K, Maclaurin T, Powell D. Assessment of food safety practices of food service food handlers (risk assessment data): testing a communication intervention (evaluation of tools). J Food Prot 2010; 73(6): 1101-7.
15. Christison CA, Lindsay D, von Holy A. Microbiological surveys of ready-to-eat foods and associated preparation surfaces in retail delicatessens, Johannesburg, South Africa. J Food Control 2008; 19(7): 727-33. doi: 10.1016/j.foodcont.2007.07.004.
16. Tavakoli HR, Karimi Zarchi AA, Izadi M. A survey on bacterial contamination of consumpted foods in belonging centers of Baqiyatallah University of Medical Sciences. Journal of Military Medicine 2007; 9(2) 89-95. [In Persian].
17. Salek Moghadam A, Forouhesh Tehrani H, Mozafari NA, Ansari H. Prevalence of virulence factors among *E. coli* isolated from food materials from Iran University of Medical Sciences' food microbial laboratory. Feyz 2000; 4(3): 32-40. [In Persian].
18. Fadaei AM, Jamshidi A, Kheiri S. Comparison of bacterial contamination of raw and pasteurized milk used in Shahrekord in 2006. Journal of Shahrekord University of Medical Sciences 2008; 10(2): 37-44. [In Persian].
19. Salek S. Microbial food intake of medical centers [dissertation]. Tehran: Shahid Beheshti University; 1999. [In Persian].
20. Tavakoli H, Riazipour M. Microbial quality of cooked meat foods in Tehran University's restaurants. Pak J Med Sci 2008; 24(4): 595-9.
21. Institute of Standards and Industrial Research of Iran.2946. Microbiology of food and animal feeding stuffs - Detection and enumeration of presumptive *Escherichia coli* - most probable number technique. Karaj: Institute of Standards and Industrial Research of Iran; 2005. [In Persian].
22. Institute of Standards and Industrial Research of Iran. Microbiology of food and animal feeding stuff-horizontal method for the enumeration of positive staphylococci coagulase (number: 6806). Karaj: Institute of Standards and Industrial Research of Iran; 2005. [In Persian].
23. Institute of Standards and Industrial Research of Iran. Microbiology of food and animal feeding stuffs - Detection and enumeration of presumptive *Escherichia coli* - Most probable number technique (number: 2946). 2nd ed. Karaj: Institute o Standards and Industrial Research of Iran; 2005. [In Persian].
24. Institute of Standards and Industrial Research of Iran. Microbiology of food and animal feeding stuffs-horizontal method for detection of *Salmonella* (number: 1810). 3rd ed. Karaj: Institute of Standards and Industrial Research of Iran; 2005. [In Persian].
25. Institute of Standards and Industrial Research of Iran. Microbiology of food and animal feeding stuffs horizontal method for the detection of *Shigella* spp (number: 2627). 2nd ed. Karaj: Institute Of Standards and Industrial Research of Iran; 2005. [In Persian].
26. Institute of Standards and Industrial Research of Iran. Microbiology of foods and foodstuffs – Detection and enumeration of *Enterococcus* in food (number: 2198). Karaj: Institute of Standards and Industrial Research of Iran; 2005. [In Persian].
27. Mirzabeygi M, Posti F, Rahbar Arasteh H. Study of

Staphylococcus aureus contamination in dairy and confectionery products from west of Tehran. Iranian Congress of Microbiology; 4-6 March 2008; Kerman. [In Persian].
28. Soltan Dallal MM, Sharifi Yazdi MK, Mirzaei N, Kalantar E. Prevalence of *Salmonella* spp. in packed and unpacked red meat and chicken in South of Tehran. Jundishapur J Microbiol 2014; 7(4): e9254. doi: 10.5812/jjm.9254 .
29. Tavakoli HR, Farhang K, Karimi Zarchi A, Heydari E. Bacteriological quality of ready to eat food in four military restaurants. Iranian Journal of Military Medicine 2012; 13(4): 207-212. [In Persian].
30. Faramarzi T, Jonidi Jafari A, Dehghani S, Mirzabeygi M, Naseh M, Arasteh RH. A survey of bacterial contamination of food supply in the West of Tehran. Journal of Fasa University of Medical Sciences 2012; 2(1): 12-18. [In Persian].
31. Aycicek H, Cakiroglu S, Stevenson TH. Incidence of *Staphylococcus aureus* in ready-to-eat meals from military cafeterias in Ankara, Turkey. J Food Control 2005; 16(6): 531-4. doi: 10.1016/j.foodcont.2004.04.005.
32. Meldrum RJ, Little CL, Sagoo S, Mithani V, de Pinna E. Assessment of the microbiological safety of salad vegetables and sauces from kebab take-away restaurants in the United Kingdom. J Food Microbiol 2009; 26(6): 573-7. doi: 10.1016/j.fm.2009.03.013.
33. Sagoo SK, Little CL, Mitchell RT. Microbiological quality of open ready-to-eat salad vegetables: effectiveness of food hygiene training of management. J Food Prot 2003; 66(9): 1581-6.
34. Young RE, Young MK, Yoon KS. Survival of pathogenic enterohemorrhagic *Escherichia coli* (EHEC) and control with calcium oxide in frozen meat products. Food Microbiol 2015; 49: 203-10. doi: 10.1016/j.fm.2015.02.010.

12

Acute toxicity effect of glyphosate on survival rate of common carp, *Cyprinus carpio*

Mohammad Forouhar Vajargah[1*], Ahmad Mohamadi Yalsuyi[2], Masoud Sattari[1,3], Aliakbar Hedayati[4]

[1]Department of Fisheries, School of Natural Resources, University of Guilan Sowmehsara, Sowmehsara, Iran
[2]Department of Aquaculture, School of Fisheries and Environment, Gorgan University of Agricultural Sciences and Natural Resources, Gorgan, Iran
[3]Department of Marine Sciences, Caspian Sea Basin Research Center, University of Guilan, Rasht, Iran
[4]Department of Aquatic Production and Exploitation, School of Fisheries and Environment, Gorgan University of Agricultural Sciences and Natural Resources, Gorgan, Iran

Abstract
Background: Herbicides are usually used to control weeds and some of them like glyphosate are non-selective herbicides. Aquatic environments are usually the last destinations of agricultural pesticides, which disrupt the metabolic processes of organisms. Thus, the aim of this study was to evaluate acute toxicity of glyphosate on the survival rate of common carp, *Cyprinus carpio*.
Methods: A total of 135 common carp averaged 7 ± 0.8 g in weight were exposed to 0, 25, 50, 75, 100, 125, 150, 175 and 200 mL.L^{-1} glyphosate (15 fish in each treatment, with triplicates) for 96 hours. The aquariums capacity was 98 L in volume (80 × 35 × 35 cm) and physicochemical parameters were the same for all groups (pH 7.4-8, temperature = 26 ± 1°C, DO = 7 mg.L^{-1} and total hardness of 190 mg $CaCO_3$). LC_{10}, LC_{20}, LC_{30}, LC_{40}, LC_{50}, LC_{60}, LC_{70}, LC_{80}, LC_{90} and LC_{95} of glyphosate were calculated at 24, 48, 72 and 96 hours after adding glyphosate using probit test.
Results: Mortality was observed in all treatments which exposed to higher than 50 mL.L^{-1} after 96 hours. The results showed that 96-hour LC_{50} of glyphosate for common carp was 92.71 mL.L^{-1}. The fish exposed to different concentrations of glyphosate showed clinical signs such as increased mucus secretion, skin darkening and death with mouth open.
Conclusion: Glyphosate disrupts the synthesis of amino acids in plants by inhibiting enzymatic activity of 5-enolpyruvylshikimate-3-phosphate synthase (EPSP). This enzyme is absent in animals. However, glyphosate is toxic for common carp.
Keywords: Animals, Herbicides, Glyphosate, Carps, Excitatory postsynaptic potentials

***Correspondence to:**
Mohammad Forouhar Vajargah
Email:
mohammad.forouhar@yahoo.com

Introduction

In recent years, the use of agricultural pesticides has been increased significantly (1). Various types of agricultural pesticides such as herbicides, insecticides and fungicides are commonly used globally (2); these pesticides usually spread in the aquatic environments through various ways such as rainfall and soil erosion (3). In other words, aquatic ecosystems are the ultimate destinations of agricultural pesticides (4). Aquatic organisms contact with their environment through physiological surfaces and pesticides can penetrate through the skin, gills and mouth into their body, and affect liver, kidneys, gonads and other organs (5). Contamination and accumulation of pesticides in the aquatic environment can lead to food poisoning and mortality in humans (1,2).

Herbicides are commonly used in farms to control weeds (6). In the meantime, glyphosate (glyphosate 41% SL) is one of the most widely used herbicides in many countries, especially developing countries (1,7). The use of glyphosate had the fastest growth rate compared to other herbicides (8). Two-thirds of the total volume of glyphosate has been sprayed in the recent decades (9). Glyphosate inhibits the 5-enolpyruvylshikimate-3-phosphate synthase (EPSP) activity in plants and impairs the synthesis of the aromatic amino acids (10). EPSP is found only in plants and some bacteria (11).

Glyphosate is highly soluble in water (10500 mL.L^{-1}) and its half-life, depending on the environmental conditions, is between 3.5 and 70 days (12). However, Souza et al (13) pointed out that the half-life of glyphosate in freshwater was between 28 and 87 days. It was thought that since EPSP enzyme was not found in animals, so glyphosate is not toxic to them. However, the results of previous studies showed that it was toxic to fish species (10,14). Loro et al (15) reported that glyphosate-based herbicide was toxic to *Rhamdia quelen* and *Leporinus obtusidens*. Sandun et al (16) reported that 96-hour LC_{50} of glyphosate to *Oreochromis niloticus* was 16.7 $mg.L^{-1}$; Da Cruz et al (17) also pointed out that glyphosate-based herbicide was toxic to fish as an aquatic organism.

Fish, as aquatic organisms, can be used as biomarkers in toxicology and biological studies (18). So fish often have been used as experimental biological models for exhibiting environmental impacts of toxins (19). Toxicological studies on lethal concentration of toxins are very important (20), and one of the methods is to determine 96-hour LC_{50} of pesticides on fish (21,22). Toxicological studies like those determining 96-hour LC_{50} of toxins on fish can provide better management of water resources as a method for detection of biological effects of pollutants (23). Finally, these studies can also be useful in determining the limits of toxins in nature and human food safety (24).

Common Carp, *Cyprinus carpio* Linnaeus, 1758, as a commercially- important fish species in aquaculture (25) is found in most temperate regions of the world (26). It is omnivorous (27) and often searches bottom of the pond for getting food (28). Feeding habits, high growth rate, reproduction in captivity, adaptation to commercial diets and density are reasons for the common carp popularity in aquaculture industries (29). However, human activities and environmental pollutants can disrupt the life cycle of common carp (30). The use of herbicides such as glyphosate in addition to the destruction of macrophytes may affect non-target organisms such as common carp through destruction of habitats and food (31,32). For example Zebrafish, *Danio rerio*, needs a substrate full of plants for spawning and reproduction (33), so the pollutants may have negative effects on breeding of this species through the destruction of non-target aquatic plants.

There is limited information about the toxicity of glyphosate. It is also true for the maintenance of carp in ponds and reservoirs as well as its long half-life in the aquatic environments. So, the aim of the present study was to assess acute toxicity of glyphosate on survival rate of common carp, *C. carpio* as an animal model.

Methods

The experiment was performed according to Yalsuyi and Vajargah (2) and Montajami et al (34).

Sample preparation

200 common carp averaged 7 ± 0.8 g in weight were prepared from some farms in Guilan province and transferred to the laboratory in Faculty of Natural Resources, University of Guilan, Guilan province, Iran, and divided into four 250-L tanks (50 fish in each tank). Fish were maintained in these tanks for two weeks in order to acclimate with laboratory conditions. Fish were fed a commercial diet (produced by Faradaneh Co. Tehran, Iran) at 3% of body weight 3 times a day. Physicochemical parameters of water in all tanks were the same (pH 7.4-8, temperature = 26 ± 1°C, DO =7 $mg.L^{-1}$ and total hardness = 190 mg $CaCO_3$).

Toxicity tests

After adaptation, 135 fish were selected randomly and divided into 9 treatment groups (0, 25, 50, 75, 100, 125, 150, 175 and 200 $mL.L^{-1}$ glyphosate) in triplicates into 27 aquariums (80 × 35 × 35 cm, capacity 85 l). Fish were exposed to different concentrations of glyphosate (Glyphosate Aria 41% SL) for 96 hours. Mortality rates of fish were recorded at 24, 48, 72 and 96 hours after adding glyphosate. Animals then were transferred into aquariums 16 hours before the toxicity test and feeding was stopped 24 hours before the experiment. Water physicochemical parameters were the same as the adaptation time (pH 7.4-8, temperature = 26 ± 1°C, DO = 7 $mg.L^{-1}$ and total hardness = 190 mg $CaCO_3$).

Data analysis

Toxicity of glyphosate was estimated using the method proposed by Vajargah and Hedayati (35). Lethal concentrations of glyphosate for 50% of the population at 24, 48, 72 and 96 hLC50 were calculated using probit test (with a 95% CI) by IBM SPSS 20. Spearman test (two-tailed test) was used to determine the correlation between different concentrations of glyphosate and fish mortality.

Results

Mortality was not observed in the adaptation period. The results of toxicity tests showed that there was a significant correlation ($P < 0.01$) between concentration of glyphosate and fish mortality. All fish died after 96 hours exposure to the concentrations higher than 150 $mL.L^{-1}$ glyphosate, while in concentration of 200 $mL.L^{-1}$, all fish died after 24 hours (Table 1).

96-h LC_{50} of glyphosate for common carp was 92.711 $mL.L^{-1}$. LC_{10}, LC_{20}, LC_{30}, LC_{40}, LC_{50}, LC_{60}, LC_{70}, LC_{80}, LC_{90} and LC_{95} of glyphosate within 24, 48, 72 and 96 hours are demonstrated in Table 2. The fish exposed to different concentrations of glyphosate showed clinical signs such as increased mucus secretion, skin darkening, fast swimming, increased movements of operculum and death with mouth open.

Discussion

As it is estimated that the world population increases up to 9 billion persons by 2050 (36), therefore, food supply needs to be increased by productivity (37); and

Table 1. Mortality rate of common carp, *Cyprinus carpio* exposed to different concentrations of glyphosate (n=15 in each treatment)

Concentration (mg.L^{-1})	Number	No. of mortality			
		24 h	48 h	72 h	96 h
0	15	0	0	0	0
25	15	0	0	0	0
50	15	0	0	0	1
75	15	1	3	4	6
100	15	2	5	7	9
125	15	2	6	8	12
150	15	3	8	13	15
175	15	6	10	14	15
200	15	15	15	15	15

All fish died at concentrations higher than 150 mL.L^{-1}.

Table 2. Lethal concentration of glyphosate for common carp, *Cyprinus carpio*

Point	Concentration (mg.L^{-1})			
	24 h	48 h	72 h	96 h
LC_{10}	109.420	71.438	63.006	52.731
LC_{20}	128.898	93.337	79.563	66.455
LC_{30}	142.943	109.130	91.501	76.352
LC_{40}	154.944	122.624	101.702	84.808
LC_{50}	**166.161**	**135.236**	**111.237**	**92.711**
LC_{60}	177.378	147.848	120.771	100.615
LC_{70}	189.379	161.342	130.972	109.071
LC_{80}	203.425	177.135	142.911	118.967
LC_{90}	222..903	199.036	159.467	132.691
LC_{95}	238.988	217.122	173.40	144.025

agricultural growth requires an increase in productivity through the use of a variety of nutrients for plants and soil, improving agricultural techniques, and the use of high-yielding plant varieties and pesticides (38). Glyphosate is widely used in agriculture (9). According to the World Health Organization (WHO) (39), application of glyphosate has increased annually. It has also long half-life in aquatic environments (13) and its residues can remain stable in foods for a year or even more, even if the foods are frozen, dried or processed (40). It also damages macrophytes as well as non-target organisms such as common carp through deterioration offish habitats and food (31). Hence, one of the main challenges concerning the widespread application of agricultural pesticides can be related to their devastating impact on non-target organisms (41).

Akinsorotan (42) reported that the 96-h LC_{50} of dizensate (glyphosate) on fingerlings of *Clarias gariepinus*, as an aquatic organism, was 18.07 mg.L^{-1}. It was also found that dizensate can reduce the survival rate of the fish, which is consistent with the results of the present study.

Micah et al (43) studied behavioral responses of *Heteroclarias* (hybrid) exposed to two types of glyphosate and found that it was toxic to *Heteroclarias* (hybrid) as an aquatic organism and its 96-hour LC_{50} was 6.838 mg.L^{-1}. They also reported that glyphosate had some clinical signs such as increased opercular ventilation and also caudal fin damage, which was consistent with the results of the present study.

Da Cruz et al (17) investigated sensitivity, ecotoxicity and histopathological effects on some Neotropical fish exposed to glyphosate alone and with surfactant. Their results showed that glyphosate was toxic to these species and there was significant correlation between mortality rate of fish and concentration of glyphosate ($P<0.01$). It also reduced the survival rate of fish as non- target organism and had harmful effects on fish, which was also similar to the results of the present study.

Jofré et al (12) studied toxicity of two commercial glyphosate on survival rate of two fish species (*Danio rerio* and *Poecilia reticulata*). The results of their study indicated that both herbicides may produce potential environmental damages, which is similar to the results of the present study.

Henao Muñoz et al (44) studied acute toxicity and sub-lethal effects of the mixture glyphosate (Roundup® Active and Cosmo-Flux 411F) to anuran embryos and tadpoles of four Colombian species. The results showed that 96-hour LC_{50} of glyphosate to embryos and tadpoles was between 2.2-3.9 μg.L^{-1} and 1.4-2.8 μg.L^{-1}, respectively. Tadpoles of

Hypsiboas crepitans was the most sensitive and glyphosate was toxic to aquatic organisms, which is consistent with the results of the present study.

By comparing the results of the present study and Jofré et al (12), Akinsorotan (42), Micah et al (43) and Henao Muñoz et al (44), it was found that the toxicity of glyphosate depends on the size, species and physicochemical parameters of the environment.

Conclusion

According to the results, although glyphosate inhibits the enzyme EPSP and this enzyme has been observed only in plants and some bacteria, but glyphosate was toxic to *C. carpio* as a non-target organism. The results of the present study can be useful for further ecotoxicological studies. On the other hand, agricultural pesticides are associated with materials which have different combinations such as salts and a surfactant called polyethylene amine (POEA). These compounds in some cases, can increase the toxicity of pesticides. For example, Peyote®, which is one of the glyphosate compounds, is more toxic than glyphosate. POEA is also toxic to aquatics (45). The present study can also be useful for further investigations on the toxicity of POEA to the other aquatics.

Acknowledgments

The present study was carried out by laboratory facilities and research equipment of Guilan University. The authors would like to gratitude Dr. Rasoul Ghorbani for his help and guide. We also thank all personnel of University of Guilan who helped us to carry out this laboratory examinations.

Competing interests

The authors declare that they have no competing interests.

Authors' contributions

Authors were participated in all aspects of this research work, like data collection, analysis, interpretation and manuscript approval.

References

1. de Oliveira JL, Campos EV, Bakshi M, Abhilash PC, Fraceto LF. Application of nanotechnology for the encapsulation of botanical insecticides for sustainable agriculture: prospects and promises. Biotechnol Adv 2014; 32(8): 1550-61. doi: 10.1016/j.biotechadv.2014.10.010.
2. Mohamadi Yalsuyi A, Forouhar Vajargah M. Acute toxicity of silver nanoparticles in Roach (*Rutilus rutilus*) and Goldfish (*Carassius auratus*). J Environ Treat Tech 2017; 5(1): 1-4.
3. Larras F, Montuelle B, Bouchez A. Assessment of toxicity thresholds in aquatic environments: does benthic growth of diatoms affect their exposure and sensitivity to herbicides? Sci Total Environ 2013; 463-464: 469-77. doi: 10.1016/j.scitotenv.2013.06.063.
4. Hedayati A, Forouhar Vajargah M, Mohamadi Yalsuyi A, Abarghouei S, Hajiahmadyan M. Acute toxicity test of pesticide abamectin on common carp (*Cyprinus carpio*). J Coast Life Med 2014; 2(11): 841-44. doi: 10.12980/JCLM.2.201414J44.
5. Ibrahim AT, Harabawy AS. Sublethal toxicity of carbofuran on the African catfish *Clarias gariepinus*: Hormonal, enzymatic and antioxidant responses. Ecotoxicol Environ Saf 2014; 106: 33-9. doi: 10.1016/j.ecoenv.2014.04.032.
6. Dentzman K, Gunderson R, Jussaume R. Techno-optimism as a barrier to overcoming herbicide resistance: Comparing farmer perceptions of the future potential of herbicides. J Rural Stud 2016; 48: 22-32. doi: 10.1016/j.jrurstud.2016.09.006.
7. Poiger T, Buerge IJ, Bachli A, Muller MD, Balmer ME. Occurrence of the herbicide glyphosate and its metabolite AMPA in surface waters in Switzerland determined with on-line solid phase extraction LC-MS/MS. Environ Sci Pollut Res Int 2017; 24(2): 1588-96. doi: 10.1007/s11356-016-7835-2.
8. Myers JP, Antoniou MN, Blumberg B, Carroll L, Colborn T, Everett LG, et al. Concerns over use of glyphosate-based herbicides and risks associated with exposures: a consensus statement. Environ Health 2016; 15: 19. doi: 10.1186/s12940-016-0117-0.
9. Benbrook CM. Trends in glyphosate herbicide use in the United States and globally. Environ Sci Eur 2016; 28(1): 3. doi: 10.1186/s12302-016-0070-0.
10. Tian YS, Xu J, Xing XJ, Zhao W, Fu XY, Peng RH, et al. Improved glyphosate resistance of 5-enolpyruvylshikimate-3-phosphate synthase from *Vitis vinifera* in transgenic *Arabidopsis* and rice by DNA shuffling. Mol Breed 2015; 35(7): 148. doi: 10.1007/s11032-015-0327-0.
11. Tohge T, Watanabe M, Hoefgen R, Fernie AR. Shikimate and phenylalanine biosynthesis in the green lineage. Front Plant Sci 2013; 4: 62. doi: 10.3389/fpls.2013.00062.
12. Jofré DM, Garcia MJ, Salcedo R, Morales M, Alvarez M, Enriz D, et al. Fish toxicity of commercial herbicides formulated with glyphosate. J Environ Anal Toxicol 2013; 4(1): 1-3. doi: 10.4172/2161-0525.1000199.
13. Souza EL, Foloni LL, Filho JT, Velini ED, Siono LM. Silva JR. Half-life of glyphosate on the control of water hyacinths in water tanks. J Water Resource Prot 2017; 9(5): 470-81. doi: 10.4236/jwarp.2017.95030.
14. Bohn T, Rover CM, Semenchuk PR. Daphnia magna negatively affected by chronic exposure to purified Cry-toxins. Food Chem Toxicol 2016; 91: 130-40. doi: 10.1016/j.fct.2016.03.009.
15. Loro VL, Glusczak L, Moraes BS, Leal CAM, Menezes

C, Murussi CR, et al. Glyphosate-based herbicide affects biochemical parameters in *Rhamdia quelen* (Quoy & Gaimard, 1824 and) *Leporinus obtusidens* (Valenciennes, 1837). Neotrop Ichthyol 2015; 13(1): 229-36. doi: 10.1590/1982-0224-20140082.

16. Sandun KV, Bandara N, Amarasinghe US. Effect of glyphosate-based herbicide, Roundup™ on territory deference of male *Oreochromis mossambicus* (Osteichthyes, Cichlidae) associated with mating behaviour. Sri Lanka J Soc Sci 2015; 20(1): 1-10. doi: 10.4038/sljas.v20i1.7451.
17. Da Cruz C, Carraschi SP, Shiogiri NS, Da Silva AF, Pitelli RA, Machado MR. Sensitivity, ecotoxicity and histopathological effects on neotropical fish exposed to glyphosate alone and associated to surfactant. Journal of Environmental Chemistry and Ecotoxicology 2016; 8(3): 25-33. doi: 10.5897/JECE2015.0362.
18. Ullah S, Zorriehzahra MJ. Ecotoxicology: a review of pesticides induced toxicity in Fish. Adv Anim Vet Sci 2014; 3(1): 40-57. doi: 10.14737/journal.aavs/2015/3.1.40.57.
19. Palanikumar L, Kumaraguru AK, Ramakritinan CM, Anand M. Toxicity, biochemical and clastogenic response of chlorpyrifos and carbendazim in milkfish *Chanos chanos*. Int J Environ Sci Technol 2014; 11(3): 765-74. doi: 10.1007/s13762-013-0264-6.
20. Arome D, Chinedu E. The importance of toxicity testing. J Pharm Biosci 2013; 4: 146-48.
21. Mohamadi Yalsuyi A, Forouhar Vajargah M. Recent advance on aspect of fisheries: A review. J Coast Life Med 2017; 5(4): 141-48. doi: 10.12980/jclm.5.2017J6-226.
22. Forouhar Vajargah M, Hedayati A, Mohamadi Yalsuyi A, Abarghouei S, Gerami MH, Ghaffari farsani H. Acute toxicity of Butachlor to Caspian Kutum (*Rutilus frisii kutum* Kamensky, 1991). J Environ Treat Tech 2014; 2(4): 155-57.
23. Forouhar Vajargah M, Hedayati A. Acute toxicity of trichlorofon on four viviparous fish: *Poecilia latipinna, Poecilia reticulata, Gambusia holbrooki* and *Xiphophorus helleri* (Cyprinodontiformes: Poecilidae). J Coast Life Med 2014; 2(7): 511-14. doi: 10.12980/JCLM.2.2014J11.
24. Khan A, Shah N, Gul A, Sahar N, Ismail A, Muhammad M, et al. Comparative study of toxicological impinge of glyphosate and atrazine (herbicide) on stress biomarkers; blood biochemical and haematological parameters of the freshwater common carp (*Cyprinus carpio*). Polish Journal of Environmental Studies 2016; 25(5): 1995-2001. doi: 10.15244/pjoes/62698.
25. Shirali S, Erfani Majd N, Mesbah M, Seifi MR. Histological studies of common carp ovarian development during breeding season in Khouzestan province, Iran. World Journal of Fish and Marine Sciences 2012; 4(2): 159-64. doi: 10.5829/idosi.wjfms.2012.04.02.56406.
26. Xu P, Zhang X, Wang X, Li J, Liu G, Kuang Y, et al. Genome sequence and genetic diversity of the common carp, *Cyprinus carpio*. Nat Genet 2014; 46(11): 1212-9. doi: 10.1038/ng.3098.
27. Schultz S, Koussoroplis AM, Changizi-Magrhoor Z, Watzke J, Kainz MJ. Fish oil–based finishing diets strongly increase long-chain polyunsaturated fatty acid concentrations in farm-raised common carp (*Cyprinus carpio* L.). Aquac Res 2015; 46(9): 2174-84. doi: doi:10.1111/are.12373.
28. Khan MN, Shahzad K, Chatta A, Sohail M, Piria M, Treer T. A review of introduction of common carp *Cyprinus carpio* in Pakistan: origin, purpose, impact and management. Croatian Journal of Fisheries 2016; 74(2): 71-80. doi: 10.1515/cjf-2016-0016.
29. Macklin R, Brazier B, Harrison S, Chapman DV, Vilizzi L. A review of the status and range expansion of common carp (*Cyprinus carpio* L.) in Ireland. Aquatic Invasions 2016; 11(1): 75-82. doi: 10.3391/ai.2016.11.1.08.
30. Sfakianakis DG, Renieri E, Kentouri M, Tsatsakis AM. Effect of heavy metals on fish larvae deformities: a review. Environ Res 2015; 137: 246-55. doi: 10.1016/j.envres.2014.12.014.
31. Segner H, Schmitt-Jansen M, Sabater S. Assessing the impact of multiple stressors on aquatic biota: the receptor's side matters. Environ Sci Technol 2014; 48(14): 7690-6. doi: 10.1021/es405082t.
32. Sinhorin VD, Sinhorin AP, Teixeira JM, Mileski KM, Hansen PC, Moreira PS, et al. Effects of the acute exposition to glyphosate-based herbicide on oxidative stress parameters and antioxidant responses in a hybrid Amazon fish surubim (*Pseudoplatystoma* sp). Ecotoxicol Environ Saf 2014; 106: 181-7. doi: 10.1016/j.ecoenv.2014.04.040.
33. Hoo JY, Kumari Y, Shaikh MF, Hue SM, Goh BH. Zebrafish: a versatile animal model for fertility research. 2016; 2016: 9732780. doi: 10.1155/2016/9732780.
34. Montajami S, Hajiahmadyan M, Forouhar Vajargah M, Hosseini Zarandeh AS, Shirood Mirzaie F, Hosseini SA. Effect of symbiotic (*Biomin imbo*) on Growth performance and survival rate of Texas cichlid (*Herichthys cyanoguttatus*) larvae. Global Veterinaria 2012; 9(3): 358-61. doi: 10.5829/idosi.gv.2012.9.3.6568.
35. Forouhar Vajargah M, Hedayati A. Toxicity effects of cadmium in grass carp (*Ctenopharyngodon idella*) and Big Head Carp (*Hypophthalmichthys nobilis*). Transylv Rev Syst Ecol Res 2017; 19(1): 43-8. doi: 10.1515/trser-2017-0004.
36. Bene C, Barange M, Subasinghe R, Pinstrup-Andersen P, Merino G, Hemre GI, et al. Feeding 9 billion by 2050 – Putting fish back on the menu. Food Secur 2015; 7(2): 261-74. doi: 10.1007/s12571-015-0427-z.
37. Bajzelj B, Richards K, Allwood JM, Smith P, Dennis JS, Curmi E, et al. Importance of food-demand management for climate mitigation. Nat Clim Chang 2014; 4(10): 924-29. doi: 10.1038/nclimate2353.
38. Sekhon BS. Nanotechnology in agri-food production: an overview. Nanotechnol Sci Appl 2014; 7: 31-53. doi: 10.2147/nsa.s39406.
39. World Health Organization. World health statistics monitoring health for the SDGs, sustainable development goals. Geneva: WHO; 2016.
40. Kruger M, Schledorn P, Schrodl W, Hoppe HW, Lutz W, Shehata AA. Detection of glyphosate residues in animals and humans. J Environ Anal Toxicol 2014; 4(2): 1-5. doi: 10.4172/2161-0525.1000210.
41. Kaur Gil lH, Garg H. Pesticides: environmental impacts

and management strategies. In: Soloneski S, ed. Pesticides-Toxic Aspects. InTech; 2014. p. 188-230. doi: 10.5772/57399.

42. Akinsorotan AM. Toxicity of dizensate (glyphosate herbicide) on *Clarias gariepinus* fingerlings. Adv Res Biol Sci 2014; 2(1): 1-5.
43. Micah AD, Adakole JA, Yusuf A, Mohammed NA. Acute effects of Glyphosate on the behavioural and hematological characteristics of hetero *Clarias* (hybrid) fingerlings. J Aquac Eng Fish Res 2017; 3(1): 13-18. doi: 10.3153/JAEFR17003.
44. Henao Munoz LM, Montes Rojas CM, Bernal Bautista MH. Acute toxicity and sublethal effects of the mixture glyphosate (Roundup Active) and Cosmo-Flux 411F to anuran embryos and tadpoles of four Colombian species. Rev Biol Trop 2015; 63(1): 223-33.
45. Szekacs I, Fejes A, Klatyik S, Takacs E, Patko D, Pomothy J, et al. Environmental and toxicological impacts of glyphosate with its formulating adjuvant. International Journal of Biological Veterinary Agricultural and Food Engineering 2014; 8(3): 219-24.
46. Environmental Protection Agency. Ecological effects test guidelines; fish acute toxicity test, freshwater and marine. Washington, USA: United Environmental Protection Agency; 1996.

13

Bioremediation of methyl tertiary-butyl ether (MTBE) by three pure bacterial cultures

Zabihollah Yousefi[1*], Zeinab Tahernezhad[1], Seyed Noroddin Mousavinasab[2], Reza Safari[3], Ahmadreza Bekhradnia[4]

[1]Department of Environmental Health Engineering, School of Public Health, Mazandaran University of Medical Sciences, Sari, Iran
[2]Department of Biostatistics, School of Public Health, Mazandaran University of Medical Sciences, Sari, Iran
[3]Iranian Fisheries Science Research Institute (IFSRI), Caspian Sea Ecology Research Center, Agricultural Research Education and Extension Organization (AREEO), Sari, Iran
[4]Department of Medicinal Chemistry, Pharmaceutical Sciences Research Center, Mazandaran University of Medical Sciences, Sari, Iran

Abstract
Background: Bioremediation of groundwater and soil contamination is more economical than physicochemical remediation. The present study focused on the bioremediation capability of two bacterial species (*Klebsiella planticola* and *Enterobacter cloacae*) from the family Enterobacteriaceae. These bacteria have been identified as new species with capability of degrading methyl tertiary-butyl ether (MTBE). In order to enhance their degradation capability, selected concentrations and retention time were investigated.
Methods: The bacteria were cultured on the nutrient agar (NA) medium at room temperature. pH of the medium was adjusted to 7. The medium was autoclaved at 121°C for 15 minutes and incubated for 24 hours at 35°C. After 24 hours, the mixture was inoculated into 50 mL of Luria Bertani (LB) liquid medium containing 50 and 150 ppm MTBE. The cultures were incubated for 2 and 5 days at 35°C and shacked on a shaker at 150 rpm. Cell concentrations of the bacteria in pure culture were determined from the optical density at 600 nm using a UV–VIS spectrophotometer. Then, the culture was centrifuged at 3800 rpm for 20 minutes. In the next step, the MTBE concentration in the supernatant was measured by gas chromatography/mass spectrometry (GC/MS, Agilent Technologies, 5975, US10304411, 5.02.07).
Results: The results showed that both strains are able to grow in the presence of 50 and 150 ppm MTBE. In the best conditions, when cell density was 3×108 CFU/mL during 5 days, the highest rate of MTBE degradation for *K. planticola* and *E. cloacae*, was 43% and 40%, respectively. It was also revealed that *Escherichia coli* can degrade 50 and 150 ppm MTBE about 19.8% and 13.65%, respectively.
Conclusion: It seems that *E. coli* can be a good candidate for MTBE degradation at high concentrations for a time longer than that in the present study. It was also found that the species have high performance at 50 ppm than 150 ppm. So, these bacteria can remove MTBE from the environment.
Keywords: Biodegradation, *Klebsiella planticola, Enterobacter cloacae, Escherichia coli*, methyl tertiary-butyl ether

***Correspondence to:**
Zabihollah Yousefi
Email: zyousefi2004@gmail.com

Introduction

Unleaded gasoline consists hydrocarbons and different chemical compounds such as methyl tertiary-butyl ether (MTBE) (1,2). MTBE ($C_5H_{12}O$) is an oxygenate organic compound, that has been used as additive in gasoline since the late 1970s, to replace tetraethyl lead (TEL) and other toxic chemicals (3-5). MTBE is a persistent compound in the environment because it is highly soluble in water, poorly adsorbed by soil and is biologically and chemically stable against degradation (6). Accidental fuel leakage during storage or transportation is the main source of environmental contamination with MTBE (7). Therefore, the presence of MTBE in water is responsible for taste and odor related issues, genotoxicity and skin and eye irritation. Taste and odor thresholds for MTBE are 20-40 ppb (8,9). Generally, MTBE is the most common oxygenate compound, because it is cost-effective and easy-to-use (7). Due to its economic benefits, bioremediation with 99% efficiency, is a more attractive option than physicochemical remediation technologies such as ozone utilization, activated carbon, vaporization extraction and other methods (3,7,10-12). All microorganisms are not able to degrade MTBE easily (13). Some bacteria such as *Pseudomonas, Rhodococcus, Mycobacterium, Enterobacter,* and *Achromobacter* are capable of degrading MTBE co-metabolically but not tert-Butyl Alcohol (TBA) (1). A few bacterial strains such as *Methylibium petroleiphilum* PM1, *Hydrogenophaga flava* ENV735, *Achromobacter xylosoxidans* MCM 1/11, *Pseudomonas* sp., *Bacillus* sp., and *Streptococcus* sp. can utilize MTBE as the sole source of carbon and energy (14-18). Two bacterial isolates (IsoSL1 and Iso2A) degraded MTBE in both nutrient-rich and nutrient-limited media. The highest rate of MTBE degradation was reported 29.6% and 27.8%, respectively, in 28 days (19). Researchers reported that bacteria such as *A. xylosoxidans* MCM 1/11 can use MTBE in 7 days (17). In this study, bioremediation of MTBE by *Klebsiella planticola* and *Enterobacter cloacae* at laboratory conditions was investigated. On the other hand, according to the abundance of *Escherichia coli* and its capability to utilize a wide range of hydrocarbons while the engineered E. coli was used for bioremediation, therefore, MTBE-degrading capacity of this bacterium was also compared. MTBE is one of the gasoline components that, nowadays, is spreading in the environment and can pollute soil, water, and groundwater. The influence of microbial degradation of organic substances and MTBE is well known (17-19). Many studies have been conducted on the MTBE biodegradation by pure bacterial cultures such as *Bacillus cereus* and *Klebsiella terrigena*, *Enterobacter* sp. NKNUO2, and other microorganisms (7,14-17,20). The first step in bioremediation is selecting the best bacteria because only some bacteria can use MTBE as a source of carbon and energy. A few pure or mixed bacterial cultures can grow on MTBE and use it as a carbon and energy source and some strains grow slowly on this oxygenated compound with low cell yields (21). Due to the complex molecular structure of MTBE, this compound is resistant to biodegradation because its ether bond and tertiary carbon atom are relatively unreactive (21-23). The toxic effects of products produced during metabolism can cause it. The intermediate products of MTBE biodegradation are tert-butoxy methanol (TBM), formaldehyde and TBA, respectively (23-25). Steffan et al demonstrated that the growth rates of propane-oxidizing bacteria on MTBE is very slow. Numerous microorganisms including EVN 735, *Variovorax paradoxus* CL-8, *Chryseobacterium* sp. A-3, *B. cereus*, *K. terrigena*, *Enterobacter* sp., and NKNUO2, have also the capability to remove MTBE from the environment (12,20,26-30). The biological degradation of MTBE and most of the organic matter is nowadays known in science (31,32). In a study by Salanitro et al, biomass yields (gram of dry weight cells per gram of MTBE) were 0.21 to 0.28 (32). Some studies have also investigated MTBE biodegradation by Mycobacterium (33,34). But so far, no study has been conducted to investigate the role of K. planticola in bioremediation of MTBE, while some species of Klebsiella have been found to be capable of utilizing MTBE, n-hexadecane, and other hydrocarbons contaminating soil (20,35,36).

Materials and Methods

Materials

MTBE (GC purity ≥98%) was purchased from Persian Type Culture Collection (PTCC). Other chemicals were analytical grade and purchased from Merck (Darmstadt, Germany).

After sterilization and passing through a 2-mm mesh sieve, specific concentrations of MTBE were added to 10 g of soil, and the growth rate of microorganisms and the concentration of MTBE were measured.

Microorganisms and incubation conditions

In order to determine a strain capable of growing on MTBE, two concentrations and two retention time were examined. *K. planticola* and *E. cloacae* were purchased from the PTCC. Then, these bacteria were cultured on the nutrient agar (NA) medium at room temperature. The composition of NA was as follows (gr^{-1}): 0.5% Peptone, 0.3% beef extract/yeast extract, 1.5% agar, 0.5% sodium chloride, and distilled water. pH of the medium was adjusted to 7. The medium was autoclaved at 121°C for 15 minutes. In the next step, the cultures were incubated for 24 hours at 35°C. After 24 hours, the inoculum density at the beginning of the test were 1.5×10^8 CFU/mL and 3×10^8 CFU/mL, the mixture were then inoculated into 50 mL of Luria Bertani (LB) liquid medium containing 50 and 150 ppm MTBE (based on pretest) (12). LB medium was composed of (g/L): 10 g/L Trypton, 5 g/L yeast extraction, and 10 g/L NaCl. Then, the medium was autoclaved at 121°C for 15 minutes at pH 7. The cultures were incubated 2-5 days at 35°C in a shaker incubator at 150 rpm. Cell concentrations of *K. planticola* and *E. cloacae* in pure culture were determined from the optical density at 600 nm using a UV–VIS spectrophotometer (Hach model). Then, the culture was centrifuged in sealed tubes and cells were harvested from the medium by centrifugation at 3800 rpm for 20 minutes. Afterwards, the MTBE concentration in the supernatant was measured by gas chromatography/mass spectrometry (GC/MS, Agilent Technologies, 5975, US10304411, 5.02.07). The conditions for the GC analysis were as follows: 45°C held for 4 minutes, temperature ramped from 16°C/min to 70°C for 4.37 minutes, from 22°C/min to 100°C for 1.36 minutes, and 28°C/min to 220°C for 4.28 minutes (1,18,22). Helium was used as the carrier gas with an approximate flow rate of 1.10 mL/min. The sample without microorganisms was applied as blank in all tests. All specimens were tested two times. In this study, 38 samples were evaluated. Data were analyzed using statistical tests such as ANOVA, correlation, regression, and etc.

Results

During the incubation periods (2 and 5 days), *K. planticola* and *E. cloacae* were capable of growing on MTBE, as the source of carbon and energy, while initial concentrations of MTBE were studied. The removal rate of MTBE by two

Table 1. Biodegradation of MTBE by *Klebsiella planticola* and *Enterobacter cloacae*

Bacterial species	Initial concentration of MTBE (ppm)	Initial amount of bacteria (CFU/ mL)	Time: 2 days		Time: 5 days	
			Removal percentage (%)	Residual value of concentration (ppm)	Removal percentage (%)	Residual value of concentration (ppm)
K. planticola	50	1.5×10^8	11.8	44.1	19	40.5
		3×10^8	29	35.5	43	21.5
	150	1.5×10^8	6.95	139.5	12.96	130.5
		3×10^8	24.3	12.5	33.5	99.5
E. cloacae	50	1.5×10^8	9.1	45.45	16.3	41.85
		3×10^8	24.6	37.7	40	30.05
	150	1.5×10^8	5.3	142	11.9	132.15
		3×10^8	15.95	126	30.95	103.5
E. coli	50	3×10^8	24.3	12.5	33.5	99.5
		1.5×10^8	9.1	45.45	16.3	41.85
	150	3×10^8	24.6	37.7	40	30.05
		1.5×10^8	5.3	142	11.9	132.15

pure bacterial cultures and the growth rate of two bacterial species at different concentrations of MTBE included in soil samples are shown in Table 1.

Biodegradation of 50 ppm MTBE by *K. planticola* and *E. cloacae* with inoculum sizes of 3×10^8 CFU/mL, is displayed in Figure 1. As shown in Figure 1, *K. planticola* and *E. cloacae* respectively indicated 43% and 40% MTBE degradation, in 120 hours detention time. In addition, the bacteria showed 24.6% and 29% MTBE degradation after 48 hours.

Biodegradation of 150 ppm MTBE by *K. planticola* and *E. cloacae* with inoculum size of 3×10^8 CFU/mL, is displayed in Figure 2. As shown in Figure 2, *K. planticola* and *E. cloacae* respectively indicated 30.95% and 33.50% MTBE degradation, in 120 hours detention time. The bacteria also showed 19.95% and 24.30% MTBE degradation after 48 hours.

Biodegradation of 150 ppm MTBE by *E. coli* with inoculum size of 3×10^8 CFU/mL, is presented in Figure 3. As presented in Figure 3, E.coli with different inoculum sizes of 1.5×10^8 and 3×10^8 CFU/mL showed 13% and 19.8% MTBE degradation, respectively, in 120 hours detention time. The bacteria also showed 9% and 6.5% MTBE degradation after 48 hours.

Discussion

The bacteria were capable to grow in all samples while the growth rate of the bacteria and MTBE degradation rate were different. The results showed that both bacterial species, in the similar conditions, could use initial MTBE concentration of 50 ppm better than the concentration of 150 ppm. In a similar study by Okeke et al, concentration

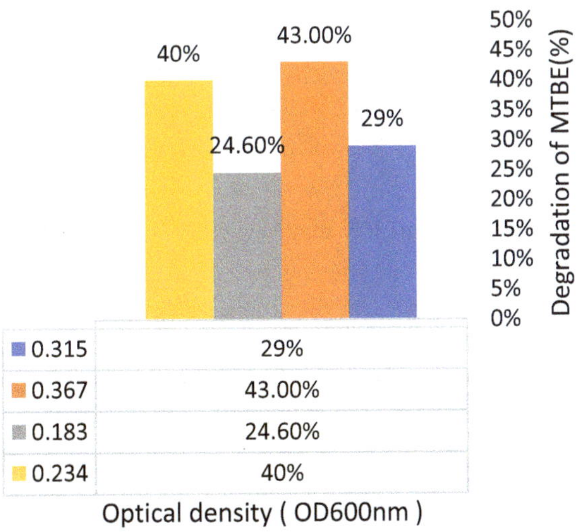

Figure 1. Biodegradation of 50 ppm MTBE by *Klebsiella planticola* and *Enterobacter cloacae* with inoculum size of 3×10^8 CFU/mL. White column, optical density of *K. planticola* after 48 and 120 hours and black column, optical density of *E. cloacae* after 48 and 120 hours.

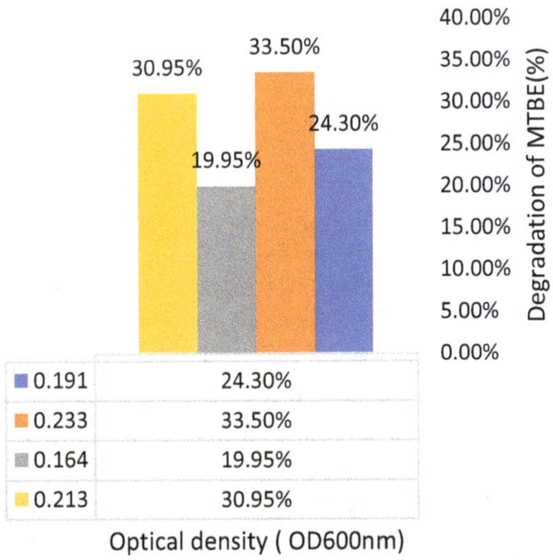

Figure 2. Biodegradation of 150 ppm MTBE by *Klebsiella planticola* and *Enterobacter cloacae* with inoculum size of 3×108 CFU/mL. White column, optical density of *K. planticola* after 48 and 120 hours and black column, optical density of *E. cloacae* after 48 and 120 hours.

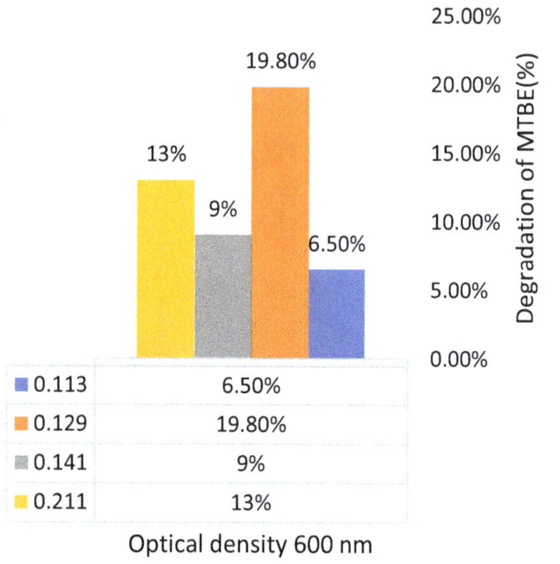

Figure 3. Biodegradation of 150 ppm MTBE by *E. coli* with different inoculum sizes of 1.5×108 and 3×108 CFU/mL. White column, optical density of *E. coli* after 48 hours. .

of 50 ppm has been reported as the best concentration of MTBE. It seems that toxicity increases at higher concentrations (18). Also, in the study by Zhang et al, on the bioremediation of MTBE-contaminated soil, the results showed that MTBE degradation rate increased from 50 to below 100 ppm (12). Another study also showed that *Staphylococcus saprophyticus* 6sy and *Pseudomonas* sp. 24p were capable of degrading 25 µg/mL MTBE better than 125 µg/mL in 21 days. Other researchers insisted on the role of different concentrations of MTBE on bioremediation of MTBE (37). Abbaspour et al showed that *Bacillus cereus* strain RJ1 can survive at different concentrations of MTBE while the initial concentration of 200 ppm is rapidly degraded (38). In this study, the highest rate of MTBE degradation was recorded after 5 days while there were no significant MTBE disappearances in the blank samples. It was also revealed that pure culture of *K. planticola* is more capable of degrading MTBE in the initial concentration of 50 ppm comparing with *E. cloacae*, especially after the end of the period. *K. planticola* showed a significant difference (student's *t* test) in different concentrations (P=0.005) compared to *E. cloacae* (P=0.0117). The initial absorbance at 600 nm was 0.1 and the inoculum size was 3×10^8 CFU/mL. According to Figure 1, MTBE degradation rate by both strains increased with increasing the microbial density. The results are consistent with the results of the study by Zhang et al (12). They reported that there is a direct relationship between the removal of MTBE and time. According to Figures 1 to 3, all bacterial species had the potential for degradation of 50 ppm and 150 ppm MTBE. Biodegradation rate of MTBE was 29% and 43% while the absorbance at a wavelength of 600 nm was 0.315 and 0.367, respectively (Figure 1). *E. cloacae* is also a good candidate. Jose Barbera et al confirmed that *E. cloacae* species play an important role in the MTBE biodegradation. They also showed that *E. cloacae* MCM2/1 has a high potential for utilizing MTBE (39). In the first hours, degradation rate by *K. planticola* was higher than other strains, and it seems that *E. coli* needs more time for degrading MTBE (Figure 3), it can be due to the complex molecular structure of MTBE, while the cultures containing yeast extract, this compound makes a good condition for better growth of the strains (19). Generally, there was no difference in the growth rate of both strains (*K. planticola* and *E. cloacae*) at different concentrations of MTBE. Besides, degradation rate was lower when the inoculum size was 1.5×10^8 CFU/mL (Table 1). The results of this study show that there is a direct relation between inoculum size and MTBE degradation. It should be noted that when the inoculum size increases, it uses more oxygen (12), which is consistent with the study by Rui-Ling et al. They reported that when cell density was 2×10^8 CFU/mL, the species had better performance than when it was 4.5×10^8 CFU/mL.

Conclusion

Klebsiella planticola, E. cloacae and *E. coli* could degrade MTBE at different concentrations and different cell densities in different times. Therefore, these strains are good candidates for removing MTBE from the environment. However, further studies using optimized media with other compounds for MTBE removal by these strains are suggested.

Acknowledgments

The authors would like to gratitude the Research Deputy of Mazandaran University of Medical Sciences for funding this study. And special thanks to P. Gil, Masoumeh Eslamifar and Masoumali Movahedi who helped us as research co-operators to perform this research.

Competing interests

The authors declare that they have no conflicts of interests.

Authors' contribution

All authors contributed in data collection, analysis, and interpretation. All authors reviewed, refined, and approved the manuscript.

References

1. Guisado IM, Purswani J, Gonzalez-Lopez J, Pozo C. Physiological and genetic screening methods for the isolation of methyl tert-butyl ether-degrading bacteria for

bioremediation purposes. Int Biodeterior Biodegradation 2015; 97: 67-74. doi: 10.1016/j.ibiod.2014.11.008.

2. Schmidt TC, Haderlein SB, Pfister R, Forster R. Occurrence and fate modeling of MTBE and BTEX compounds in a Swiss Lake used as drinking water supply. Water Res 2004; 38(6): 1520-9. doi: 10.1016/j.watres.2003.12.027.
3. Levchuk I, Bhatnagar A, Sillanpaa M. Overview of technologies for removal of methyl tert-butyl ether (MTBE) from water. Sci Total Environ 2014; 476-477: 415-33. doi: 10.1016/j.scitotenv.2014.01.037.
4. The U.S. Environmental Protection Agency. MTBE in Fuels [cited 2017 Oct 23]. Available from: http://www.epa.gov/mtbe/gas.htm.
5. Morse PM. Producers brace for MTBE Phaseout. Chem Eng News 1999; 77(15): 26-7. doi: 10.1021/cen-v077n015.p026.
6. Soltani B, Moheb A. Ultrasound irradiation facilitated adsorption of MTBE from aqueous solution using exfoliated graphite. Chem Eng Technol 2010; 33(7): 1107-11. doi: 10.1002/ceat.200900345.
7. Chen CS, Tien CJ, Zhan KV. Evaluation of intrinsic bioremediation of methyl tert-butyl ether (MTBE) contaminated groundwater. Journal of Soil and Groundwater Environment 2014; 19(5): 9-17. doi: 10.7857/JSGE.2014.19.5.009.
8. Moreels D, Bastiaens L, Ollevier F, Merckx R, Diels L, Springael D. Evaluation of the intrinsic methyl tert-butyl ether (MTBE) biodegradation potential of hydrocarbon contaminated subsurface soils in batch microcosm systems. FEMS Microbiol Ecol 2004; 49(1): 121-8. doi: 10.1016/j.femsec.2004.02.016.
9. Young WF, Horth H, Crane R, Ogden T, Arnott M. Taste and odour threshold concentrations of potential potable water contaminants. Wat Res 1996; 30(2): 331-40. doi: 10.1016/0043-1354(95)00173-5.
10. Nau A, Kohl S, Zanthoff HW, Wiederhold H, Vogel H. Ozonized activated carbon as catalyst for MTBE-cleavage. Appl Catal A Gen 2011; 397: 103-111.
11. U.S. Environmental Protection Agency. Technologies for Treating MTBE and Other Fuel Oxygenates. Washington, DC: Agency Office of Solid Waste and Emergency Response Office of Superfund Remediation and Technology Innovation; 2004.
12. Zhang RL, Huang GQ, Lian JY, Li XG. Degradation of MTBE and TBA by a new isolate from MTBE-contaminated soil. J Environ Sci (China) 2007; 19(9): 1120-4.
13. Davis LC, Erickson LE. A review of bioremediation and natural attenuation of MTBE. Environmental Progress 2004; 23(3): 243-52. doi: 10.1002/ep.10028.
14. Nakatsu CH, Hristova K, Hanada S, Meng XY, Hanson JR, Scow KM, et al. *Methylibium petroleiphilum* gen. nov., sp. nov., a novel methyl tert-butyl ether-degrading methylotroph of the *Betaproteobacteria*. Int J Syst Evol Microbiol 2006; 56(Pt 5): 983-9. doi: 10.1099/ijs.0.63524-0.
15. Streger SH, Vainberg S, Dong H, Hatzinger PB. Enhancing transport of hydrogenophaga flava ENV735 for bioaugmentation of aquifers contaminated with methyl tert-butyl ether. Appl Environ Microbiol 2002; 68(11): 5571-9.
16. Lee EH, Cho KS. Effect of substrate interaction on the degradation of methyl tert-butyl ether, benzene, toluene, ethylbenzene, and xylene by *Rhodococcus* sp. J Hazard Mater 2009; 167(1-3): 669-74. doi: 10.1016/j.jhazmat.2009.01.035.
17. Eixarch H, Constanti M. Biodegradation of MTBE by *Achromobacter xylosoxidans* MCM1/1 induces synthesis of proteins that may be related to cell survival. Process Biochem 2010; 45(5): 794-8. doi: 10.1016/j.procbio.2009.12.015.
18. Okeke BC, Frankenberger WT Jr. Biodegradation of methyl tertiary butyl ether (MTBE) by a bacterial enrichment consortia and its monoculture isolates. Microbiol Res 2003; 158(2): 99-106. doi: 10.1078/0944-5013-00181.
19. Makut MD, Ishaya P. Bacterial species associated with soils contaminated with used petroleum products in Keffi town, Nigeria. Afr J Microbiol Res 2010; 4(16): 1698-702.
20. Nasrollahzadeh HS, Najafpour GD, Aghamohammadi N. Biodegradation of phenanthrene by mixed culture consortia in batch bioreactor using central composite face-entered design. Int J Environ Res 2007; 1(2): 80-87.
21. Talaie AR, Jafaarzahe N, Talaie MR, Beheshti M. Biodegradation of aromatic compounds in crude oil by isolated microorganisms from environment. J Zanjan Univ Med Sci 2010; 18(70): 68-80. [In Persian].
22. Arabi R, Bemanian SH, Taherzadeh MJ. Rapid biodegradation of Methyl tert - Butyl Ether (MTBE) by pure bacterial cultures. Iran J Chem Chem Eng 2007; 26(1): 1-7.
23. Francois A, Mathis H, Godefroy D, Piveteau P, Fayolle F, Monot F. Biodegradation of methyl tert-butyl ether and other fuel oxygenates by a new strain, *Mycobacterium austroafricanum* IFP 2012. Appl Environ Microbiol 2002; 68(6): 2754-62.
24. Smith CA, O'Reilly KT, Hyman MR. Characterization of the initial reactions during the cometabolic oxidation of methyl tert-butyl ether by propane-grown *Mycobacterium vaccae* JOB5. Appl Environ Microbiol 2003; 69(2): 796-804.
25. HHatzinger PB, MCclay K, Vainberg S, Tugusheva M, Condee CW, Steffan RJ. Biodegradation of Methyl tert -Butyl Ether by a pure bacterial culture. Appl Environ Microbiol 2001; 67(12): 5601-7. doi: 10.1128/AEM.67.12.5601–5607.2001
26. Zaitsev GM, Uotila JS, Haggblom MM. Biodegradation of methyl tert-butyl ether by cold-adapted mixed and pure bacterial cultures. Appl Microbiol Biotechnol 2007; 74(5): 1092-102. doi: 10.1007/s00253-006-0737-3.
27. Chen SC, Chen CS, Zhan KV, Yang KH, Chien CC, Shieh BS, et al. Biodegradation of methyl tert-butyl ether (MTBE) by *Enterobacter* sp. NKNU02. J Hazard Mater 2011; 186(2-3): 1744-50. doi: 10.1016/j.jhazmat.2010.12.079.
28. Hanson JR, Ackerman CE, Scow KM. Biodegradation of methyl tert-butyl ether by a bacterial pure culture. Appl Environ Microbiol 1999; 65(11): 4788-92.
29. Hatzinger PB, McClay K, Vainberg S, Tugusheva M, Condee CW, Steffan RJ. Biodegradation of methyl tert-butyl ether by a pure bacterial culture. Appl Environ Microbiol 2001; 67(12): 5601-7. doi: 10.1128/aem.67.12.5601-5607.2001.
30. Steffan RJ, McClay K, Vainberg S, Condee CW, Zhang D. Biodegradation of the gasoline oxygenates methyl tert-butyl ether, ethyl tert-butyl ether, and tert-amyl methyl ether by propane-oxidizing bacteria. Appl Environ Microbiol 1997; 63(11): 4216-22.

31. Mo K, Lora CO, Wanken AE, Javanmardian M, Yang X, Kulpa CF. Biodegradation of methyl t-butyl ether by pure bacterial cultures. Appl Microbiol Biotechnol 1997; 47: 69–72.
32. Salanitro JP, Diaz LA, Williams MP, Wisniewski HL. Isolation of a bacterial culture that degrades methyl t-Butyl ether. Appl Environ Microbiol 1994; 60(7): 2593-6.
33. Fayolle F, Vandecasteele JP, Monot F. Microbial degradation and fate in the environment of methyl tert-butyl ether and related fuel oxygenates. Appl Microbiol Biotechnol 2001; 56(3-4): 339-49.
34. Alfonso-Gordillo G, Flores-Ortiz CM, Morales-Barrera L, Cristiani-Urbina E. Biodegradation of methyl tertiary butyl ether (MTBE) by a microbial consortium in a continuous up-flow packed-bed biofilm reactor: kinetic study, metabolite identification and toxicity bioassays. PLoS One 2016; 11(12): e0167494. doi: 10.1371/journal.pone.0167494.
35. Nduka JK, Umeh LN, Okerulu IO, Umedum LN, Okoye HN. Utilization of different microbes in bioremediation of hydrocarbon contaminated soils stimulated with inorganic and organic fertilizers. J Pet Environ Biotechnol 2012; 3(2): 1-9. doi: 10.4172/2157-7463.1000116.
36. Dutra ES, Pascon RC, Vallim MA. Sao Paulo Zoo composting as a source of bacteria with bioremediation potential. Afr J Microbiol Res 2013; 7(45): 5200-6. doi: 10.5897/AJMR2013.5874.
37. Lalevic B, Raicevic V, Kikovic D, Jovanovic L, Surlan-Momirovic G, Jovic J, et al. Biodegradation of MTBE by bacteria isolated from oil hydrocarbons- contaminated environments. Int J Environ Res 2012; 6(1): 81-6. doi: 10.22059/ijer.2011.474.
38. Abbaspour M, Javid AH, Jalilzadeh Yengjeh R, Hassani AH, Ghavam Mostafavi P. The Biodegradation of methyl tert-Butyl ether (MTBE) by indigenous *Bacillus cereus* strain RJ1 isolated from soil. Petroleum Science and Technology 2013; 31(18): 1835-41. doi: 10.1080/10916466.2011.611562.
39. Jose Barbera M, Mateo E, Monkaityte R, Constanti M. Biodegradation of methyl tert-butyl ether by newly identified soil microorganisms in a simple mineral solution. World J Microbiol Biotechnol 2011; 27(4): 813-21. doi: 10.1007/s11274-010-0522-4.

14

Effect of UV light on pentachlorophenol removal in the electro-Fenton process

Zahra Heidari[1], Mohsen Motevasel[1], Nematollah Jaafarzadeh[2*]

[1]Department of Chemical Engineering, Petroleum University of Technology, Abadan, Iran
[2]Environmental Technologies Research Center, Ahvaz Jundishapur University of Medical Sciences, Ahvaz, Iran

Abstract
Background: This research studied the effect of UV light on pentachlorophenol (PCP) removal in the electro-Fenton (EF) process.
Methods: PCP was used as the pollutant in this study. The effects of Fenton's reagent, i.e. hydrogen peroxide concentration, solution pH, and treatment time by EF (EF) and photoelectro-Fenton (PEF) processes, were studied to determine rates of PCP removal. The results showed that a better performance and a high removal efficiency were achieved by coupling UV radiation and the EF process.
Results: EF processes required more time to remove PCP, while after a reaction time of 10 minutes, the PEF achieved a removal efficiency of 90.4%; this value is higher than the maximum efficiency of the EF process (83.44% after 40 minutes). The kinetic mechanisms of both processes were examined and compared. The rate constants at optimum conditions were 0.0455 and 0.0579 min^{-1} for EF and PEF processes, respectively.
Conclusion: Removal efficiency was obtained in the order of PEF > EF.
Keywords: Ultraviolet rays, Reaction Time, Kinetics.

***Correspondence to:**
Nematollah Jaafarzadeh
Email: jaafarzadeh-n@ajums.ac.ir

Introduction

The presence of phenol compounds in the environment has acute toxicity for mankind. Due to five chlorines on the pentachlorophenol (PCP) structure, it is the most toxic agent of chlorophenols (1). PCP can affect the nervous, digestive, and respiratory systems and lead to cancer in humans. It is used in pesticides, disinfectants, and wood preservatives (2). PCP remains in the environment because of the unsuitable disposal of industrial wastes containing PCP and its pertinacity. Thus, the treatment of phenolic pollutants before disposal is very important. It is necessary to find a highly effective method to treat PCP waste (3). Advanced oxidation processes (AOPs) are more efficient than conventional methods. They are able to oxidize and mineralize most organic compounds, including bio-recalcitrant ones, by producing highly reactive and non-selective oxidants called hydroxyl radicals (HO) (4). AOPs include two steps of oxidation: the formation of hydroxyl radicals, and the reaction of these radicals with an organic compound (5).

Conventional biological wastewater treatment processes are inefficient for the removal of recalcitrant organic compounds that are the main sources of pollutants in industrial effluent. The electro-Fenton (EF) process is known as a powerful and environmentally-friendly technology for the removal of this compound from wastewaters (6). In the EF process, highly oxidative hydroxyl radicals are formed from the reaction between H_2O_2 and Fe^{2+} (7). The Fenton process includes the following reactions (8,9):

$H_2O_2 + Fe^{2+} \rightarrow OH^{\bullet} + OH^- + Fe^{3+}$ [1]

$OH^{\bullet} + RH \rightarrow R^{\bullet} + H_2O$ [2]

$R^{\bullet} + H_2O_2 \rightarrow ROH + OH^{\bullet}$ [3]

$OH^{\bullet} + H_2O_2 \rightarrow HO_2^{\bullet} + H_2O$ [4]

$Fe^{3+} + HO2^{\bullet} \rightarrow Fe^{2+} + H^+ + O_2$ [5]

$Fe^{2+} + HO2^{\bullet} \rightarrow Fe^{3+} + HO2^-$ [6]

$Fe^{2+} + OH^{\bullet} \rightarrow Fe^{3+} + OH^-$ [7]

$H_2O_2 + Fe^{2+} \rightarrow FeO^{2+} + H_2O$ [8]

$FeO^{2+} + H_2O_2 \rightarrow O_2 + H_2O$ [9]

In the Fenton process Fe^{2+} is consumed faster than it is produced. The EF method solved this problem by regenerating Fe^{2+} in the cathode according to the following reaction (10):

$Fe^{3+} + e^- \rightarrow Fe^{2+}$ [10]

The photoelectron-Fenton (PEF) process can regenerate a large amount of Fe^{2+} by solution irradiation with UV light by the following reaction (11):

$(Fe\text{–}OH)^{2+} + hv \rightarrow Fe^{2+} + OH^{\bullet}$ [11]

Furthermore, in the PEF mechanism, hydroxyl radicals can be produced from H_2O_2 in the presence of UV radiation (11,12):

$H_2O_2 + hv \rightarrow 2OH^{\bullet}$ [12]

Recently, different usages for the EF process have been found, for example, the treatment of landfill leachate (13), phenol degradation (14), the effect of UV light on acetaminophen degradation in the EF process (15), COD and color removal from landfill leachate (16-18). According to our previous study (19,20), PCP has been successfully removed in the EF and sonoelectro-Fenton processes, but the effect of UV light on PCP removal in the EF process has not yet been studied. Thus, the current study investigated the effects of UV radiation on PCP removal in the EF process. The influence of operating parameters such as H_2O_2 concentration, pH, and treatment time of PCP on degradation was investigated. The reaction kinetics were studied to find the removal mechanism and compare it with the EF results.

Methods

PCP 98.5% and H_2O_2 (30%) were purchased from Merck. Sodium sulfate 99.5% (used as an electrolyte), H_2SO_4, and NAOH were obtained from Merck. Concentrated hydrochloric acid was used for electrode washing. Chemical oxygen demand (COD) was determined using the open reflux method (21). The efficiencies of PCP degradation and COD removal were defined as:

COD removal efficiency $= \Delta\,[COD]\,/COD_0 = ([COD_f\text{-}COD_0]\,/COD_0) \times 100$

where $[COD]_0$ and $[COD]_f$ are the COD concentrations in the solution at 0 minute and at the end of each reaction, respectively. A divided double-electrode electrochemical cell was used in this study. The reactor was a glass beaker with a volume of 400 mL. The cathodes and anodes of the reactors were a piece of steal (st37). The same experimental set-up as the EF process was used in the photoelectro-Fenton (PEF) process. The addition of eight UVC lamps with a frequency of 247 nm was used. The pH of the solutions was adjusted using concentrated sulfuric acid (H_2SO_4) and sodium hydroxide (0.1 M). A DC power supply used to provide reasonable voltage was connected to the electrodes, and 250 mL solution was prepared by determining the initial PCP concentration (15 mg/L) and then adding sodium sulfate as the electrolyte (2000 mg/L). The initial pH of the solutions was set. The conductivity of the medium was fixed by adding Na_2SO_4 (2000 mg/L). Then, 250 mL of sample was transferred to the E-F reactor. After adding the required amount of H_2O_2, 8-watt UVC lights were turned on and the PEF experiment was started. The EF set-up was the same as the PEF process but without UV lights.

Results

Figure 1 shows the effect of initial H_2O_2 concentration on PCP removal efficiency at a constant PCP concentration of 15 mg/L, voltage of 24 V, and pH = 3 after a reaction time of 40 minutes by EF and PEF processes. Under these operational conditions, the PCP removal efficiency rates in both processes were increased with increases in H_2O_2 concentration. The effect of pH (3–7) on PCP removal was studied using both processes, and the results are shown in Figure 2. Experiments were performed using an initial PCP concentration of 15 mg/L, reaction time of 40 minutes, and H_2O_2 concentration of 200 m mole/L. A voltage of 24 V was maintained for the EF and PEF processes. The effects of treatment time on PCP removal efficiency at an initial PCP concentration of 15 mg/L, pH of 3, and H_2O_2 concentration of 200 m mole/L at a voltage of 24 V in the EF and PEF processes are shown in Figure 3. In the kinetics study, the zero-, first-, and second-order models were analyzed separately to determine the behavior of PEF reactions. Modeling of PCP removal by pseudo-first-order, pseudo-second-order, and zero-order equations is shown in Figures 4, 5, and 6, respectively. The results indicate that the removal kinetics followed the

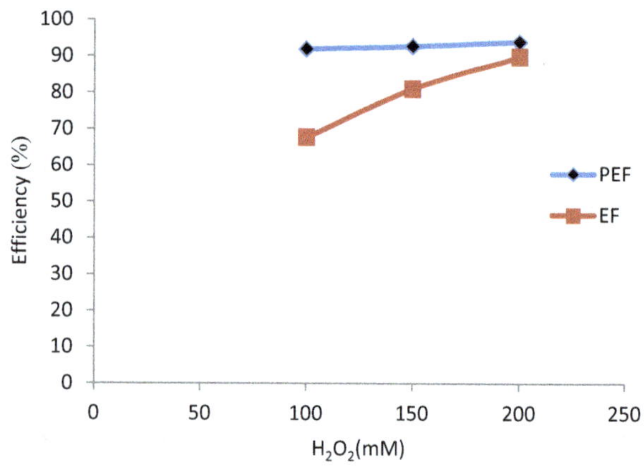

Figure 1. Effect of initial H_2O_2 concentration on PCP removal efficiency in the EF and PEF processes.

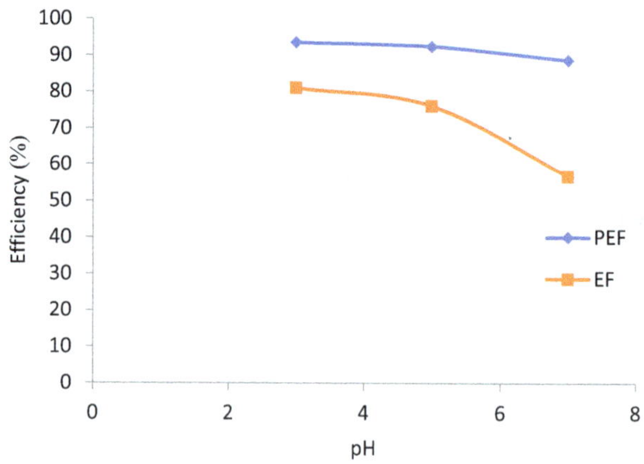

Figure 2. Effect of pH on PCP removal efficiency in the EF and PEF processes.

first-order reaction.

Discussion

Effect of H_2O_2 concentration

The highest removal of PCP presented at an H_2O_2 concentration of 200 mM in both processes. The maximum

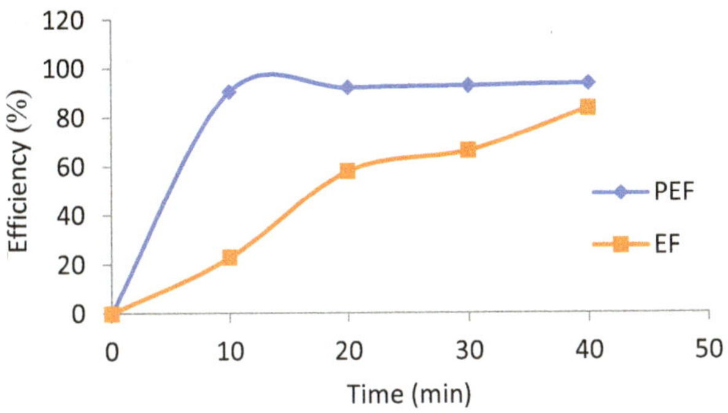

Figure 3. Effect of treatment time on PCP removal efficiency in the EF and PEF processes.

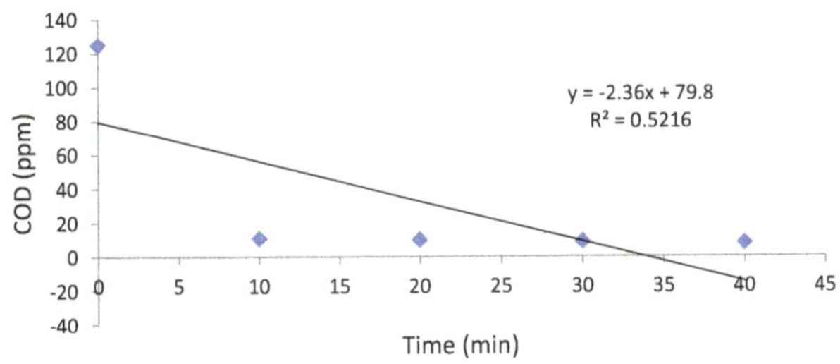

Figure 4. Zero-order kinetics modeling of PCP removal using PEF.

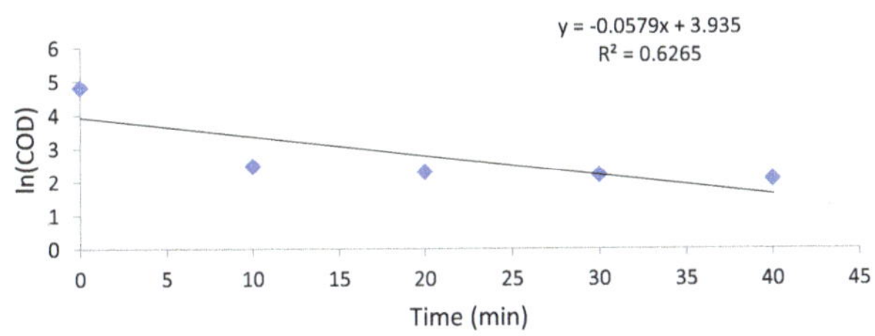

Figure 5. First-order kinetics modeling of PCP removal using PEF.

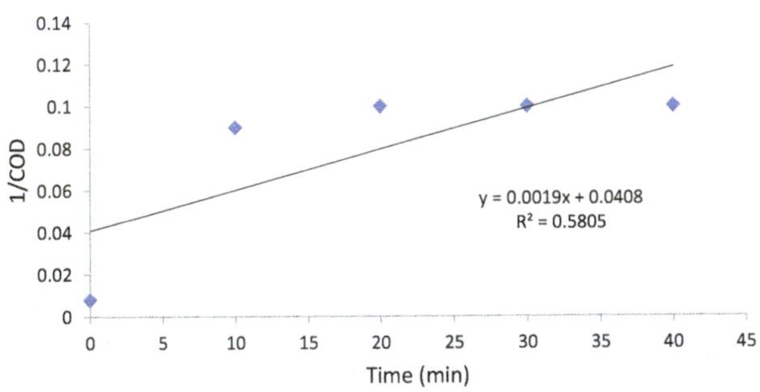

Figure 6. Second-order kinetic modeling of PCP removal using PEF.

PCP removal efficiency of 90% was observed in the EF process at the H_2O_2 concentration of 200 mM, while a removal efficiency of 92% was observed in the PEF at an H_2O_2 concentration of 100 mM. This phenomenon was due to an OH• production from reactions 11 and 12. The difference in PCP removal efficiency was insignificant in the PEF processes. Thus, high efficiency can be achieved by adding the lowest amount of H_2O_2 concentration in the PEF process, and it is economical. In the AOP, H_2O_2 is the main source of hydroxyl radical production according to reaction 1. The excess amount of H_2O_2 has a scavenger effect, so finding the lowest concentration of H_2O_2 for higher removal efficiency is very important (1,10,11,22). In the PEF process, UV light reduces the scavenging effect and generates a greater amount of hydroxyl radicals according to Eq. [12] (1). This result was observed in several other studies, including the effect of UV light on acetaminophen degradation in the EF process (10) and treatment of landfill leachate by PEF process (11).

Effect of pH

It is well known that advanced oxidation reactions occur in low pH values (13). Hydroxyl radicals have high oxidation ability in acidic mediums (1). The results showed that PCP removal efficiency is significantly affected by pH. The maximum PCP removal was observed at pH 3 (93.6% in PEF process). Increasing pH from 3 to 7 reduced the amount of PCP removed for both process. This is due to the reduction in hydroxyl oxidation potential in high pH values. At high pH values, ferric hydroxide was formed and caused the low generation of hydroxyl radicals (1,20). At higher pH values, electro-coagulation starts in the reactor because of the conversion of Fe^{2+} and Fe^{3+} to Fe (OH)n-type structures (1,13). Increasing pH to a value beyond 3 affected the removal efficiency because of the transformation of ferrous ions (Fe^{2+}) to ferric iron (Fe^{3+}). By adding UV light radiation to the EF process, it is possible to reduce Fe^{3+} to Fe^{2+} and generate hydroxyl radicals according to the following reaction (3):

$$Fe(OH)^{2+hv} \rightarrow Fe^{2+} + {}^{\bullet}OH \qquad [13]$$

Hydroxyl radicals produced in these reactions are used for PCP removal at higher pH values. In this situation, PEF processes could be used at a near neutral pH and reduce the problems created by acidic effluent treatment (1). This result was observed in several other studies, including advanced oxidation of phenol by EF and SEF process (1), COD and color removal from synthetic textile wastewater by SEF process (22), and PCP removal by SEF (20).

Effect of treatment time

As shown in Figure 3, the PCP removal efficiency of the EF and PEF processes was increased by increasing the reaction time; in the PEF process, a removal efficiency of 90.4% was obtained after a reaction time of 10 minutes; this value is higher than the maximum efficiency of the EF process (83.44% after 40 minutes). These phenomena can be a result of the greater amount of hydroxyl radical produced, according to Eq. [12] (1). In the studies of Babuponnusami et al (1), and Altin (11), similar results were observed.

Kinetics of pentachlorophenol removal

According to our previous studies, the removal of PCP by the EF process can be represented as (20):

PCP + OH• → Oxidation products [14]

As described in our previous study, the zero-order, first-order, and second-order reaction kinetics, respectively, can be written as shown below, and the removal of PCP by the EF process followed the pseudo-first-order kinetics (20):

$C = C0 - k0t$ [15]

$\ln C - \ln C_0 = - k_{app} t$ [16]

$1/C = 1/C0 - Kt$ [17]

The correlation coefficients for the PCP removal kinetics of zero-, pseudo-first, and second order were 0.5216, 0.6265, and 0.5805, respectively. The comparison of the correlation coefficients indicated a good agreement between the removal kinetics and the pseudo-first order models. The results of zero-, first-, and second-order reaction kinetics for PCP removal in EF and PEF processes are summarized in Table 1.

Figure 7 shows the comparison of the results of the first-order kinetics models for both the EF and the PEF method, and it shows that the rate constants of the EF and PEF processes are 0.0455 and 0.0579, respectively. The same results were reported by other studies (1,10,20).

Conclusion

This study investigated the effects of UV radiation combined with EF for the removal of PCP from aqueous solutions. The results indicated that both the EF and PEF processes were effective in removing PCP from wastewater. The effects of changing the H_2O_2 concentration was clearer in the PEF process than in the EF process. At low H_2O_2 injection amounts, adding UVA irradiation enhanced the PCP removal rate in the PEF process because of the greater production of OH• in the PEF process. Another advantage of combining UV and EF was that it could act at high pH values near the neutral pH and solve the problems associated with acidic effluent. From the kinetic studies, both processes followed the first-order reaction. The rate constant values at optimum conditions were equal to 0.0455 and 0.0579 min^{-1} for the EF and PEF processes, respectively. The following items are recommended as subjects for further research: studying the efficiency of PCP removal from aqueous solutions by sequential sono-photoelecro-Fenton; repeating this process for real wastewater.

Table 1. The regression coefficients for zero-, first-, and second-order kinetics

Oxidation process	Zero-order	First-order	Second-order
EF	0.9045	0.9707	0.9418
PEF	0.5216	0.6265	0.5805

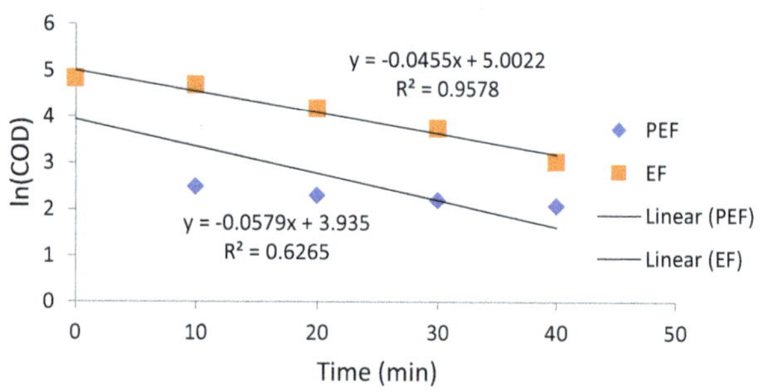

Figure 7. Pseudo-first-order kinetics plot under the EF and PEF processes under optimum conditions (H_2O_2=200 mM, voltage = 24 V, PCP=15 mg/L, and pH = 3)

Acknowledgments

The authors would like to thank the Petroleum University of Technology for providing financial support for this study.

Competing interests

The authors declare that no competing interests exist.

Authors' contributions

All authors contributed equally to the study, and all authors participated in data acquisition, analysis, and interpretation. All authors critically reviewed, refined, and approved the manuscript.

References

1. Babuponnusami A, Muthukumar K. Advanced oxidation of phenol: A comparison between Fenton, electro-Fenton, sono-electro-Fenton and photo-electro-Fenton processes. Chem Eng J 2012; 183: 1-9. doi: 10.1016/j.cej.2011.12.010.
2. Kumar Y, Popat KM, Brahmbhatt H, Ganguly B, Bhattacharya A. Pentachlorophenol removal from water using surfactant-enhanced filtration through low-pressure thin film composite membranes. J Hazard Mater 2008; 154(1-3): 426-31. doi: 10.1016/j.jhazmat.2007.10.060.
3. Zhang J, Ye P, Chen S, Wang W. Removal of pentachlorophenol by immobilized horseradish peroxidase. Int Biodeterior Biodegradation 2007; 59(4): 307-14. doi: 10.1016/j.ibiod.2006.09.003.
4. Moreira FC, Vilar VJP, Ferreira ACC, dos Santos FRA, Dezotti M, Sousa MA, et al. Treatment of a pesticide-containing wastewater using combined biological and solar-driven AOPs at pilot scale. Chem Eng J 2012; 209: 429-41. doi: 10.1016/j.cej.2012.08.009.
5. Amri N, Nasuha N, Halim SFA, Ngah K. Degradation of Reactive Black 5 dye by CWPO using Fe/mining sand

under photo-Fenton process. AIP Conference Proceedings 2015; 1660(1): 070094. doi: 10.1063/1.4915811.

6. Nidheesh PV, Gandhimathi R. Trends in electro-Fenton process for water and wastewater treatment: An overview. Desalination 2012; 299: 1-15. doi: 10.1016/j.desal.2012.05.011.
7. Huang YH, Chou S, Perng MG, Huang GH, Cheng SS. Case study on the bioeffluent of petrochemical wastewater by electro-fenton method. Water Sci Technol 1999; 39(10-11): 145-9. doi: 10.1016/S0273-1223(99)00265-6.
8. Neyens E, Baeyens J. A review of classic Fenton's peroxidation as an advanced oxidation technique. J Hazard Mater 2003; 98(1-3): 33-50. doi: 10.1016/S0304-3894(02)00282-0.
9. Ma J, Song W, Chen C, Ma W, Zhao J, Tang Y. Fenton Degradation of Organic Compounds Promoted by Dyes under Visible Irradiation. Environ Sci Technol 2005; 39(15): 5810-5. doi: 10.1021/es050001x.
10. Jaafarzadeh N, Ghanbari F, Ahmadi M, Omidinasab M. Efficient integrated processes for pulp and paper wastewater treatment and phytotoxicity reduction: Permanganate, electro-Fenton and Co3O4/UV/peroxymonosulfate. Chem Eng J 2017; 308: 142-50. doi: 10.1016/j.cej.2016.09.015.
11. Altin A. An alternative type of photoelectro-Fenton process for the treatment of landfill leachate. Sep Purif Technol 2008; 61(3): 391-7. doi: 10.1016/j.seppur.2007.12.004.
12. Ruiz EJ, Hernández-Ramírez A, Peralta-Hernández JM, Arias C, Brillas E. Application of solar photoelectro-Fenton technology to azo dyes mineralization: Effect of current density, Fe2+ and dye concentrations. Chem Eng J 2011; 171(2): 385-92. doi: 10.1016/j.cej.2011.03.004.
13. Atmaca E. Treatment of landfill leachate by using electro-Fenton method. J Hazard Mater 2009; 163(1): 109-14. doi: 10.1016/j.jhazmat.2008.06.067.
14. Pimentel M, Oturan N, Dezotti M, Oturan MA. Phenol degradation by advanced electrochemical oxidation process electro-Fenton using a carbon felt cathode. Appl Catal B 2008; 83(1): 140-9. doi: 10.1016/j.apcatb.2008.02.011.
15. Su CC, Cada CA, Dalida MLP, Lu MC. Effect of UV light on acetaminophen degradation in the electro-Fenton process. Sep Purif Technol 2013; 120: 43-51. doi: 10.1016/j.seppur.2013.09.034.
16. Daud Z, Hanafi NFM, Awang H. Optimization of COD and Colour Removal from Landfill Leachate by Electro-Fenton Method. Aust J Basic Appl Sci 2013; 7(8): 263-8.
17. Peralta-Hernández JM, Martínez-Huitle CA, Guzmán-Mar JL, Hernandez-Ramirez A. Recent Advances in the application of electro-Fenton and photoelectro-Fenton process for removal of synthetic dyes in waste water treatmen. J Environ Eng Manage 2009; 19(5): 257-65.
18. Özcan A, Şahin Y, Oturan MA. Complete removal of the insecticide azinphos-methyl from water by the electro-Fenton method – A kinetic and mechanistic study. Water Res 2013; 47(3): 1470-9. doi: 10.1016/j.watres.2012.12.016.
19. Heidari Z, Motavasel M, Jaafarzadeh N. Application of Electro-Fenton (EF) process to the removal of pentachlorophenol from aqueous solutions. Iranian Journal of Oil Gas Science and Technology 2015; 4(4): 76-87. doi: 10.22050/ijogst.2016.12481
20. Heidari Z, Motevasel M, Jaafarzadeh N. Advanced oxidation of pentachlorophenol: A comparison between electro-Fenton, sono electro-Fenton processes. American Journal of Oil and Chemical Technologies 2017; 5(2): 141-9. doi: 10.1016/j.cej.2011.12.010.
21. APHA. Standard Method for Examination of Water and Wastewater. 17th ed. Washington, DC: American Public Health Association; 1989.
22. Şahinkaya S. COD and color removal from synthetic textile wastewater by ultrasound assisted electro-Fenton oxidation process. Ind Eng Chem 2013; 19(2): 601-5. doi: 10.1016/j.jiec.2012.09.023.

15

Investigation of formaldehyde removal from synthetic contaminated air by using human hair

Amirreza Talaiekhozani[1*], Mohammad Reza Talaei[2], Mehdi Yazdan[3], Seyed Masoud Mir[3]

[1]Assistant Professor, Department of Civil Engineering, Jami Institute of Technology, Isfahan, Iran
[2]Associate Professor, Department of Chemical Engineering, Faculty of Engineering, University of Isfahan, Isfahan, Iran
[3]BSc Student, Department of Chemical Engineering, Jami Institute of Technology, Isfahan, Iran

Abstract

Background: Human hair can be used as an inexpensive and accessible adsorbent to remove a variety of pollutants from air. Although several studies have been done on removal of formaldehyde from wastewater by human hair, to date no study has investigated using hair to remove formaldehyde from air. Therefore, the aim of this study was to remove formaldehyde from synthetic contaminated air by a reactor packed with human hair.

Methods: Air contaminated with formaldehyde was introduced into a cylindrical reactor packed with human hair at the initial concentration of 8500 mg/L. Formaldehyde concentration was measured in the influent and effluent of the reactor to indicate formaldehyde removal efficiency. Other measurements of parameters effective on formaldehyde removal were taken including amount of human hair and environmental temperature.

Results: Results of this study revealed that each gram of human hair was able to remove 0.13 to 0.49 g of formaldehyde from air. Human hair adsorbed 98% of formaldehyde from synthetic contaminated air under 20°C. These results demonstrate that increased temperature had a negative effect on formaldehyde removal.

Conclusion: Results of this study show that human hair can be applied as a simple and inexpensive adsorbent to remove formaldehyde from industrial air exhaust. In addition, results of these tests can be considered as a small step to promote better air quality.

Keyword: Formaldehyde, Human hair, Adsorption process, Air treatment

***Correspondence to:**
Amirreza Talaiekhozani
Email: atalaie@jami.ac.ir

Introduction

Nowadays, industry produces many different pollutants in the form of gases, liquids and solids, which are released into the environment (1-3). Therefore, it is essential to control emissions of wastewater, exhausted gases and solid waste by developing treatments methods for application before they are released (2,4,5). Exhausted gases emitted from industry contribute to air pollution (6). Several air pollutants are harmful to humans by causing cancer or infertility (7). Air treatment is more complex than wastewater or solid waste treatment and needs more developed technology (8,9). Formaldehyde is widely used in industry and released into the atmosphere where it is a pollutant (10). Formaldehyde is a highly toxic, teratogenic, carcinogenic and mutagenic substance and thousands of tons are released into the atmosphere yearly (11). Formaldehyde can be absorbed from the air into seas and oceans where it generates water pollution. Formaldehyde is a basic chemical used in the production of keratin-based hair smoothing products. Formaldehyde is a listed dangerous chemical (1-3). This causes some manufacturers, importers, or distributors use other terms for chemical formaldehyde on their product information. There are many alternative terms used for formaldehyde including methylene glycol, formalin, methylene oxide, paraform, formic aldehyde, methanal, oxomethane, oxymethylene, timonacic acid or CAS No. 50-00-0 (12). These alternative terms mean that some products are labeled and marketed as formaldehyde free. Workers in beauty salons breathe in the formaldehyde released from such hair smoothing products or they may absorb it through their skin. Workers in beauty salons are exposed to formaldehyde during all hair straightening processes, particularly if the temperature is increased by use of tools such as during blow-drying or flat ironing processes (1). Occupational Safety and Health Administration (OSHA) recommends the maximum concentration of formaldehyde in air at 0.15 and 8 hours exposure is 2 and 0.5 ppm, respectively (13). In addition, the American Conference of Governmental Industrial Hygienists reports the threshold limit value ceiling of formaldehyde at 0.3 ppm (11).

Although several studies have been done on formaldehyde removal from wastewater (9); there has been very little research on removal of this dangerous substance from air. Methods of formaldehyde removal from air can be divided into three categories; physical, chemical and biological methods. In physical methods, formaldehyde is degraded to water and carbon dioxide by increasing the temperature to above 550°C. Although this method is effective to remove formaldehyde from the air, it is expensive and generates secondary pollutants such as carbon dioxide (5). Biological methods have also been used to remove formaldehyde from air. In biological methods, microorganisms are adapted to consume formaldehyde as their sole source of carbon. Biological methods are inexpensive but their operation is very complex.

Adsorption is another method for formaldehyde removal from air. Adsorption is an effective method and partially inexpensive for formaldehyde removal from air such that its operation is not as complex as biological methods. Various adsorbents have been introduced to remove pollutants from air and research has shown that human hair can be applied a natural adsorbent. Talaie et al applied human hair to remove formaldehyde from industrial wastewater (1). It was reported that this hazardous substance was adsorbed chemically onto human hair (1). Ghanbarnejad et al reports that both sheep wool and human hair were suitable for removing formaldehyde from water (9). They also report that formaldehyde was chemically adsorbed onto both sheep wool and human hair. In addition, increasing temperature had a destructive effect on adsorption of formaldehyde onto sheep wool and human hair (9). Rostami reports an investigation of removal of cadmium and lead from aquatic environments by human hair (14). This result showed that adsorption of cadmium onto human hair was higher than that of lead. Rostami reports that human hair was able to remove 38 mg cadmium per each gram human hair. It was reported that treatment of human hair by 0.1 M NaOH and Na_2S solution significantly increased adsorption of both cadmium and lead (14). However, treatment of human hair by this solution had some disadvantages such as a malodorous emission and caused breaking - up of human hair.

Although several of studies have been done on formaldehyde removal from wastewater by human hair, it has not been tested to date as an adsorbent to remove formaldehyde from air. Therefore, the aim of this study was to investigate removal of formaldehyde from air and to determine its effective factors including amount of hair and temperature. In this study, an adsorption reactor containing human hair was prepared and synthetic contaminated air was introduced to evaluate formaldehyde removal from air.

Methods and Materials

The pilot plant

The pilot plant used in this study is depicted in Figure 1. Formaldehyde-contaminated air was synthesized by bubbling fresh air through 37% formaldehyde solution. The bubble column was maintained until the outgoing air stream became saturated with formaldehyde. The synthetic contaminated air was passed through an adsorption bed packed with human hair. Formaldehyde was adsorbed onto the human hair, and the treated air then left the adsorption bed column. Flow rate of the incoming air stream was measured using a flow meter. The adsorption column was a polyethylene cylinder 50 cm long and 8 cm in diameter. The adsorption reactor temperature was adjusted by a water batch (Figure 1). The water batch temperature was maintained at the desired value by an electrical temperature controller with accuracy of ±1°C.

The effects of influencing parameters

In this study, the effects of the parameters amount of human

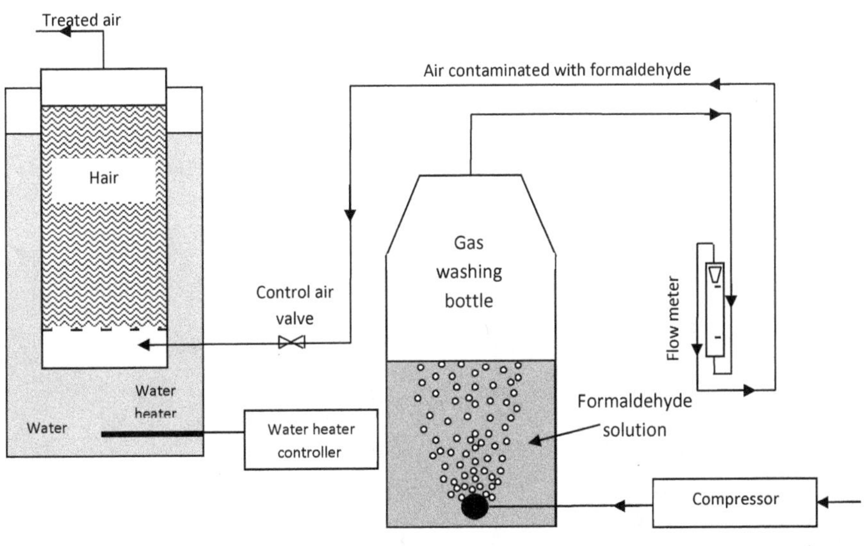

Figure 1. Schematic of the pilot planet.

hair and temperature were evaluated on formaldehyde removal. This evaluation is explained in the following section. There was no replicate for the experiments in this study.

Amount of human hair

The amount of human hair used in the adsorption reactor was changed to investigate its effect on formaldehyde removal. The formaldehyde removal efficiency of adsorption reactor containing 20, 30, 40 and 50 g of human hair was determined in 100 minutes. Eq. 1 was used to calculate formaldehyde removal efficiency.

$$RE = \left(\frac{C_{out} - C_{in}}{C_{out}}\right) \times 100 \quad (1)$$

where, RE is formaldehyde removal efficiency in %, C_{in} is formaldehyde concentration in influent air in mg/L and C_{out} is formaldehyde concentration in effluent air in mg/L.

Temperature

Figure 1 shows the adsorption reactor immersed into a water tank equipped with a temperature controller. Temperature of adsorption reactor was adjusted on the 20, 30, 40 and 50°C. Formaldehyde removal efficiency was determined for all temperatures.

Batch experiment

The removal of formaldehyde using human hair was investigated in batch mode. A special bottle was prepared for the batch experiment (Figure 2). The bottle was loaded by a given mass of human hair that was initially placed in an enclosed and sealed storage tank with a remote control opening door. When the remote control door opened, then the human hair was exposed to the air captured in the bottle, and the adsorption process began. Two steps were taken for the batch experiment; the first step was continual injection of synthetic air contaminated by formaldehyde into a bottle for 5 minutes to sweep all initial fresh air inside the bottle and the second step was release of human hair into the bottle by opening the remote control door to begin the adsorption process. A continuous record was made of formaldehyde concentration equilibrium by digital hydrocarbon meter.

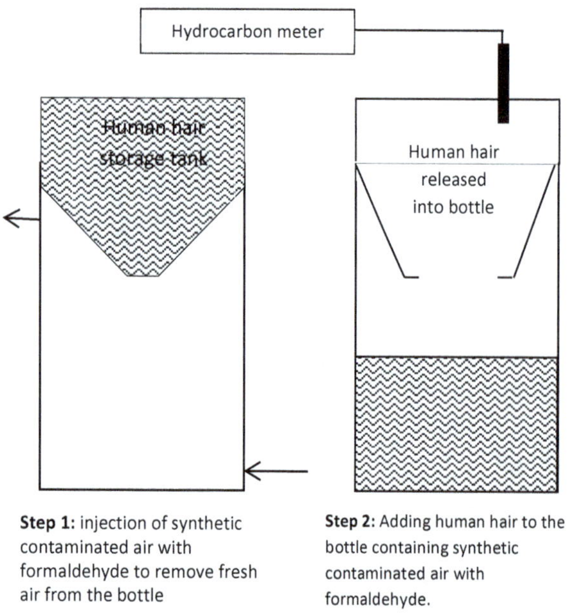

Figure 2. Schematic of batch experiment.

Analytical methods

Formaldehyde concentration was measured in the air streams by a digital hydrocarbon meter Testo 330-1G-KIT4. Ambient temperature was determined by alcoholic thermometer. Microsoft Excel was used for plotting the graphs and mathematical calculations.

Results

Continuous mode

Figure 3 shows the break-through curves obtained for hair mass loadings of 20 to 40 g. It is common knowledge that the break-through curve is independent of the adsorbent mass of loading if all conditions; flow rate, temperature, bed void fraction and inlet concentration are the same. However, the fact remains that when the bed length allows the mass transfer zone then there is ample time for the development process. As can be seen in this figure the break-through curves for adsorbent masses of 20 and 30 g were different with those of 40 and 50 g. Also, the break-through curves obtained for adsorbent mass of 40 g was very close to that of 50 g. This demonstrates that for an adsorbent mass of 40 g or more then there was adequate time for mass transfer zone to be developed.

The temperature of the adsorption reactor containing human hair was adjusted on the 20, 30, 40 and 50°C to evaluate its effect on formaldehyde removal. The results of temperature effect on formaldehyde removal are shown in Figure 4 as a break-through curve. As can be seen in this figure, an increase in temperature had an adverse effect on formaldehyde removal.

Batch mode

In the batch experiment, the aim was to obtain an isotherm for formaldehyde-human hair adsorption system in the

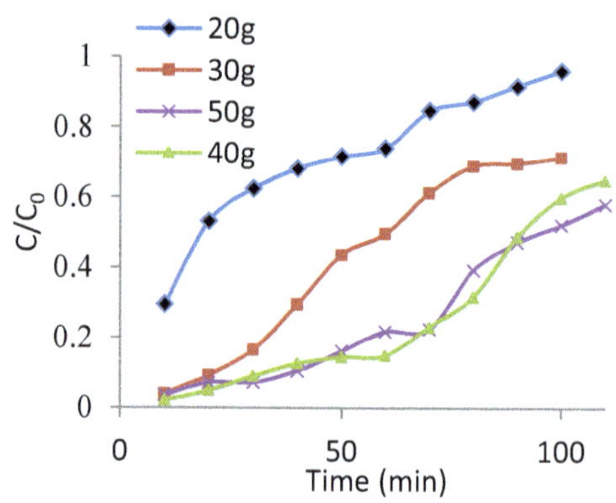

Figure 3. The break-through curve of the continuous adsorption process in a packed bed for different masses of human hair.

gas phase. The result of this study is shown in Figure 5 as an isotherm at temperature of 20°C.

Discussion

The results of this study reveal that the saturation adsorption capacity of human hair ranged from 0.049 to 0.13 g formaldehyde/g of hair; and results were dependent on temperature. It is the maximum capacity and may not always be attainable in practice. The continuous adsorption process was carried out using a bed packed with a load of

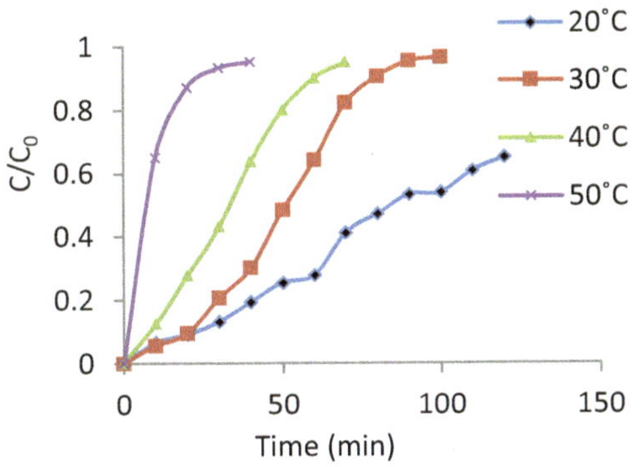

Figure 4. Break-through curve of the continuous adsorption process in a packed bed for different temperature.

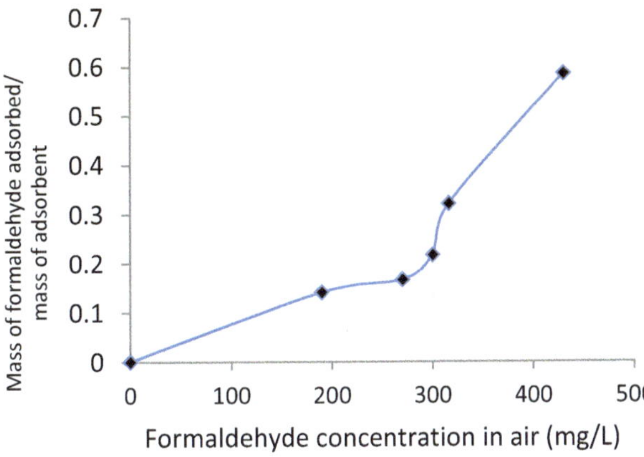

Figure 5. Mass of formaldehyde adsorbed/mass of adsorbent versus formaldehyde concentration in air.

adsorbent. When the adsorption process had begun, the mass transfer zone started forming and after complete development (which will occur if the bed has adequate length) it moves through the bed. When this zone reaches the end of the bed the pollutant concentration starts rising and ends up as inlet concentration. Saturation occurs when the outlet concentration becomes close to that of the inlet concentration. However, if there is a restriction on the outlet concentration, then the operation should stop well before this time. It means that when the operation ceases, the bed is not completely saturated. The complete continuous adsorption process is performed though successive adsorption-regeneration cycles. Unfortunately, no documents have been published to date on methods of human hair adsorbent regeneration. Therefore, human hair must be frequently replaced to maintain the formaldehyde removal efficiency at its highest level. As such, the results shown in Figure 3 reveal that, under the conditions applied in this experiment, at least 40 g of human hair must be used for mass transfer zone to be developed.

Hair is composed of a protein known as keratin. Formaldehyde has a high reactivity towards proteins (1). Formaldehyde is able to react with different side chains of amino acids such as the amino groups of lysine, arginine, glutamine and asparagine. Formaldehyde can form crosslinks with keratin, such as NH-CH_2-NH bridges, and between N-terminal cysteine and amine groups -S-CH_2-NH (15). The best pH for the reaction between formaldehyde and keratin is 6 to 7. Amide derivatives of aspartic acid and glutamic acid react with formaldehyde. Some of these reactions can be bi-functional and mono-functional. The simple crosslinks are CH_2. It is very difficult to locate the active sites and the extent of formaldehyde keratin reactions because most modified side chains of amino acids are not stable to hydrolytic reaction conditions (16). Reaction between keratin and formaldehyde was divided into two steps. The first step involved amino groups and formaldehyde and produced an unstable product (aminomethylol derivative). The second reaction led to a stable methylene bridge (17). The vapor pressure of the formaldehyde at 20°C is 3285

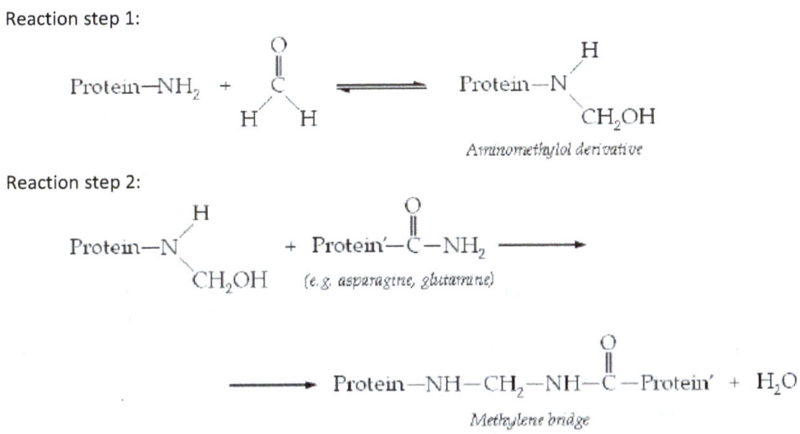

mm Hg. This means that there was no opportunity for the formaldehyde vapor to be condensed in the conditions applied throughout the experiments. Thus, formaldehyde removal was not by condensation.

The results shown in Figure 4 demonstrate that adsorption capacity increased as temperature was reduced. This fact is in line with the characteristics of physical adsorption, which is in contrast with the literature provided in the preceding section. In other words, in a chemical adsorption process, adsorption capacity is usually decreased by temperature. However, chemical adsorption can be considered as a two-step process. In the first step, contamination is adsorbed on the surface of an adsorbent physically in the form of adsorbate. Then, adsorbate undergoes a series of reactions with human keratin as afore-mentioned. Therefore, if the rate of the first step was controlling, then the adsorption capacity can be reduced by temperature even though the adsorption process falls into the category of chemical adsorption.

Based on these results, an empirical equation was developed to calculate the amount of human hair needed for removal of formaldehyde from an air stream (Eq. 2).

$$w = r \times Q \times c \times t \quad (2)$$

where, r is the amount of formaldehyde which can be removed by 1 g of human hair in g/g, w is the mass of human hair that is utilized for removal of formaldehyde from an air stream in g, Q is air flow rate in m^3/h, c is inlet formaldehyde concentration in g/m^3 and t is desired filtering time in hour. The coefficient of r was obtained ranging from 0.049 to 0.13 and can be estimated by Eq. 3, as follows:

$$r = 9 \times 10^{-6} \times T^3 + 0.008 \times T^2 - 2.44 \times T + 244.8 \quad (3)$$

where, T is temperature in K. It should be mentioned that Eq. 3 is valid only for temperatures between 20 and 60 °C.

Conclusion

Formaldehyde is a toxic, mutagenic, teratogenic and suspected carcinogenic chemical that is highly reactive with proteins such as keratin. Therefore, formaldehyde can be removed from air by an adsorption reactor packed with human hair. Results of this study revealed that each gram of human hair was able to remove from 0.13 to 0.49 g of formaldehyde from air. Human hair adsorbed 98% of formaldehyde form synthetic contaminated air under 20 °C. In addition, results illustrated that increased temperature had a distractive effect on formaldehyde removal by human hair. Although formaldehyde removal by human hair presents an effective method to treat contaminated air, economic calculations are needed to reveal determine whether or not this process is economically viable on a larger scale.

Acknowledgments

This article has been extracted from a Bachelor of Science dissertation in field of chemical engineering at Jami Institute of Technology, Isfahan, Iran. The authors of this article appreciate the Jami Institute of Technology for its financial and moral support, which enabled completion of this dissertation.

Competing interests

The authors declare that there is no conflict of interest that would prejudice the impartiality of this scientific work.

Authors' contributions

All authors of this study have a complete contribution for data collection, data analyses and manuscript writing.

References

1. Talaie AR, Bagheri M, Ghotbinasab S, Talaie MR. Evaluation of formaldehyde wastewater adsorption on human hair. Health Syst Res 2011; 6(4): 735-743. [In Persian].
2. Talaiekhozani A, Talaie MR, Fulazzaky MA. Evaluation of formaldehyde removal from contaminated air by using a biotrickling filter reactor in a continuous condition. Journal of Air Pollution and Health. 2016;1(2):69-76.
3. Talaiekhozani A, Masomi B, Hashemi SMJ. Evaluation of gaseous pollutants emission rate from Marvdasht landfills. J Adv Med Sci Appl Tech 2016; 2(1): 162-75.
4. Talaiekhozani A, Bagheri M, Najafabadi NR, Borna E. Effect of nearly one hundred percent of municipal solid waste recycling in najafabad city on improving of its air quality. J Air Pollut Health 2016; 1(2): 111-22.
5. Talaiekhozani A, Bagheri M, Goli A, Talaie Khoozani MR. An overview of principles of odor production, emission, and control methods in wastewater collection and treatment systems. J Environ Manage 2016; 170: 186-206. doi: 10.1016/j.jenvman.2016.01.021.
6. Talaiekhozani A, Ali Fulazzaky M, Ponraj M, Abd Majid M. Removal of formaldehyde from polluted air in a biotrickling filter reactor. Desalination and Water Treatment 2014; 52(19-21): 3663-71. doi: 10.1080/19443994.2013.854002.
7. Alaee S, Talaiekhozani A, Ziaei GR, Lohrasbi P. Evaluation of Iranian college students' awareness about infertility risk factors. Jundishapur J Health Sci 2016; 8(2): e34172. doi: 10.17795/jjhs-34172.
8. Fulazzaky MA, Talaiekhozani A, Ponraj M, Abd Majid MZ, Hadibarata T, Goli A. Biofiltration process as an ideal approach to remove pollutants from polluted air. Desalination and Water Treatment 2013; 52(19-21): 3600-15. doi: 10.1080/19443994.2013.854102.
9. Ghanbarnejad P, Goli A, Bayat B, Barzkar H, Talaiekhozani A, Bagheri M, et al. Evaluation of formaldehyde adsorption by human hair and sheep wool in industrial wastewater with high concentration. J Environ Treat Tech 2014; 2(1): 12-7.
10. Fulazzaky MA, Talaiekhozani A, Hadibarata T. Calculation of optimal gas retention time using a logarithmic equation applied to a bio-trickling filter reactor for formaldehyde removal from synthetic contaminated air. RSC Adv 2013; 3(15): 5100-7. doi: 10.1039/C3RA22753G.
11. Talaiekhozani A, Fulazzaky MA, Ponraj M, Majid

ZA. Formaldehyde from production to application. 3rd Conference of Application of Chemistry in Novel Technologies; November 7, 2013; Isfahan. Iran. p. 1-16.

12. Hazard Alert: Hair Smoothing Products That Could Release Formaldehyde. OSHA; 2016 [cited 10 September 2016]. Available from: https://www.osha.gov/SLTC/formaldehyde/hazard_alert.html.
13. Formaldehyde Program: Environmental Health and Safety at UVM. UVM; 2016 [cited 10 September 2016]. Available from: http://www.uvm.edu/safety/formaldehyde.
14. Rostami S. Application of human hair to remove heavy metals from aquatic environments (Cadmium and lead) [dissertation]. Isfahan: Jami Institute of Technology; 2001.
15. Hinton EH. A survey and critique of the literature on crosslinking agents and mechanisms as related to wool keratin. Text Res J 1974; 44(4): 233-92. doi: 10.1177/004051757404400401.
16. Simpson WS. Wool chemistry. Wool. A volume in Woodhead Publishing Series in Textiles. 2002; 130-159. doi: 10.1533/9781855737648.130.
17. Wortmann G, Sweredjuk Thome R, Sweredjuk G, Zwiener G, Wortmann FJ. Chemisorption of protein reactive indoor air pollutants by wool. 12th International Conference on Renewable Resources and Plant Biotechnology. June 12-13, 2006, Magdeburg, Germany.

16

Sulfur dioxide emissions in Iran and environmental impacts of sulfur recovery plant in Tabriz Oil Refinery

Shokufeh Delfi[1], Mohammad Mosaferi[2*], Ali Khalafi[3], Khaled Zoroufchi Benis[4]

[1]Department of Environmental Health Engineering, School of Health, Tabriz University of Medical Sciences, Tabriz, Iran
[2]Health and Environment Research Center, Tabriz University of Medical Sciences, Tabriz, Iran
[3]Department of Chemical Engineering, School of Chemical Engineering, University of Tehran, Tehran, Iran
[4]Department of Chemical Engineering, School of Chemical Engineering, Sahand University of Technology, Tabriz, Iran

Abstract
Background: Combustion of fossil fuels contributes to sulfur dioxide (SO_2) emissions. To deal with this issue, the government of Iran has appointed the oil refineries to upgrade their installations and produce high quality fuels. Thus, this study investigated the status of SO_2 emissions in Iran and the capability of advanced technologies to control SO_2 emissions.
Methods: The status of SO_2 emissions was reviewed and discussed through national online reports. Meanwhile, the environmental impacts of sulfur recovery and tail gas treatment (TGT) plant (STP) were assessed by applying rapid impact assessment matrix (RIAM) for implementation and non-implementation alternatives in Tabriz Oil Refinery Company (TORC).
Results: SO_2 emissions have been increased by 2.1 times during 2004-2014 in Iran. Power plants and transportation play a significant role in this regard and overall contribute 82% of emissions. Among the other fossil fuels, fuel oil and gasoil account for 95% of SO_2 emissions. Based on the environmental impact assessments (EIAs), sulfur recovery management and enhancing sulfur removal efficiency from flue gas up to 99.9% are two main positive environmental aspects of STP project that would enable TORC to prevent 87 600 tons of SO_2 emissions, annually. Nevertheless, flue gas and sour gas streams which have been determined as probable pollution sources of process, should be managed through proper monitoring framework.
Conclusion: The increasing trend of SO_2 emissions and significant role of fuel oil and gasoil has required Iranian oil refineries to enhance the quality of fuels by employing clean and cost-effective technologies.
Keywords: Air pollution, Fossil fuels, Oil and gas industry, Environmental assessment, Tabriz

***Correspondence to:**
Mohammad Mosaferi
Email: mosaferim@tbzmed.ac.ir

Introduction

Sulfur dioxide (SO_2), emitting from either natural or anthropogenic sources, is one of the important air pollutants leading to acid precipitations, climatic changes and health problems. Previous studies showed that short- or long-term exposure to SO_2 contributes to increase of hospital admissions and mortality due to respiratory and cardiac problems including chronic obstructive pulmonary disease and acute myocardial infraction (1-3). More than 70% of global SO_2 emissions is accounted for anthropogenic sources including power plants, refineries and vehicles (4). Fioletov et al detected 491 emitting sources via ozone monitoring instrument and suggested that the oil and gas industries are the second anthropogenic sources of SO_2 emissions over the globe (5). Sulfur oxides along with other pollutants such as nitrogen oxides (NO_2), volatile organic compounds (VOCs) and carbon monoxide (CO) are the group of pollutants generated from the operations of oil industries. Sulfur content of crude oil varies from 0.05 to 6 by weight percentage, approximately (6).

The investigations indicate that global SO_2 emission has followed an increasing trend during 2000 to 2005 and has been resulted from industrial activities development in Asian countries, particularly in China and India. Despite the fact that flue gas desulfurization (FGD) and some other practical measures in power plants of China, the United States and Europe have resulted in great decline of emissions rate since 2006 (7-10), the emissions from fuel combustion have remained constant since 1980 (10,11). To achieve health benefits from improved outdoor air quality (12), sulfur-limit transportation fuels like diesel oil and gasoline, have been gradually restricted, in Germany. For instance, diesel fuel standards have been decreased from 5000 to 350 ppm while in the United States, it has been changed from 500 in 1993 to 15 ppm since 2006 (13). In this regard, the government of Iran has appointed oil refinery companies to upgrade their installations and provide high quality fuels by the end of 2019. These stringent standards require gas plants and crude oil refineries to employ reliable and cost-effective technologies for advanced sulfur recovery (14,15). Among biodesulfurization, surface adsorption and oxidation, hydrodesulfurization (HDS) is the most common process applied to eliminate sulfur from crude oil in petroleum industry. In this process, sulfur containing compounds react with hydrogen on Mo/Al_2O_3_Co or Mo/Al_2O_3-Ni catalysts to yield hydrocarbons and H_2S (16).

East Azerbaijan province with a population of 3724620 people had gasoil consumption of 950 million liters in 2015 and have ranked 23rd in the country (17). Tabriz Oil Refinery Company (TORC) is located in the northwest of Iran, near the city of Tabriz (Figure 1). This refinery has a nominal capacity of 110000 barrels per day producing 6 types of fuels including gasoil, fuel oil, gasoline, liquid petroleum gas (LPG) and kerosene (18). Currently, 35.5 by weight percentage of refined crude oil is converted to gasoil in TORC. Sulfur content of crude oil needed to be reduced from 150 to ≤50 ppm to provide Euro 4 gasoil, utilizing gasoil hydrotreating plant (GHP). This process would enable TORC to produce 4.77 million liters Euro 4 gasoil daily, comprising 19.87% of the total gasoil produced in the country. Nevertheless, the prospective sour gas streams of this plant would impose exceeded burden on the sulfur recovery unit (SRU).

To address this problem, employing sulfur treatment plant (STP) technology is expected to bring about the following advantages:

1) Raise liquid sulfur recovery capacity from 80 up to 190 tons per day
2) Raise sulfur removal efficiency from sour and acid gas streams up to 99.9%
3) Minimize hydrogen sulfur (H_2S) emissions from flue gas

Figure 2 describes the procedure of sulfur recovery process in STP; the sour and acid gas streams from Amine treatment unit (ATU), sour water stripping unit (SWSU) and GHP are collected and sent to SRU with clause process. Claus process is a main technique for processing high amount of acid streams and involves two reactions; initially, SO_2 is generated through the combustion of H_2S using air or O_2, thereafter, the reaction of SO_2 with H_2S will

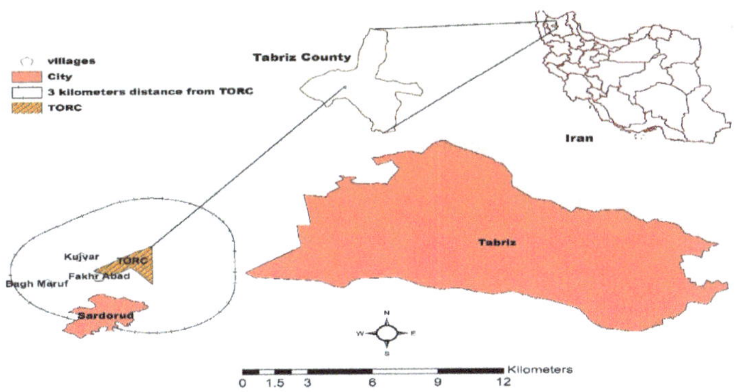

Figure 1. Location of Tabriz Oil Refinery Company.

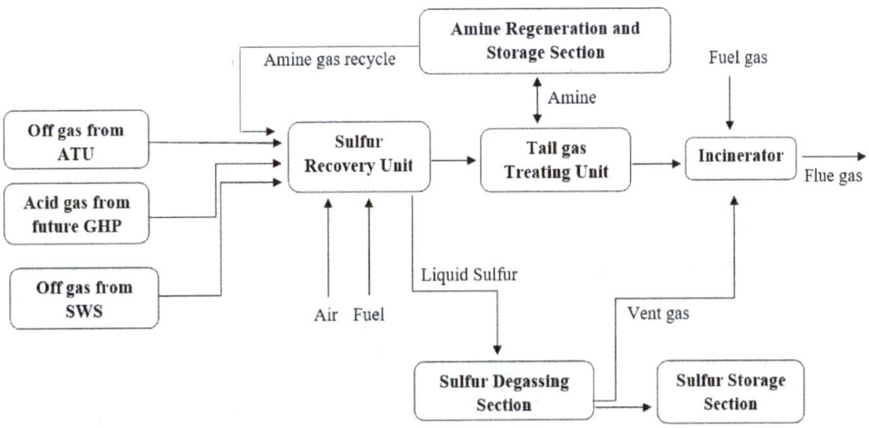

Figure 2. Sulfur recovery and tail gas treating plant diagram.

produce liquid sulfur which would finally store in solid form. Stream of sulfur oxides (H_2S, CS_2, SO_2 and COS) generated through Claus process would sent to tail gas treatment plant (TGT). Incorporation of high temperature and hydrogen in advanced treatment, will convert these compounds to H_2S gas. After absorption of H_2S by amine solution, treated tail gas will be finally sent to incinerator (19,20).

Based on the national environmental regulations, all industrial plants are subjected to environmental impact assessment (EIA). EIA is defined as the systematic identification and evaluation of potential impacts of proposed projects, plans, programs, or legislative actions relative to the physical, chemical, biological, cultural, and socio-economic components of the total environment. EIA is an environmental management tool aiming at identifying environmental issues and providing solutions to prevent or minimize these problems to desired levels. It also provides an environmental management plan, which includes a monitoring program. Rapid impact assessment matrix (RIAM) is one of the useful impact assessment tools that has been employed in many case studies for various purposes including landfills, water management, etc. (21-23).

Present study was conducted to provide an overview of SO_2 emissions in Iran through online national reports and assess the environmental impact of STP process by applying RIAM method. Indeed, the overall approach of this paper was to investigate the participation rate of different sectors and fuels in SO_2 emissions and also the capability of advanced technologies to control emissions.

Methods

SO2 emissions in Iran

To provide an overview of SO_2 emissions status in Iran, the latest online documents published by the Ministry of Energy were investigated. The trend of SO_2 emissions was reviewed during 2001 to 2014, whilst the contribution of sources has been investigated during 2014. Findings provided us with both SO_2 emissions trend and share of different energy sectors and fuels in this regard.

RIAM description for STP

RIAM provides a transparent and permanent record of the analysis process while at the same time organizing the EIA procedure, which in turn reduces the time spent on executing EIAs. The simple structured form of RIAM allows reanalysis and in-depth analysis of the selected components in a rapid and precise manner. In addition, the capability of comparing different options makes this method flexible which provides decision makers with transparent judgments (24).

RIAM is based on the standard definition of assessment criteria including importance, magnitude, permanence, reversibility and cumulative. Each criterion involves a range of values with specific description (Table 1).

Table 1. Assessment criteria of rapid impact assessment matrix

Criteria	Scale	Description
A_1	0	No importance
	1	Important only to the local condition
	2	Important to the areas immediately
	3	Important to national interests
	4	Important to international interest
A_2	+3	Major positive benefits
	+2	Significant improvement in status quo
	+1	Improvement in status quo
	0	No change
	-1	Negative change to status quo
	-2	Significant negative impacts
	-3	Major negative impacts
B_1	1	No change
	2	Temporary
	3	Permanent
B_2	1	No change
	2	Reversible
	3	Irreversible
B_3	1	No change
	2	Non-cumulative
	3	Cumulative

The values are selected based on the overall predicted impacts of activities on the environmental components. Thereafter, the selected values will undergo the following mathematical calculations (24):

$$A1 \times A2 = aT$$

$$B1 + B2 + B3 = bT$$

$$aT \times bT = ES$$

The scores of importance (A_1) and magnitude (A_2) are the criteria that can individually change the score, so the application of a multiplier ensures that the weight of each score is counted. While, the scores of permanence (B_1), reversibility (B_2) and cumulative (B_3) are added together to ensure that the individual score wouldn't affect the obtained score (bT). Multiplying (aT) and (bT) scores together, will provide a final environmental score (ES) for each environmental component (24). To provide a more certain assessment, ES values will be set into one of the range bands described in Table 2. In this study, the scores of assessment criteria were estimated based on the location, scale and the nature of desulphurization process of STP and assessment carried out according to the range bands. Finally, all positive and negative impacts were presented in graphical form and discussed (24).

STP would operate in an area of about 0.4 hectares beyond the existing sulfur recovery plant. This location is sand-filled and devoid of any vegetation or special habitat. Meanwhile, most of the required facilities including access roads, energy sources, and wastewater management system are available in place. Hence, the impact assessment was conducted for implementation (construction and

Table 2. Conversion of environmental scores to range bands

ES	RB	Description
72 to 108	E	Major positive impacts
36 to 71	D	Significant positive impacts
19 to 35	C	Moderately positive impacts
10 to 18	B	Positive impacts
1 to 9	A	Slightly positive impacts
0	N	No change
-1 to -9	-A	Slightly negative impacts
-10 to -18	-B	Negative impacts
-19 to -35	-C	Moderately negative impacts
-36 to -71	-D	Significant negative impacts
-72 to -108	-E	Major negative impacts

Abbreviations: RB, range bands; ES, environmental score.

operation phases) and non-implementation alternatives separately based on the following assumptions:
1. The prospective sour gas stream from GHP will impose additional burden on SRU in case of non-implementation alternatives
2. STP technology is an environmentally friendly approach which deals with the additional sour gas streams with minimum pollution in case of implementation alternatives
The impacts of STP were evaluated against 15 various environmental components. Environmental impacts were categorized into 4 groups including physical, biological, cultural and socioeconomic environments. Physical components focus on the changes in the quality and quantity of water sources and air pollutants. Biological components refer to the existed fauna and flora, while the cultural and socioeconomic components are mainly concerned with human life quality.

Results

General trend of SO_2 emissions is represented in Figure 3 (25), which was positive during 2001-2014; emission rate has started to increase from 2004 and after a steep slope between 2006-2007, it has reached the highest level of 678078 tons in 2009 and after a rapid decrease in 2010, it started to increase with a mild slope up until 2013, however, the emission rate was partially decreased about 130,246 tons by 2014. Figure 4 indicates the share of various sectors in SO_2 emissions as follows: Power plants > transportation > industry > agriculture > (public, domestic, commercial). Power plants and transportation overall contribute 82% of the emissions. Fuel oil together with gasoil account for 95% of SO_2 emissions, while the remained 5 % belongs to gasoline, heavy jet oil (ATK), kerosene and natural gas, totally (Figure 5).
Table 3 and Figure 6 represent the final yields of the assessment for both non-implementation and implementation alternatives. The results of assessment showed that non-implementation alternatives kept 86 % of the environment safe and stable. Nevertheless, incomplete treatment and discharge of prospective additional sour gas stream from GHP would pose negative impact on air quality. Surface water pollution is another undesired impact caused by solid sulfur washing.
The project implementation alternatives did not have any positive or negative impact on 70 % of the environment. 16% of the entire impacts of implementation alternatives were described as slightly negative impacts (-A) which mainly resulted from construction activities including embankment, excavation and transportation of construction materials or staff. These activities affect soil, air and surface water quality as well as road traffic. However, they are predicted to be temporary and

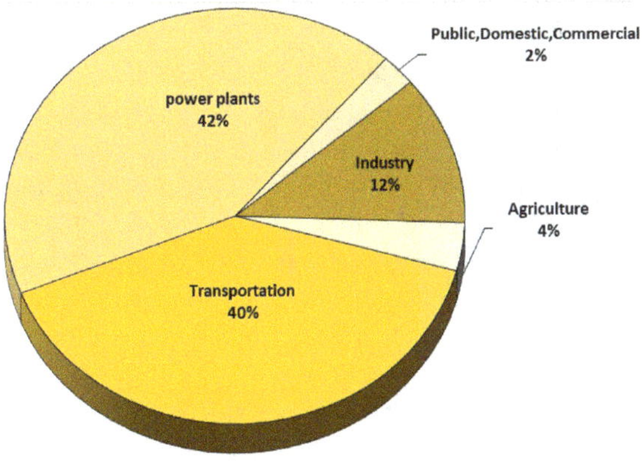

Figure 4. Share of different sectors in SO_2 emissions during 2014 in Iran.

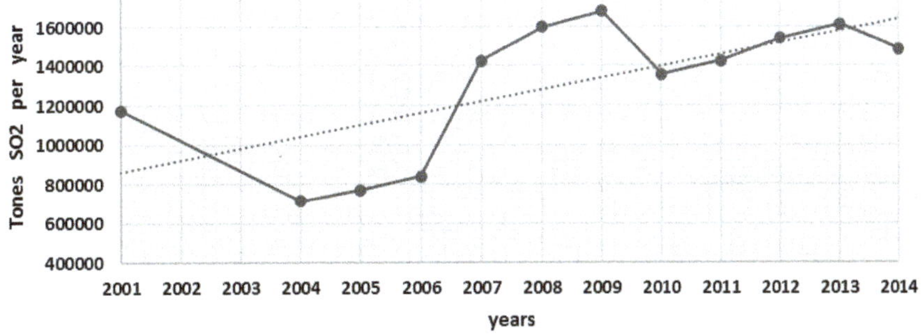

Figure 3. Trend of SO_2 emissions from all energy-consuming sectors including power plants, refineries, transportation, agriculture, etc. during 2001-2014 in Iran

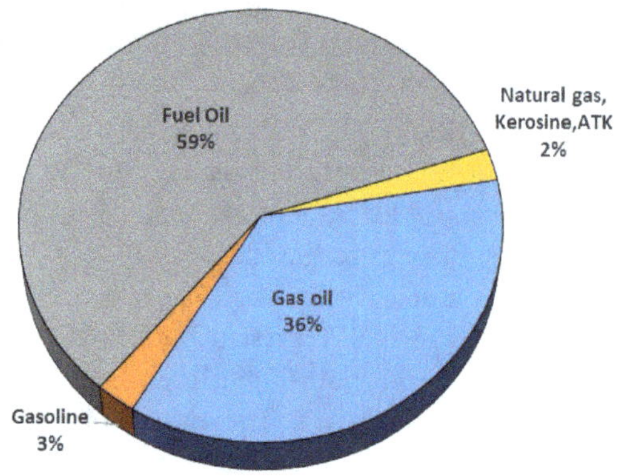

Figure 5. Share of different fuels in SO_2 emissions during 2014 in Iran

reversible. The remained 14% of positive impacts are completely associated with air quality; employment of novel technology for advanced treatment of tail gas and SO_2 which will be able to convert the ES of air quality from -28 to 30. Besides, providing job opportunity and industrial application of land were classified as slightly positive impacts (A) of STP employment. The overall identified impacts of this project were concerned with physical and socioeconomic environments. However, biological and cultural environments were not affected by the implementation or non-implementation alternatives.

Discussion

SO_2 emissions

Results of the present study revealed that SO_2 emissions followed a growing trend during 2001-2014 (Figure 3). Among all energy consuming sectors, power plants and transportation have more contribution to emissions, respectively. However, compared to previous years, the share of power plants (42%) was almost equal to that of transportation (40%) in 2014, which probably implies the alternative utilization of clean fuel in power industries (Figure 4).

Generally, natural gas, fuel oil and gasoil are the main sources of energy for electricity generation in Iran's power plants. According to Mazandarani et al studies, consumption of natural gas, diesel and fuel oil have been respectively increased by 18.6, 3.1 and 8.4 times in power plants during 1979-2008 (26) and consequently, given the eleven-time increase in electricity consumption, nominal capacity reached up to 56 181 MW by 2009 and more than 96 % of electricity has produced by fossil fuel-based power plants during the year (27). This report is greatly in line with general trend of SO_2 emissions (Figure 3) and interestingly expresses the peak of emission rates in 2009. Actually, the economic growth of Iran depends on oil and gas industries. However, beyond the supply side of the energy, the problem of pollutant emissions over local and global atmosphere should be addressed (28). As Figure 5 indicates, fuel oil and gasoil account for 82% of SO_2 emissions in 2014. On the other hand, gasoil (diesel fuel) and gasoline are two important fuels in transportation sector but gasoline has negligible share in SO_2 emissions compared to gasoil (Figure 5). Consequently, due to its extensive utilization both in power industry and transportation, the sulfur content of diesel fuels can be considered as a key factor of fuel standards (29).

It is well known that sulfur content of fuels plays a significant role in SO_2 emissions; Nazari et al reported that fuel oils consumed in Iranian steam power plants contain an average of 2.8 weight percentage of sulfur which makes their SO_2 emission factors to be 4 and 7 times higher than that of gas turbines and combined cycle power plants, respectively (30). Relevantly, Tan et al suggested that physical and chemical properties of diesel fuels have important influence on exhaust emissions. SO_2 emission continuously increases along with the engine load, and

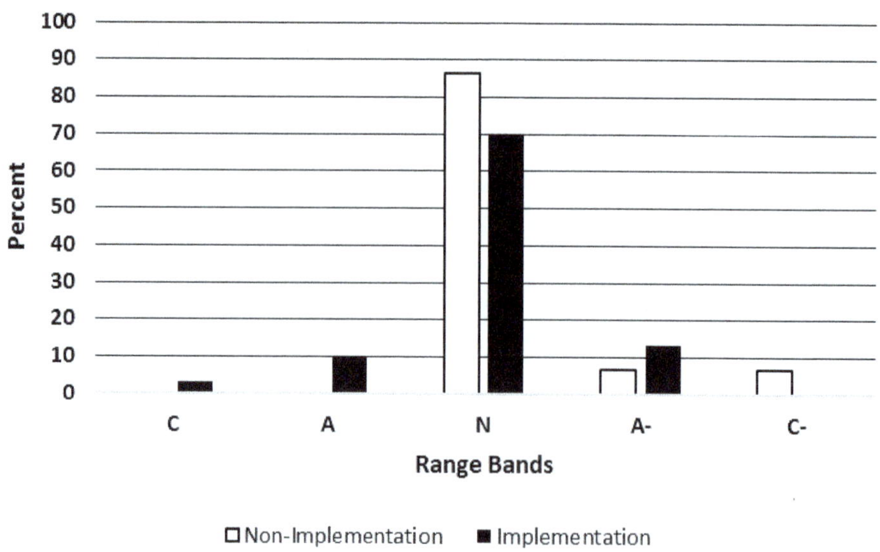

Figure 6. Comparison of Non-implementation and implementation alternatives for STP.

Table 3. Environmental impact assessment of STP for Non-implementation (NI), construction and operation

Environmental Components		Phase	Criteria						
			A_1	A_2	B_1	B_2	B_3	ES	RB
Physical Environment	Climate	NI	0	0	1	1	1	0	N
		Construction	0	0	1	1	1	0	N
		Operation	0	0	1	1	1	0	N
	Air	NI	2	-2	3	1	3	-28	-C
		Construction	1	-1	1	2	1	-4	-A
		Operation	3	+2	3	1	1	30	C
	Soil	NI	0	0	1	1	1	0	N
		Construction	1	-1	3	3	1	-7	-A
		Operation	0	0	1	1	1	0	N
	Surface water	NI	2	-1	1	1	1	-3	-A
		Construction	2	-1	1	1	1	-6	-A
		Operation	2	-1	1	1	1	-6	-A
	Ground water	NI	0	0	1	1	1	0	N
		Construction	0	0	1	1	1	0	N
		Operation	0	0	1	1	1	0	N
Biological Environment	Vegetation	NI	0	0	1	1	1	0	N
		Construction	0	0	1	1	1	0	N
		Operation	0	0	1	1	1	0	N
	Animals	NI	0	0	1	1	1	0	N
		Construction	0	0	1	1	1	0	N
		Operation	0	0	1	1	1	0	N
	Habitat	NI	0	0	1	1	1	0	N
		Construction	0	0	1	1	1	0	N
		Operation	0	0	1	1	1	0	N
	Protected areas	NI	0	0	1	1	1	0	N
		Construction	0	0	1	1	1	0	N
		Operation	0	0	1	1	1	0	N
Socioeconomic	Employment	NI	0	0	1	1	1	0	N
		Construction	1	+1	1	2	1	4	A
		Operation	1	+1	1	2	1	4	A
	Land application	NI	0	0	1	1	1	0	N
		Construction	0	0	1	1	1	0	N
		Operation	1	+1	3	1	1	5	A
	Road traffic	NI	0	0	1	1	1	0	N
		Construction	1	-1	1	1	3	-5	-A
		Operation	0	-1	2	1	3	0	N
	Migration	NI	0	0	1	1	1	0	N
		Construction	0	0	1	1	1	0	N
		Operation	0	0	1	1	1	0	N
Culture	Religious beliefs	NI	0	0	1	1	1	0	N
		Construction	0	0	1	1	1	0	N
		Operation	0	0	1	1	1	0	N
	Cultural heritage	NI	0	0	1	1	1	0	N
		Construction	0	0	1	1	1	0	N
		Operation	0	0	1	1	1	0	N

linearly varies with the fuel sulfur contents (31). Zhang et al also stated that sulfur content of crude oil fields and employment of advanced desulfurization technologies, were crucial factors in sulfur content of diesel and gasoline fuels in River delta regions (32).

Environmental impact assessment of STP

The overall analysis of EIA indicated that STP process is an environmentally friendly technology, aiming at enhancing sulfur removal efficiency from acid gas streams with minimum emissions. Moreover, the advanced treatment of tail gas would enable the extension of sulfur recovery level to 200 tons per day which is equivalent to prevention of 240 tons of SO_2 emissions daily. The entire process will increase sulfur recovery capacity up to 439 585 tons per year. On the other hand, undesirable impacts of STP project can be effectively managed based on the recommended mitigation measures mentioned in Table 4. Desulphurization facilities occupy a small part of the refinery, which, if properly utilized, they won't threaten

Table 4. Mitigation measures and management program for construction activities and operation system of STP

Construction Phase	
Air quality	Selecting roof and proper location for trash dumping Water spraying of trash in regular intervals to reduce dust release Observing the speed limit by drivers
Water quality	Constructing drainage canal for run-off control Dedicating construction activities during low-rain seasons
Noise pollution control	Selecting the proper equipment with minimum level of noise Regular maintenance and servicing of equipment and installations
Waste management	Meeting source reduction, source segregation, reuse and recycling principles Using proper waste containers Regular collection and disposal
Operation System Control	
Sulfur recovery and TGT section	The whole STP performance should meet the environmental agency standards for acceptable level of emissions. Minimum 96 % conversion at the end of run should be achieved within the entire Claus plant. All processes of advanced treatment including hydrogenation, quench section, filters, amine absorbing and regeneration section should be performed; SO_2 leakage and lean amine temperature are two key factors of TGT section that should be controlled. Appropriate analyzers (H_2S and H_2) for quench and absorber towers should be considered. Maximum CS_2 and COS hydrolysis should be achieved in hydrogenation section.
Incineration section	Oxidation of SO_2 should be completely done at proper temperature levels to reduce H_2S emissions to less than 10 ppm. Concentration of flue gas pollutants should be measured and monitored, continually.
Pipes and installations	Performance of installations and the pipes should be controlled and managed in order to prevent SO_2 and H_2S emissions and solid sulfur leakage.

public health of nearby residential areas, located within 3 km away from refinery (Figure 1). However, emissions of H_2S and SO_2 during the process should be repeatedly monitored through the environmental management system. This system assists the operators to achieve a safe operation based on the identification of pollution source and its magnitude; in case of STP, for instance, the flue gas of incinerator and release of sulfur gas from installations are considered as the main pollution sources. To control these pollutants, SO_2 and H_2S levels should be recorded applying fixed detectors near the furnace or reactors. Besides, the staff should be equipped with portable detectors to be aware of exceeded level of sulfur gases at working area.

Conclusion

Generally, Power plants are defined as the major contributors to SO_2 emissions. However, desulfurization of flue gas and progressive utilization of clean fuels in electricity industries over recent years, is going to draw attentions toward transportation fuels. Due to extensive utilization of gasoil in transportation and power plants, more emphasis should be placed on its quality. In this regard, Iranian oil refineries aim at producing Euro 4 gasoil, employing clean and cost-effective technologies. It is estimated that employing hydro-desulfurization combined with STP technology in TORC, will extend sulfur recovery capacity up to 73 000 tons yearly which will subsequently result in preventing 87 600 tons of SO_2 emissions, annually.

Acknowledgments

This research was conducted at Environmental Health Engineering Department, Tabriz University of Medical Sciences, Tabriz, Iran. The authors would like to gratitude Tabriz Oil Refinery Company (TORC) for its financial support (grant number: 92-52).

Competing interests

The authors declare that they have no competing interests.

Authors' contributions

All authors equally participated in data collection, analysis and reviewing the manuscript.

References

1. Kermani M, Fallah Jokandan S, Aghaei M, Bahrami Asl F, Karimzadeh S, Dowlati M. Estimation of the number of excess hospitalizations attributed to sulfur dioxide in six major cities of Iran. Health Scope 2016; 5(4): e38736. doi: 10.17795/jhealthscope-38736.
2. Ghanbari Ghozikali M, Mosaferi M, Safari GH, Jaafari J. Effect of exposure to O3, NO2, and SO2 on chronic obstructive pulmonary disease hospitalizations in Tabriz, Iran. Environmental Science and Pollution Research 2015; 22(4): 2817-23. doi: 10.1007/s11356-014-3512-5.

3. Goudarzi G, Geravandi S, Idani E, Hosseini SA, Baneshi MM, Yari AR, et al. An evaluation of hospital admission respiratory disease attributed to sulfur dioxide ambient concentration in Ahvaz from 2011 through 2013. Environ Sci Pollut Res Int 2016; 23(21): 22001-7. doi: 10.1007/s11356-016-7447-x.
4. Lu Z, Streets DG, Zhang Q, Wang S, Carmichael GR, Cheng YF, et al. Sulfur dioxide emissions in China and sulfur trends in East Asia since 2000. Atmos Chem Phys 2010; 10(13): 6311-31. doi: 10.5194/acp-10-6311-2010.
5. Fioletov VE, McLinden CA, Krotkov N, Li C, Joiner J, Theys N, et al. A global catalogue of large SO2 sources and emissions derived from the ozone monitoring instrument. Atmos Chem Phys 2016; 16(18): 11497-519. doi: 10.5194/acp-16-11497-2016.
6. Jafarinejad S. Control and treatment of sulfur compounds specially sulfur oxides (SOx) emissions from the petroleum industry: a review. Chem Int 2016; 2(4): 242-53.
7. Klimont Z, Smith SJ, Cofala J. The last decade of global anthropogenic sulfur dioxide: 2000–2011 emissions. Environ Res Lett 2013; 8(1): 014003. doi: 10.1088/1748-9326/8/1/014003.
8. Kurokawa J, Ohara T, Morikawa T, Hanayama S, Janssens-Maenhout G, Fukui T, et al. Emissions of air pollutants and greenhouse gases over Asian regions during 2000–2008. Regional Emission inventory in ASia (REAS) version 2. Atmos Chem Phys 2013; 13(21): 11019-58. doi: 10.5194/acp-13-11019-2013.
9. Stern DI. Global sulfur emissions from 1850 to 2000. Chemosphere 2005; 58(2): 163-75. doi: 10.1016/j.chemosphere.2004.08.022.
10. Smith SJ, van Aardenne J, Klimont Z, Andres RJ, Volke A, Delgado Arias S. Anthropogenic sulfur dioxide emissions: 1850–2005. Atmos Chem Phys 2011; 11(3): 1101-16. doi: 10.5194/acp-11-1101-2011.
11. Smith SJ, Pitcher H, Wigley TM. Global and regional anthropogenic sulfur dioxide emissions. Glob Planet Change 2001; 29(1): 99-119. doi: 10.1016/S0921-8181(00)00057-6.
12. Li S, Williams G, Guo Y. Health benefits from improved outdoor air quality and intervention in China. Environ Pollut 2016; 214: 17-25. doi: 10.1016/j.envpol.2016.03.066.
13. Eßer J, Wasserscheid P, Jess A. Deep desulfurization of oil refinery streams by extraction with ionic liquids. Green Chem 2004; 6(7): 316-22. doi: 10.1039/b407028c
14. Jangra S, Bhardwaj A. Sulphur recovery by tail gas treating technology (Mcrc process) maximum Claus. Int J Sci Environ Technol 2014; 3(4): 1609-13.
15. Babich IV, Moulijn JA. Science and technology of novel processes for deep desulfurization of oil refinery streams: a review. Fuel 2003; 82(6): 607-31. doi: 10.1016/S0016-2361(02)00324-1.
16. Garcia-Cruz I, Valencia D, Klimova T, Oviedo-Roa R, Martinez-Magadan JM, Gomez-Balderas R, et al. Proton affinity of S-containing aromatic compounds: implications for crude oil hydrodesulfurization. J Mol Catal A Chem 2008; 281(1-2): 79-84. doi: 10.1016/j.molcata.2007.08.031.
17. Mosavi Khah R. Energy consumption statistics for energy products. Tehran: publication department of National Iranian Oil Products Distribution Company; 2015. [In Persian].
18. Natioan Iranian Oil Refining & Distiribiution. Tabriz Oil Refining Company [2018 May 5]. Available from: http://en.niordc.ir/index.aspx?fkeyid=&siteid=77&pageid=2029.
19. Chardonneaua M, Ibrahim S, Gupta AK, AlShoaibi A. Role of toluene and carbon dioxide on sulfur recovery efficiency in a claus process. Energy Procedia 2015; 75: 3071-5. doi: 10.1016/j.egypro.2015.07.630.
20. Garmroodi Asil A, Shahsavand A, Mirzaei S. Maximization of sulfur recovery efficiency via coupled modification of GTU and SRU processes. Egypt J Petrol 2017; 26(3): 579-92. doi: 10.1016/j.ejpe.2016.08.003.
21. El-Naqa A. Environmental impact assessment using rapid impact assessment matrix (RIAM) for Russeifa landfill, Jordan. Environmental Geology 2005; 47(5): 632-9. doi: 10.1007/s00254-004-1188-8.
22. Phillips J. Applying a mathematical model of sustainability to the rapid impact assessment matrix evaluation of the coal mining tailings dumps in the Jiului Valley, Romania. Resources, Conservation and Recycling 2012; 63: 17-25. doi: 10.1016/j.resconrec.2012.03.003.
23. Gilbuena R Jr, Kawamura A, Medina R, Amaguchi H, Nakagawa N, Bui DD. Environmental impact assessment of structural flood mitigation measures by a rapid impact assessment matrix (RIAM) technique: a case study in Metro Manila, Philippines. Sci Total Environ 2013; 456-457: 137-47. doi: 10.1016/j.scitotenv.2013.03.063.
24. Pastakia CMR, Jensen A. The rapid impact assessment matrix (Riam) For eia. Environ Impact Assess Rev 1998; 18(5): 461-82. doi: 10.1016/S0195-9255(98)00018-3.
25. Ministry of Energy. Balance sheet of energy 2014. Available from: http://isn.moe.gov.ir.
26. Mazandarani A, Mahlia TM, Chong WT, Moghavvemi M. A review on the pattern of electricity generation and emission in Iran from 1967 to 2008. Renewable and Sustainable Energy Reviews 2010; 14(7): 1814-29. doi: 10.1016/j.rser.2010.03.014.
27. Mazandarani A, Mahlia TMI, Chong WT, Moghavvemi M. Fuel consumption and emission prediction by Iranian power plants until 2025. Renewable and Sustainable Energy Reviews 2011; 15(3): 1575-92. doi: 10.1016/j.rser.2010.11.043.
28. Alikhani Hessari F. Sectoral energy consumption in Iran. Renewable and Sustainable Energy Reviews 2005; 9(2): 203-14. doi: 10.1016/j.rser.2004.03.002.
29. Fanick ER. Diesel fuel keeping pace with diesel engine technology. SAE Technical Paper; 2008. doi: 10.4271/2008-01-1808.
30. Nazari S, Shahhoseini O, Sohrabi-Kashani A, Davari S, Paydar R, Delavar-Moghadam Z. Experimental determination and analysis of CO2, SO2 and NOx emission factors in Iran's thermal power plants. Energy 2010; 35(7): 2992-8. doi: 10.1016/j.energy.2010.03.035.
31. Tan PQ, Hu ZY, Lou DM. Regulated and unregulated emissions from a light-duty diesel engine with different sulfur content fuels. Fuel 2009; 88(6): 1086-91. doi: 10.1016/j.fuel.2008.11.031.
32. Zhang K, Hu J, Gao S, Liu Y, Huang X, Bao X. Sulfur content of gasoline and diesel fuels in northern China. Energy Policy 2010; 38(6): 2934-40. doi: 10.1016/j.enpol.2010.01.030.

17

Assessment of air pollution in exercise centers and health risks

Balal Oroji[1], Eisa Solgi[1*], Asghar Sadighzadeh[2]

[1]Department of Environmental Sciences, School of Natural Resources and Environmental Sciences, Malayer University, Malayer, Hamadan, Iran
[2]Nuclear Fuel Cycle Research School, Nuclear Science and Technology Research Institute, Tehran, Iran

Abstract
Background: In recent years, Tehran has faced major problems with air pollution for many reasons, and this issue has become a critical point in most of the days. However, less attention has been paid to the indoor air pollutants in exercise centers and their possible health effects. In this research, it was tried to briefly describe the characteristics and chemical composition of the aerosols present in the exercise centers of Tehran.
Methods: Sampling was carried out by a high volume sampler with a value of 1.5 m^3/min. Fiberglass filters were used to sample aerosol particles. The samples were then studied by scanning electron micrograph (SEM) method.
Results: The results showed that average concentration of aerosol particles in the indoor and outdoor sports halls was 125 and 162 $\mu g/m^3$, respectively. Therefore, there was a minor difference in the aerosols concentration inside and outside the sports venues during the competition period and in the presence of athletes. Also, chemical composition and morphology of the aerosol particles showed that there was a minor difference between the atmospheric particles inside and outside the exercise centers. Major elements found in the $PM_{2.5}$ aerosol were Si, O, C, Mg, Ca, Mn and K. In general, common major crustal elements found in the atmospheric particles over all the sites were Si, Al, and Fe.
Conclusion: It seems that many citizens of the polluted cities exercise indoor because of causes other than outdoor air pollution such as lack of time or appropriate facilities. Thus, it is necessary for all students, athletes, people and other health workers involved in sports and exercise medicine to know briefly about indoor air pollutants and its possible health effects on athletes who exercise in these environments.
Keywords: Air pollution, Athletes, Aerosols, Outdoor

***Correspondence to:**
Eisa Solgi
Email: e.solgi@yahoo.com

Introduction

Human and natural resources are the sources of particles diffusion in the atmosphere. Fossil fuels in the transportation sector, factories, and manufacturing industries are the sources of particles diffusion in the human sector (1-3). According to the World Health Organization (WHO), by reducing airborne pollutants from 70 to 20 $\mu g/m^3$ in the atmosphere, the mortality rate can be reduced by 15% (4). The aerosol particles in the atmosphere are liquid or solid. Their size varies from a fraction of a micrometer to hundreds of microns. Airborne pollutants such as particulate matter (PM) affect people more than any other types of pollutant. The main components of air suspended particles are sulfates, nitrates, ammonia, sodium chloride, black carbon, mineral particles, and water. In other words, air suspended particles are a mixture of widespread solids and liquids composed of organic and inorganic materials suspended in the air, which chronic exposure to these particles in the air causes cardiovascular and pulmonary disease, and also lung cancer (4). Hence, air pollution is one of the topics about which researchers have concerned in recent years. On the other hand, the most important issue in comprehensive public health is indoor air quality. In other words, indoor air quality is one of the important issues in public health. In fact, the clean environment is essential for human health and well-being, and it has become a global challenge (5,6). The lack of ventilation in this place causes serious damages to athletes. Indoor air pollutants have different sources. A group is the pollutants which are produced inside the buildings (internal pollutants), another group is those which are produced outside the buildings and can penetrate indoor through windows or other pores and openings, joints, and cracks in walls, floors, and ceilings (external pollutants), and finally, natural radon gas which can go inside the buildings from the ground. Another important factor that should be considered in gymnasiums is poor indoor air quality due to gathering of the large number of people in small buildings that often have poor ventilation (7). In recent years, air pollution has been a major challenge for the citizens of Tehran. The occurrence of dust storms has increased the level of suspended particles in the atmosphere. The main air pollutants in Tehran are CO, NOx, SO2, O2, HC, and PM, accounting for about 85% of the fuel used by transportation vehicles, factories and household heating equipment (8). Tall buildings, air stability and high vehicle density have increased the concentration of airborne pollutants at dangerous levels, making this a major environmental challenge (9). In these conditions, the level of environmental pollutants in exercise centers is very high. It is well accepted that exercising in the outdoor air polluted environment causes more contacts with air pollutant and has possibly more negative effects on athletes' health. However, less attention has been paid to the indoor air pollutants in exercise centers and their possible health effects. Since the many physiological changes such as air inhalation through the mouth, increasing in minute ventilation, air flow rate, and pulmonary diffusion capacity are practically in outdoor and indoor environments are essentially the same, so it can be concluded that exercise in indoor air polluted environment can have the same importance as exercising in an outdoor environment (10). In this research, it was tried to briefly describe the characteristics and chemical composition of the aerosols present in the exercise centers of Tehran.

Materials and Methods

The sampling was done at 9 exercise centers in different areas of Tehran by a high-volume air sampler (model TFIA, Staplex's Co., Brooklyn, NY). For this purpose, the filters were first placed in an oven for 24 hr at 105°C for dehumidification. After cooling in a silica gel, the distiller was weighed 0.1 mg and prepared for installation on the sampler. After sampling, the filters were placed in an oven at 105°C for 24 hours for dehumidification. Sampling was performed before, after and in the presence of athletes in the exercise centers. Sampling was done inside the exercise center at a height of 1.5 m from the ground for 2 to 6 hr. Sampling was carried out by a high volume sampler with a value of 1.5 m^3/min. Fiberglass filters were used to sample aerosol particles. The filters were weighed before and after sampling. Due to the fact that this filter collects all particles of interest or of concern has excellent performance in the field of fine particulate filtration, it is therefore considered as an efficient filter. Commonly, the efficiency is 99.95% or higher for a standard aerosol of 0.3 μm diameter. In this way, the total number of aerosol particles was also measured at the sampling time. The samples were then studied by scanning electron micrograph (SEM) method. A very thin layer of gold was deposited on the surface of the samples to make them electrically conductive using vacuum coating unit. The SEM-EDX analyses were carried out using a computer controlled field emission SEM (ZEISS EVO 18 SEM) equipped with a Bruker Quantax 200 EDS with a Peltier-cooled X Flash silicon detector.

Results

At the beginning of the work, the indoor and outdoor average concentration of particles was measured during the competition and in the presence of athletes. Different results were obtained for different locations. In the areas, where the hall was well-ventilated and new, the difference between the indoor and outdoor concentrations increased. But the average concentration of particles was 162 μg/m^3 in the city, while it was 125 μg/m^3 in the exercise centers during the review period. Therefore, there was a minor difference in the concentration of aerosols inside and outside the exercise centers during the competition period and in the presence of athletes, therefore, exercise centers cannot be considered as a healthy place to practice and conduct the competition during air pollution. The average concentration of aerosols in 9 exercise centers in Tehran is shown in Figure 1. In this figure, the effect of outdoor environment on the indoor environment is visible and cannot be ruled out. The conditions that are taking place today in major cities and cities such as Tehran are very dangerous and it is recommended that people do not work in this dangerous environment, especially children, heart and respiratory illnesses, elderly people and even athletes. Also, it seems that many citizens of this city exercise indoor because of causes other than outdoor air pollution such as lack of time or appropriate facilities. Table 1 shows the indoor and outdoor PM concentrations in the filters during 4-day tournament. The outdoor concentrations of these elements were significantly higher than the indoors, except when the outdoor wind speed increased. The higher contributions of the outdoor elements generated by traffic, soil and sea were registered.

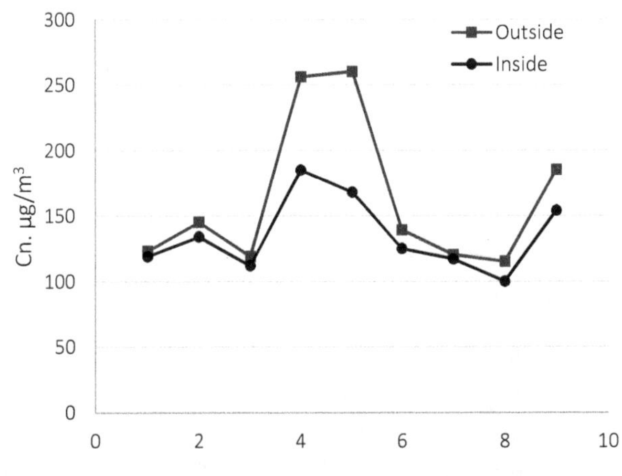

Figure 1. The average concentration of aerosol particles inside and outside the hall.

Table 1. Indoor and outdoor average aerosol concentrations in the study area (μg/m³)

	Time	PM			Time	PM	
		Indoor	Outdoor			Indoor	Outdoor
	09:00	124	146		09:00	143	165
	11:00	130	137		11:00	146	174
T1	13:00	128	142	T3	13:00	152	168
	16:00	142	144		16:00	143	167
	18:00	138	147		18:00	135	167
	09:00	110	134		09:00	138	144
	11:00	115	132		11:00	145	134
T2	13:00	113	140	T4	13:00	152	146
	16:00	123	138		16:00	149	152
	18:00	125	142		18:00	145	144

Abbreviation: PM, particulate matter.

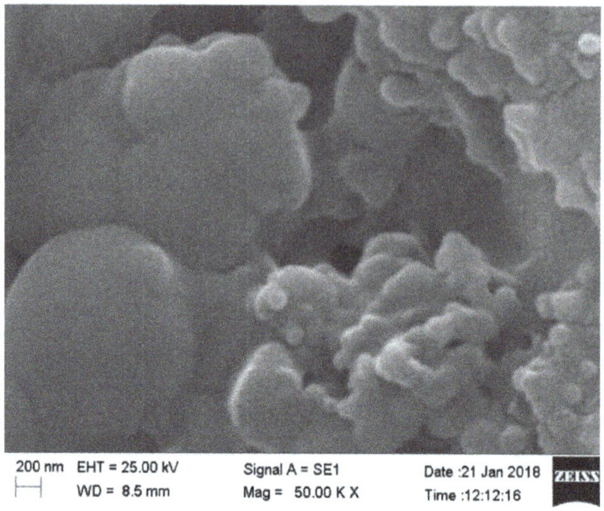

Figure 2. SEM image of aerosol particles in the size range of $PM_{2.5}$.

Table 2. Concentrations of elements of aerosols in the size range of $PM_{2.5}$ in a sports hall

Elements	Weight (%)
C	23.46
O	46.51
Na	4.14
Al	1.92
Si	16.39
K	1.72
Ca	1.92
Zn	1.91
Ti	2.03

Discussion

The analysis of the samples showed that there were physiochemical differences in aerosol particles in sports centers in and outside the city center. Hence, in urban areas, elements (except predominant elements) such as chlorine, calcium, iron and particles rich in silicon, aluminum, potassium and magnesium were determined. The findings indicate the presence of soil particles in this regional case study. A SEM image of the aerosol particles in the study area is shown in Figure 2. Also, analysis of SEM images of PM<1 micron showed that these particles are spherical, crystalline, transparent and irregular. On the other hand, in the images of SEM, it was observed that particles were 2.5 microns in size, and had an irregular, cluster and spherical shape. In the studied images, calcium was considered as the dominant particle among others, which can be considered as a calcium carbonate form associated with calcite phase. An example of the chemical composition of aerosol particles in the sports centers located in the western regions of Tehran is shown in Table 2. The main elements of $PM_{2.5}$ include silicon, oxygen, magnesium, calcium, manganese and potassium. These elements were observed in different samples proportions. In general, the main elements of the main shell of atmospheric particles at all stations were silicon, aluminum, and iron. Mineral particles are usually derived from natural sources, including the recovery of roads dust (crust dust). Other particles produced and distributed in the city by human activities, such as combustion of fuel by vehicles, industries and factories, roads and urban development, and wearing metals, present in the sports halls due to its inadequate ventilation. On the other hand, the lack of ventilation in some gyms is a real challenge to the problem. The condition was also more severe in older sports halls with high burnout.

These particles are generally recognized by their coarse and irregular shape. Based on these results, different concentrations of zinc, titanium, iron and carbon elements along with aluminum and silicon were observed throughout the region, especially in the central regions of the study area. This can be referred to as a gray source. There was also the presence of pollution sources in the composition of particles. The SEM image of a particle is shown in Figure 3. Also, Table 3 shows chemical composition of these particles. These particles can be related to construction, regional transportation of the urban areas, agricultural activities (burning plants), natural dust, as well as the activity of sand production workshops. The particles are mainly composed of feldspar (calcium, silicon and aluminum) and clay (aluminum, iron and silicon), mainly originating from crust, but they can also lead to erosion of construction materials and production of road dust caused by transport. Other elements were present in a small concentration of alumino-silicate particles, which include magnesium, sodium, titanium and zinc. According to the reports from Department of Environmental and Air Quality Control Company subsidiary of Tehran municipality, in most of the days, pollutants in the atmosphere of the area are close to the critical level and sometimes crossed it. Due to the large volume of construction in different parts of Tehran and lack of management of the activities of sand plants,

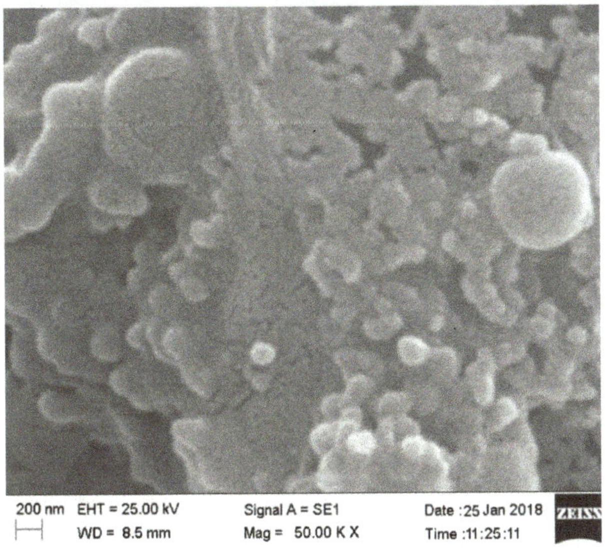

Figure 3. SEM image of aerosol particles in a sports hall located in the central regions of the study area.

Table 3. Concentrations of elements of aerosols in a sports hall located in the central regions of the study area

Element	Weight (%)
C	36.59
O	47.01
Al	1.72
Si	4.22
Ca	7.43
Ti	1.01
Fe	2.02

the level of suspended particles is high in this area. Since the factories are located in the direction of the prevailing wind in the region, hence, the emission of particles from these sources is always one of the main sources in the formation of pollutions in the atmosphere of Tehran. According to the evidence, pollutants produced in these areas affect the whole city of Tehran. It seems that in the studied area, especially in the polluted areas, lack of proper management of the sports facilities can lead to the pollution of sports halls. As a result, athletes may be at risk for health problems.

There is, in fact, a relationship between the exposure to intense concentrations of suspended particles and the increase in daily and annual concentrations. Also, if the concentrations of these pollutants are reduced, while other factors are fixed, the associated deaths are reduced, indicating that by reducing the concentration of suspended particles, the community health can be improved. Some researchers have observed the health effects of air suspended particles even at very low concentrations, which means that there is no threshold for the suspended particles to reduce the adverse health effects (11). The WHO estimates that if the average annual concentration of PM_{10} in the world is reduced from the current value of 70 $\mu g/m^3$ to the guidance level of 20 $\mu g/m^3$, the air-pollution-related deaths will decrease by about 15%. Several studies have shown that exposure to air suspended particles is associated with health effects such as cardiovascular and respiratory diseases (11,12). Researchers have shown that PM_{10} is associated with hospitalization due to respiratory disease. Also, $PM_{2.5}$ has a strong relationship with heart and respiratory diseases. Ultra-fine PM penetrates into the lower parts of the respiratory system and lungs, causing many cardiopulmonary and respiratory disease (13-16).

Conclusion

The study of the chemical composition and morphology of suspended particles in the atmosphere of Tehran revealed two important findings. Firstly, during the time of air pollution, even indoor sports facilities are also affected by pollution. Secondly, there is a pollution-related health risk for people at this time in the outdoor sports centers. It is well accepted that exercising in the outdoor air polluted environment causes more contacts with air pollutants and has possibly more negative effects on athletes' health. However, less attention has been paid to the indoor air pollutants in exercise centers and their possible health effects. Studies have shown that surface contamination of the city has a direct effect on the indoor environment quality. Therefore, it is not recommended to go to gyms for racing and physical activity on the polluted days, because damage to the athletes' health in indoor sports centers is 22% less than that in outdoors. Considering the average total particle concentration, the possible damage to the athletes' health in indoor sports centers is by 60% more than the outdoors. Depending on the indoor physical conditions and physical activity, volatile air enter into the lungs and respiratory system for respiration. Hence, extreme activity in indoor polluted, probability of exposure to airborne pollutants is far greater than when people are slowly operating in the outdoor environment. Since the effect of air pollution in the indoor and outdoor environment is the same during training, therefore, in large and industrial cities like Tehran, children, elderly people, cardiac and respiratory patients and even normal athletes It is better to stay at home and not have intense physical activity. Thus, it is necessary for all health professionals involved in sports and exercise medicine to know briefly about indoor air pollutants and its possible health effects on athletes who exercise in these environments.

Acknowledgments

The authors would like to thank the Nuclear Science and Technology Research Institute for technical support in conducting this research.

Competing interests

The authors declare that they have no competing interests.

Authors' contributions

All authors were equally involved in the collection, analysis, and interpretation of the data. All authors critically reviewed, refined, and approved the manuscript.

References

1. Superczynski SD, Christopher SA. Exploring land use and land cover effects on air quality in Central Alabama using GIS and remote sensing. Remote Sens 2011; 3(12): 2552-67. doi: 10.3390/rs3122552.
2. Molnar A, Becsi Z, Imre K, Gacser V, Ferenczi Z. Characterization of background aerosol properties during a wintertime smog episode. Aerosol Air Qual Res 2016; 16(8): 1793-804. doi: 10.4209/aaqr.2015.04.0205.
3. Jing Y, Zhang P, Chen L, Xu N. Integrated analysis of dust transport and budget in a severe Asian dust event. Aerosol Air Qual Res 2017; 17(10): 2390-400. doi: 10.4209/aaqr.2017.05.0170.
4. World Health Organization. Ambient Air Pollution: A Global Assessment of Exposure and Burden of Disease. World Health Organization; 2016.
5. European Environment Agency (EEA). Environment and human health [cited 2018 May 1]. Available from: https://www.eea.europa.eu/publications/environment-and-human-health/download.
6. Almeida SM, Silva AV, Sarmento S. Effects of exposure to particles and ozone on hospital admissions for cardiorespiratory diseases in SetuBal, Portugal. J Toxicol Environ Health A 2014; 77(14-16): 837-48. doi: 10.1080/15287394.2014.887399.
7. Ramos CA, Wolterbeek HT, Almeida SM. Exposure to indoor air pollutants during physical activity in fitness centers. Build and Environ 2014; 82: 349-60. doi: 10.1016/j.buildenv.2014.08.026.
8. Givehchi R, Arhami M, Tajrishy M. Contribution of the Middle Eastern dust source areas to PM10 levels in urban receptors: Case study of Tehran, Iran. Atmos Environ 2013; 75: 287-95. doi: 10.1016/j.atmosenv.2013.04.039.
9. Oroji B. Risk assessment radioactive aerosols with determination residence times in the atmosphere Tehran, Iran [dissertation]. Malayer: Malayer University; 2018. [In Persian].
10. Carlisle AJ, Sharp NC. Exercise and outdoor ambient air pollution. Br J Sports Med 2001; 35(4): 214-22. doi: 10.1136/bjsm.35.4.214.
11. World Health Organization (WHO). Ambient (outdoor) air quality and health. [2018 May 2] Available from: http://www.who.int/news-room/fact-sheets/detail/ambient-(outdoor)-air-quality-and-health.
12. Pope CA 3rd, Dockery DW. Health effects of fine particulate air pollution: lines that connect. J Air Waste Manag Assoc 2006; 56(6): 709-42. doi: 10.1080/10473289.2006.10464485.
13. Bell ML, HEI Health Review Committee. Assessment of the health impacts of particulate matter characteristics. Res Rep Health Eff Inst 2012; (161): 5-38.
14. Arhami M, Minguillon MC, Polidori A, Schauer JJ, Delfino RJ, Sioutas C. Organic compound characterization and source apportionment of indoor and outdoor quasi-ultrafine particulate matter in retirement homes of the Los Angeles Basin. Indoor Air 2010; 20(1): 17-30. doi: 10.1111/j.1600-0668.2009.00620.x.
15. Brunekreef B, Forsberg B. Epidemiological evidence of effects of coarse airborne particles on health. Eur Respir J 2005; 26(2): 309-18. doi: 10.1183/09031936.05.00001805.
16. Sioutas C, Delfino RJ, Singh M. Exposure assessment for atmospheric ultrafine particles (UFPs) and implications in epidemiologic research. Environ Health Perspect 2005; 113(8): 947-55. doi: 10.1289/ehp.7939.

18

Emission evaluation of CO_2 and CH_4 gases in the selected gas pressure booster station in the Bangestan field of the National Iranian Oil Company

Mehdi Ahmadi[1], Maedeh Rozkhosh[2], Nemat-allah Jaafarzadeh Haghighifard[3*]

[1]Associate Professor, Environmental Technologies Research Center, Department of Environmental Health Engineering, School of Public Health, Ahvaz Jundishapur University of Medical Sciences, Ahvaz, Iran
[2]M.Sc. of Assessment and Land Use Planning, Science and Research Branch, Islamic Azad University of Khozestan, Faculty of Environment, Ahvaz, Iran
[3]Professor, Environmental Technologies Research Center, Department of Environmental Health Engineering, School of Public Health, Ahvaz Jundishapur University of Medical Sciences, Ahvaz, Iran

Abstract
Background: Iran is located in the seventh rank in terms of CO_2 emissions resulting from the fuel combustion in the world. Gas compressor booster stations, due to the several sources of contaminants, are causing the release of large amounts of CO_2 and CH_4, which will cause climate change; therefore, estimating the emissions of the gases from oil and gas, different processing units are necessary.
Methods: In this study, the emissions factor method, provided by various organizations, was used for determining emissions of CO_2 and CH_4 from different sources.
Results: According to the results obtained, the total amount of CO_2 emissions in selected units is from the selected unit and is a significant contribution to the CH4 emissions, so that the whole amount of CO_2 emissions is equal to 7739.027 tons per day and the total amount of CH_4 emissions is 4 tons per day.
Conclusion: Burner has the highest amount of CO_2 emissions among the sources of pollutants in the fixed combustion sources; and, the highest emissions of CH_4, among the exit gas sources, belong to the process of removing water. Among the exit gas sources-compressors maintenance activities the highest emissions belong to CH_4. The amount of CO_2 emissions from indirect sources, including electrical equipment in the studied units, are from natural gas fuel which are much more than those from fuel oils for burning. CH_4 gas from volatile sources in the gas compressors have the highest emissions compared to other sources.
Keywords: Greenhouse gases, Emission factor, Gas compressor booster station of Bangestan

***Correspondence to:**
Nemat-allah Jaafarzadeh Haghighifard
Email: Jaafarzadeh-n@ajums.ac.ir

Introduction

Due to growth and expansion of industrialization, the energy demand across the globe is increasing rapidly. This growth in energy consumption has been led to environmental degradation, water and air degradation and greenhouse gases and other pollutants emission (1). Greenhouse gases include CO_2, CH_4, N_2O, HFC_S, PFC_S, and SF_6, the most important of which are respectively CO_2 and CH_4 (2). According to the evaluations of the Research Center for Energy and Environmental Studies, the share of greenhouse gas emissions in the country's oil industry the most important part of which is burned associated gases and gases burned in oil units, is about 35% of the country's total greenhouse gas emissions (3). Overview of the gas compressor booster stations shows that the major sources of greenhouse gas emissions (CO_2 and CH_4) are from various sources of these units such as burner, ray steam boiler, tanks, removing water process, electrical equipment, gas valves and compressors. These resources are of the major share of contribution in the similar units in terms of greenhouse gas emissions. Because these gases are among the most important greenhouse gases, and have a great impact on the global warming, this research becomes more important.

Totally, four types of Emission Estimation Techniques (EET_S) that can be used for estimating the emission are: sampling or direct measurement, mass balance, fuel analysis, and other engineering calculations and emission factors. Generally, the direct measurement is the most accurate method for calculating the specific emissions, but it is expensive and difficult to conduct for some resources. The calculating programs and engineering calculations often can provide the exact estimation much more than emission factors; although in some cases they may require a lot more effort. Since the entries in the program require specific data of the process, the results are specific estimations of the process (4). The emission factor is an index value that is in an attempt to link the quantity of a pollutant released in the atmosphere to an activity related to the release of related pollutants. These factors usually expressed as the weight of pollutant are classified into a unit of weight, volume, distance, or duration of an activity of contamination spread (5).

In a study to fit the quantity of reducing greenhouse gas emissions of Carbon Capture and Storage (CCS) conducted through the project guidelines, the oil and natural gas industry project, it was determined that technology for collecting carbon dioxide from large point sources, compression, transportation, and its long-term injection in the storage places provides the potential to play a key role in reducing greenhouse gas emissions and affordable energy (6). Evaluation of CO_2 emissions and the potential for reducing it in oil refining industry of Korea using energy-environment models showed that new technology and alternative scenarios can reduce carbon dioxide emissions in the national and industrial sectors respectively up to 0.048% and 0.065% (1). To estimate the amount of CO_2 in the peripheral area of a selected unit of gas and liquefied gas in the National Iranian Oil Company (NIOC) based on the analysis of fuel showed that acid gas burners with a 63% share have the most share in CO_2 emissions (7). The results of the estimation of pollutant emissions in one of the oil and gas operation units of NIOC using the Environmental Protection Agency's (EPA) emission factors indicated that the amount of CO_2 emissions and CO_2 in gas turbines and burner are far more than the amount estimated by the EPA (8).

Regarding economic justification of the project it can also be noted that the potential measurement of greenhouse emissions is considered as the first stage in the development of business support through Clean Development Mechanism (CDM). The output of this project will help decision makers to assess the possibility of entering the CDM cycle, and if there is the possibility, it can help them enjoy economic advantage arising from the reduction in the production of these gases and as a result of carbon concession sales in international markets.

Methods

In this study, one of the gas compressor booster stations of Bangestan of NIOC in Southwest Iran was investigated. The gas compressor booster stations, which have been constructed adjacent to operating plants, receive rich gases, which are separated from oil during the second, third and fourth stages of breakdown in the operating unit of oil separators. After compressing and separating liquids from them, these gases' final products in the form of gas and gas liquids are sent to the gas and liquid gas plants to receive further refining and processing. In this way in order to calculate emissions, first, the overall process of gas compressor booster station in relation to the sources of production of the pollution was detected. After identifying these sources, they were categorized as follows: fixed combustion sources, exit gas sources, repair and maintenance activities, indirect sources, and volatile sources. Type and rate of fuel consumed in the designated unit is provided by various organizations according to the emission factors, and these have been presented in the Table 1. Emissions for each of the sources spreading pollution was estimated using equation 1:

$$E = A \times EF \times [1-(ER/100)] \quad \text{(Eq. 1)}$$

Where:

E is the emission pollutant rate (the amount of pollutant mass); A is the activity rate; EF is an emission factor (the amount of pollutant mass emitted per the amount of product produced or the activity rate); ER is the overall percentage of the emission reduction the value of it is considered to be zero, due to the lack of using pollutant reduction systems in the studied unit (5). Finally, the data were examined and analyzed using Excel software by comparing a variety of sources of pollutants in a studied unit.

Characteristics of fuel used in the study unit

To estimate the amount of emissions of pollutants (CO_2 and CH_4), fuel type and the amount of fuel consumed in each resource should be determined separately. Since fuel consumed for the sources of pollutants in the study unit is fuel gas, the data contained in the gas compressor station (presented in Table 2) have been used.

Results

The amount of CO_2 and CH_4 emissions from the gas flares

The amount of emissions calculated for two gas burners with an average dB of 0.3 million cubic feet per day has been presented in Table 3.

The amount of CO_2 and CH_4 gas emissions caused by the reboiler

The amount of emissions calculated for a gas ray boiler of this unit with a dB of 0.1 million cubic feet per day has been presented in Table 4, and emissions arising from the process of removing water from gas in gas pressure booster station in Bangestan have been calculated. The amount of gas in the processing station is an average of 15 million cubic feet a day, we multiply this amount by the CO2 and CH4 molar percentage (Table 2) (To removing water, gases of all the steps of breakdown in this stage are accumulated), the amount of emissions of this source of the pollutants is obtained.

Table 1. Presents emission factors for emission sources by various reference

	References	Emission Factor			
		CH_4		CO_2	
Gas Flares	ARPEL, 1998 (lb/MMBtu) (9)	-		0.61	
	CAPP, 2003 (g/m^3 gas) (10)	1853		13.6	
	EEA, 2006 (lb/MMBtu) (11)	-		0.12	
	EIA, 2006 (lb/MMBtu) (12)	120.72		-	
	IPCC, 1996 (lb/MMBtu) (13)	141.01		-	
	NAEI, 2007 (lb/MMBtu) (14)	105.01		0.389	
	The Norwegian Oil industry Association, 1993 (lb/MMBtu) (15)	148.98		0.012	
	United Kingdom Offshore Association, 1993 (lb/MMBtu) (16)	144.76		0.61	
Reboilers	MDEQ, 2011(lb/MMscf) (17)	116.78		0.011014	
Dehydration	API, 2009 (tonnes/10^6 scf) (18)	Due to the modulus CH_4 emissions Calculated		0.0023315	
Maintenance activities Tanks	API, 2009 (tonnes/vessel-year) (18)	Due to the modulus CH_4 emissions Calculated		0.0015	
Compressors	API, 2009 (tonnes/compressor-year) (18)	Due to the modulus CH_4 emissions Calculated		2.42×10^{-2}	
Maintenance activities Compressor	API, 2009 (tonnes/compressor-year) (18)	Due to the modulus CH_4 emissions Calculated		0.1620 (Start) 0.07239 (Blodown)	
Valves/Valves-Gas	API, 2009 (tonnes/Valves-year) (18)	-		4.5×10^{-6}	
Electrical equipment	**Type of fuel**	Mazout	Natural gas	Mazout	Natural
	*AGO, 2001(tonne/MMBTU) (19)	-	0.0542	-	
	*API, 1999 (tonne/MMBTU)] (19)	0.0743	0.0531	-	-
	*API, 2009 (tonne/MMBTU)] (19)	same	same	3.17×10^{-6}	1.06×10^{-6}
	*CIEEDAC, 2001 (tonne/MMBTU)] (19)	-	0.052	-	-
	*DEFRA, 1999 (tonne/MMBTU) (19)	0.0703	0.0556	-	-
	*EPA, 1998 (lb/10^{6}scf) (19)	-	120000	-	2.3
	IPCC, 2001(tonne/MMBTU)* (19)	0.0743	0.0532	-	-
	*WRI/WBCSD, 2000 (tonne/MMBTU) (19)	-	0.0531	-	-

Table 2. Characteristics of composition of the gas used in the combustion sources and emission sources studied at different stages of differentiation in gas compressor station (20).

Characters Stages		Stages 1	Stages 2	Stages 3	Stages 4
Molly components (%)	Methane	392.3	54.1	2.2	13.6
	Ethan	76.7	26.8	5.7	3.5
	Propane	33.1	17.3	1.5	1.8
	Iso-butane	3.7	2.2	1.6	0.6
	Normal butane	9.2	5.7	1.1	2.1
	Ayzvpntan	2.3	1.5	0.7	1
	Normal pentane	2.6	1.6	0.2	1.2
	Hexane	1.7	1.1	3.5	0.9
	Normal butane	1.5	0.7	0.3	0.8
	Hydrogen sulfide	0.7	0.2	0	0
	Carbon dioxide	16.5	3.5	0	0
	Water	6.4	4.5	2.4	4.4
	The total gas flow (MMSCFD)	11.1	2.4	59.9	0.6
	The molecular weight of the gas	22.62	29.66	54.1	31.67
	Temperature (°C)	63.3	59.4	59.4	55.6
	Pressure (bar)	21.01	5.15	5.15	1.06

Table 3. Emissions of CO_2 and CH_4 from gas flares

Emission factor (tonne/day)				Reference
CO_2		CH_2		
High-pressure flares	Low-pressure flares	High-pressure flares	Low-pressure flares	
-	-	0.027	0.055	ARPEL, 1998
5.247	10.494	0.038	0.077	CAPP, 2003
-	-	0.005	0.01	EEA, 2006
5.475	10.951	-	-	EIA, 2006
6.395	12.792	-	-	IPCC, 1996
4.767	9.534	0.017	0.035	NAEI, 2007
6.757	13.515	0.0005	0.001	The Norwegian Oil industry Association, 1993
6.563	13.126	0.027	0.055	United Kingdom Offshore Association, 1993

Note: for flares efficiency of 98% is assumed.

Table 4. Emissions of CO_2 and CH_4 from reboilers and arising from removing water process

Emission factor (tonne/day)		Reference
CO_2	CH_4	
5.301×10^{-3}	4.955×10^{-7}	Re-Boilers (MDEQ, 2011)
5.761×10^{-3}	0.05	Removing water process (Reference API, 2009)

The CO_2 and CH_4 emissions resulting from repair and maintenance activities of compressor and tanks

As it can be seen in Table 5, the amount of CO2 emissions resulting from CH4 compressors, compressor and tank maintenance activities, and valves for each maintenance activity have been calculated. To calculate the amount of emissions from all kinds of valves according to the emission factors provided by API, the number of each of the various types of valves in the unit is multiplied by the relevant emission factors; thus, emissions from these sources are calculated as well. Also to calculate the amount of emissions from all kinds of valves according to the emission actors provided by API (Table 5), the number of each of the various types of valves in the unit is multiplied by the relevant emission factors; thus, emissions from these sources are calculated as well.

The CO_2 and CH_4 emissions resulting from natural gas and fuel oils for burning

To calculate emissions from indirect sources, first, we must know the amount of fuel consumed by power plants to supply the unit's electricity for every megawatt hour of electricity consumption at the unit that is 2500 MW per hour; then it is multiplied by the emission factors provided by different organizations for fuel oils and gas for burning (Table 6), and thus emissions from indirect sources, which include electrical equipment, can be calculated.

Table 5. Emissions of CO2 and CH4 from gas compressors, maintenance activities compressors, maintenance activities tanks and valves

Emission factor (tonne/day)		Reference API, 2009
CO_2	CH_4	
0.42	3.642	Emission gas compressors
0.167	1.502	Emissions maintenance activities compressors
3.713×10^{-3}	0.033	Emissions maintenance activities tanks
-	0.1	Valves

Discussion

According to the calculations and investigations performed, as it can be seen in Figure 1, a total of 7739.027 tons of CO_2 gas is released per day when indirect emissions sources, including electrical equipment, with a 94% share have the largest share of CO_2 emissions in the station. Then the rest of the sources compared to the source with a share less than 1% are awarded respectively to the gas burners, gas compressors, the process of removing water, ray boiler, and finally the exit gas resources at the time of the activity related to the repair and maintenance of compressors and reservoirs. In a study carried out to estimate the amount of CO_2, SO_2 and CO in the peripheral environment in one of the units, it was found that the estimated total amount of each of the gases SO_2, CO_2 and CO were respectively equal to 741620.49 kg/day, 3650.09 kg/day, and 1136.24 kg/day. According to the results obtained, maximum rate of emissions was related to the CO_2 gas that is consistent with the study's results so that the amount of CO_2 emissions with 7739027 kg/day is more than CH_4 gas with 4001 kg/day in the selected station (9). The results of another study to estimate the amount of CO_2 and NO_2 and CO gases in the peripheral environment in one of the units of Karun's oil and gas exploitation showed

Table 6. Emissions of CO_2 and CH_4 from electrical equipment

CO_2	CH_4	CO_2	CH_4	Reference
Mazout	Natural gas	Mazout	Natural gas	
-	7809.893	-	-	AGO, 2001 (tonne/MMBTU)
11.808	7651.292	-	-	API, 1999 (tonne/MMBTU)
11.808	7651.292	-	-	API, 2009 (tonne/MMBTU)
-	7492.791	$5.037\times^{10-4}$	0.15	CIEEDAC, 2001 (tonne/MMBTU)
11.172	8011.552	-	-	DEFRA, 1999 (tonne/MMBTU)
-	7842.093	-	-	EPA, 1998 ($lb/10^6scf$)
11.665	7665.701	-	0.15	IPCC, 2001 (tonne/MMBTU)
-	76.7.628	-	-	WRI/WBCSD, 2000 (tonne/MMBTU)

that the total amount of CO_2 emissions of the gas and liquid gas unit and gas sweetening is respectively equal to 449946.9 kg/day and 922212.97 kg/day. According to the results obtained from the amount of CO_2 emissions in the studied unit, it is more than the gas and liquid gas unit and gas sweetening with 7739027 kg/day (8).

As Figure 2 shows, totaling 4 tons per day of gas-CH_4 can

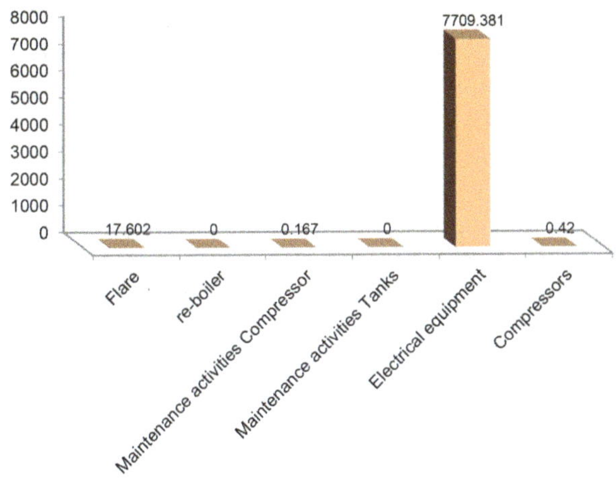

Figure 1. Comparison of the CO_2 emissions of each pollutant sources in the selected unit

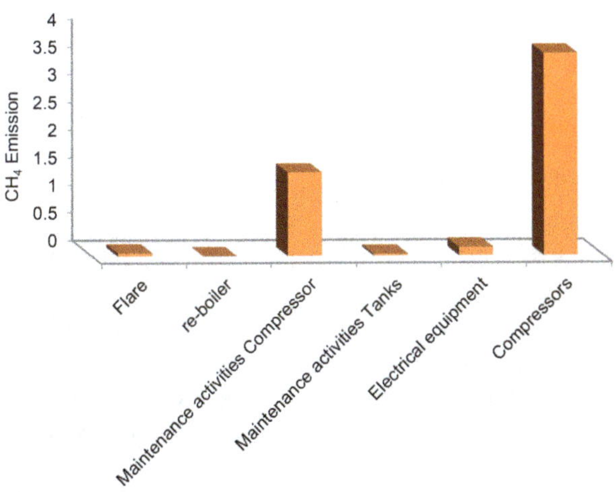

Figure 2. Compare the CH_4 emissions of each pollutant sources in the selected unit

be released from the selected station that gas compressors with 91% emissions have most emissions of CH_4 gas. Then the electrical equipment with 4%, volatile emissions from valves with 3% of emissions, burners with 1%, the other 1%, the process of removing water by 1%, and in the end ray boilers, activities related to maintenance and repair of compressors and tanks with the lowest emissions with a share close to 1% of the emissions have the lowest share in the unit. A study conducted to measure the Differential Absorption Lidar (DIAL) volatile emissions in the gas plant of Alberta, Canada showed that gas compressors are the most important source of CH_4 emissions. Then the operation of the burner in the pilot mode is another important source of emissions of this gas in the plant. According to the results obtained from the study, CH_4 emissions from compressors is 1272 kg/day and from the burners is 650.4 kg/day that is consistent with the results of the research so that the emissions from compressors of selected units with 3642 kg/day tons per day is more than burners with 57 kg/day per day (21). The results of another study entitled "test of emission factor for burners in a refinery" showed that the emission rate from burners on one of the refineries for the CO_2 and CH_4 gases, which have been calculated by EPA and API emission factors, were 124880 and 134.209 tons respectively in 2002. Compared with the results obtained from the amount of the emissions of the gases studied, it is less with 20.805 tons per year of CH_4, and 6424.73 tons per year of CO2 (22).

According to the conducted studies, the total amount of CO_2 emissions in the world is 28999. 4 million tons per year. Iran's part of the sector is 1.83% and the share of emissions of the gas from the petroleum sector in the world is 10630.8 million tons per year, 2.48 % of which is share of Iran (23). The selected gas station emits 2824806.905 tons per year or 1% of CO_2 compared to Iran's oil sector. The main focus of this section is more on carbon dioxide gas because the global warming potential of the CO_2 is more than CH_4.

Conclusion

According to the conducted calculations and inquiries,

the highest share of CO_2 emissions from indirect emission sources include electrical equipment with 99%, and the biggest share of CH_4 gas release is for the burners from fixed sources of combustion with 65%. Some of the guidelines that can be provided in order to reduce the sources of emissions mentioned in the studied unit are: the use of low-consumption light bulbs and a new system of uploading and downloading operation of electric motors, reduction or removal of the feasibility of the combustion of gases in the gas burners and ray boilers, recovery and use of emissions from oil wells, replacing a hydrogen fuel with gaseous fuel to improve the operations of maintenance and basic repair and maintenance operations in a timely manner for the equipment diffusing pollutant gases, new lighting control systems, the use of nanotechnology in the exact detection of leakage and its location, acceleration in the process of the development of CCS technology, the feasibility of CO_2 injection for the land areas, creation of awareness among the owners of the industries in order to participate in the CDM projects and benefit from the environmental benefits in the local and global levels resulting from the reduction in greenhouse gas emissions, the benefits of economic and social development for the implementation of the project in the host country, and the transfer of technology and economic benefits due to the economic progress of the related technologies to release less greenhouse gas.

Acknowledgements
Hereby the authors express thanks to the National Iranian South Oil Company's management and experts for the sake of providing basic information.

Competing interests
The authors declare that they have no competing interests.

Authors' contributions
MA, MR and NJ conceived and designed the study. MR performed the literature search and wrote the manuscript. All authors participated in the data acquisition, analysis and interpretation. All authors critically reviewed, refined and approved the manuscript.

References

1. Park S, Lee S, Jeong SJ, Song HJ, Park JW. Assessment of CO2 emissions and its reduction potential in the Korean petroleum refining industry using energy-environment models. Energy 2010; 35(6): 2419-29.
2. Kim Y, Worrell E. International comparison of CO2 emission trends in the iron and steel industry. Journal of Energy Policy 2002; 30(10): 827–38.
3. Shahhosseini M. Enjoying the benefits of clean development mechanism (CDM) in the oil and gas industries world. Journal of Exploration and Production 2010; 67: 35-39.
4. National Pollutant Inventory (NPI). Emission estimation technique manual for oil and gas extraction and production. Australia; 1999.
5. U.S. Environmental Protection Agency (EPA). Emission factor, introduction to AP 42. Volume I, Fifth edition. USA: Environmental Protection Agency, 1995.
6. Ritter K, Siveter R, Lev-on M, Shires T, Kheshgi H. Harmonizing the quantification of CCS GHG emission reduction through oil and natural gas industry project guidelines. Energy Procedia 2009; 1(1): 4451-58.
7. Jaafarzade haghighi fard N, Zoveydavi A, Glishkhani M, Maasoomi A. CO2 estimation of national Iranian south oil company gas sweetening plants by using fuel analysis method. Iran J Health & Environ 2011; 3: 321-30. [In Persian]
8. Ghilishkhani M, Jaafarzadeh N. Etimation amount of pollutant gases in units of the national iraian oil company to production oil and gas using emission coefficients EPA. Second International Symposium on Environment Engineering. Tehran, Iran, 2009
9. Regional Association of Oil and Natural Gas Companies in Latin America and the Caribbean (ARPEL). Guidelines for atmospheric emissions inventory methodologies in the petroleum industry. Alberta, Canada, 1998.
10. Canadian Association of Petroleum Producers (CAPP). Calculating greenhouse gas emissions. Global climate change, voluntary challenge guide, 2003.
11. European Environment Agency (EEA). Waste incineration, flaring in gas and oil extraction. In: emission inventory guidebook; 2006.
12. Energy Information Administration (EIA). Documentation for emissions of greenhouse gases in the United States. Washington, D.C, USA, 2006.
13. Intergovernmental Panel on Climate Change (IPCC). Guidelines for national greenhouse gas inventories, reference manual. Vol. 3. 1996.
14. National Atmospheric Emissions Inventory (NAEI). The UK emission factor database; 2007
15. The Norwegian Oil industry Association. OLF environmental program, phase II, summary report; 1993
16. United Kingdom Offshore Association Limited. Brown and root environmental atmospheric emissions from UK oil and gas exploration and production facilities in the continental shelf area; 1993.
17. Montana Department of Environmental Quality

(MDIQ). Air resources management bureau, natural gas compressor stations greenhouse gas applicability example sample calculation problems, Air resources management bureau; 2011.

18. American Petroleum Institute (API). Compendium of greenhouse gas emissions estimation methodologies for the oil and gas industry; 2009.
19. Ritter K, Nordrum S, Shires TH, Levon M. Consistency in greenhouse gas emissions estimation for oil and gas industry operations - A non-trivial pursuit. 12th International Emission Inventory Conference, San Diego, April 29 - May 1, 2003.
20. Makvandi MR. Introduction to desalting oprations, learning to production gas and LPG. Ahwaz: Training and technical proficiency testing center of Shahid Majd zade; 2005. [In Persian]
21. Martin J, Lumbreras J, Rodrigeuz ME. Testing flare emission factors for flaring in refineries. 12th Annual Emission Inventory Conference, 28-1 April, San Diego, California, 2003
22. Chambers A, Strosher M, Wootton T, Moncrieff J, McCready P. DIAL measurement of fugitive emissions from natural gas plants and the comparison with emission factor estimates. 15th Emission Inventory Conference, 15-18 May, New Orleans, 2006.
23. International Energy Agency (IEA). CO2 emissions from fuel combustion highlights; 2011.

Estimation of health effects (morbidity and mortality) attributed to PM10 and PM2.5 exposure using an Air Quality model in Bukan city, from 2015-2016 exposure using air quality model

Bahram Kamarehie[1], Mansour Ghaderpoori[1*], Ali Jafari[1], Mohammadamin Karami[1], Aliakbar Mohammadi[2], Khaled Azarshab[3], Afshin Ghaderpoury[4], Najaf Noorizadeh[5]

[1]Assistant Professor of Environmental Health, School of Health and Nutrition, Lorestan University of Medical Sciences, Khorramabad, Iran
[2]Lecturer, Department of Environmental Health Engineering, Neyshabur University of Medical Sciences, Neyshabur, Iran
[3]MSc of Water and Wastewater, Faculty of Environment, Islamic Azad University, West Tehran Branch, Tehran, Iran
[4]MSc of Environmental Health Engineering, Students Research Committee, Shahid Beheshti University of Medical Sciences, Tehran, Iran
[5]MSc of Occupational Health Engineering, Department of Occupational Health, School of Health, Shahid Beheshti University of Medical Sciences, Tehran, Iran

Abstract
Background: Air Quality software is a useful tool for assessing the health risks associated with air pollutants. Quantifying the effects of exposure to air pollutants in terms of public health has become a critical component of policy discussion. The present study purposed to quantify the health effects of particulate matters on mortality and morbidity in a Bukan city hospital from 2015-2016.
Methods: Information regarding coordinates, exposed population, number of stations used in profiling, mean and maximum concentrations (annual, winter, and summer), annual 98th percentile, baseline incidence (BI) per 100 000 per year, and relative risk was needed for use with the software.
Results: The average particulate matter concentration was higher in summer than in winter. The concentrations of PM_{10} in summer and winter were 84.37 and 74.86 µg m^{-3}, respectively. The Air Quality model predicted that total mortality rates related to PM10 and PM2.5 were 33.3 and 49.8 deaths, respectively. As a result, 3.79% of the total mortality was due to PM_{10}. In Bukan city, 2.004% of total deaths were due to cardiovascular mortality. The Air Quality model predicted that the deaths of 92.2 people were related to hospital admissions for respiratory disease.
Conclusion: The continual evaluation of air quality data is necessary for investigating the effect of pollutants on human health.
Keywords: Air pollution, Bukan, Morbidity, Particulate matter, Software, Public health

***Correspondence to:**
Mansour Ghaderpoori
Email: mghaderpoori@gmail.com

Introduction

A dust storm is defined as air turbulence which spreads a large mass of dust in the atmosphere and reduces horizontal visibility to less than a thousand meters (1). Dust storms carry a lot of various materials. Annually, dust storms transport particulate matter approximately 800 trillion grams to Asia (2). The frequent occurrence of dust storms due to drought in the Middle East is causing environmental and health problems (3,4). Particulate matter is one of the most important compounds in the atmosphere. It comprises microscopic solids or liquid matters suspended in the atmosphere (5). Furthermore, it consists of complex mixtures that may contain biological, metal, toxic, and/or acid materials (6). Sources of particulate matter can be man-made or natural (7). Particulate matter impacts climate and precipitation, has harmful effects on human health, animal health, and the environment (8-10), and constitutes the most important issues and challenges associated with air pollution (11,12). PM_{10} and $PM_{2.5}$ have average aerodynamic diameters of less than 10 and 2.5 microns, respectively (13,14). Studies show that particulate matter can be associated with increased hospital admissions, physiological changes in the body, and different diseases, especially of the respiratory (15) and cardiovascular (16) system, asthma, and lung cancer mortality (17). According to a report by the World Health Organization (WHO), particulate matter contributes to approximately 800000 premature deaths each year (6). The report also estimated that 1.5% of deaths in the world are caused by air pollution (18).

Air Quality (or Air Q) software is a useful tool for assessing the health risks associated with air pollutants. Quantifying the effects on public health of exposure to air pollution has become a critical component in policy discussion. WHO/Europe's software tool Air Q performs calculations that allow the quantification of the health effects of exposure to air pollutants, including estimations of the reduction in life expectancy. Air Q has two main parts. In the first part, the short-term effects of changes in air pollution (based on risk estimates from time-series studies) are estimated. In the second part, the long-term effects of exposure (using life-tables approach and based on risk estimates from cohort studies) are estimated (19).

Iran is a dry country, and drought has exacerbated its dryness in the past two decades. Soil erosion, uncontrolled increases in agricultural land, uncontrolled exploitation of groundwater, and the desiccation of rivers have caused an increase in dust storms. Lake Urmia is located in northwestern Iran and is one of the largest saline lakes in not only Iran, but also the world (20). Moreover, it is the largest lake in the Middle East (21,22). Bukan city is located south of Lake Urmia. Currently, most parts of the lake have dried up because of drought. In addition to dust storms, salt storms are also on the rise. Both salt storms and salty dust storms can increase the negative health effects of exposure to them. The present study aimed to quantify the health effects of particulate matter on mortality and morbidity in a hospital in Bukan city.

Methods

Location data

Bukan city is situated in West Azerbaijan province at northwest of Iran (36° 32' N, 46° 13' E). Figure 1 shows the location of the city and the nearby air quality monitoring station. At present, there is only one air quality monitoring station there. Bukan city has an area of 306.2541 km^2. According to the latest census in Iran, the city's population is 224628 persons.

Data collection and information processing

In this work, PM_{10} data was obtained from the Bukan Environmental Department. Study stages were classified into 4 steps, shown in Figure 2. In Step 1 (data collection from monitoring station), data regarding hourly PM_{10} and $PM_{2.5}$ concentrations (2015-2016) was received from the Bukan Environmental Department in a Microsoft Office Excel spreadsheet. In Step 2, the information was processed with MS Excel using the following procedure:

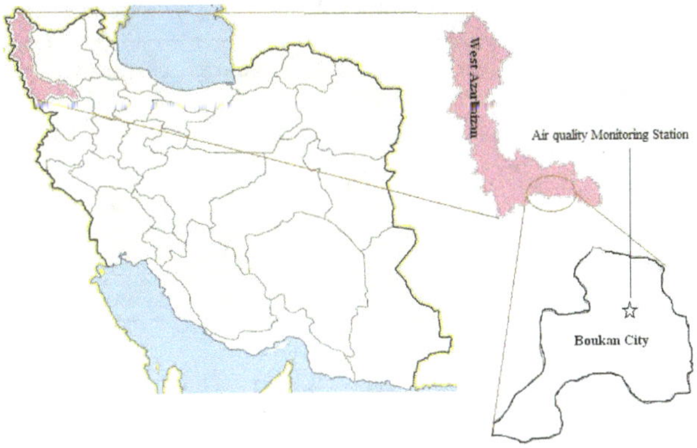

Figure 1. Location of the study area in Bukan City, West Azerbaijan, Iran.

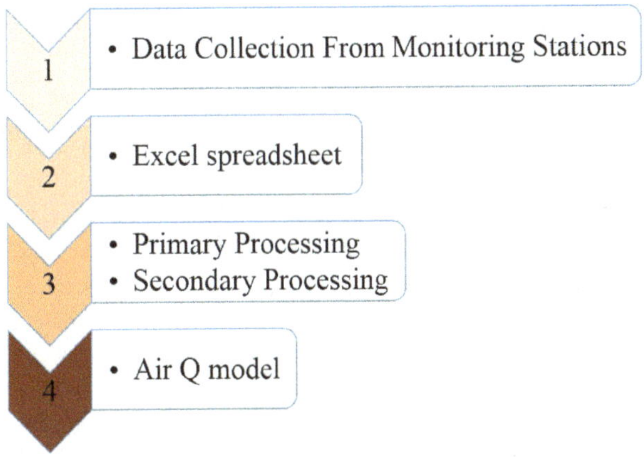

Figure 2. Flowchart of use of Air Q software (4 steps).

primary processing (removing, sheeting, integration time), secondary processing (code writing in Excel, calculating PM_{10} and $PM_{2.5}$ means, primary and secondary filtering of data). In this work, the interval of 10 µg m^{-3} was selected for assessing short-term health impacts. After data classification based on the interval of 10 µg m^{-3}, the results were entered into the software.

Air Quality software

Air Q is a software that quantifies air pollution data. This work employed Air Q software, version 2.2.3. When working with the software, one air pollutant had to be selected for the assessment of its effect on health, and the data regarding population exposure to this pollutant was entered in the program. The data entered included coordinates (latitude and longitude), exposed population, number of stations used for profiling, mean and maximum concentrations (annual, winter, and summer), annual 98th percentile, baseline incidence (BI) per 100000 per year, and relative risk (RR) (mean, lower, and upper). For the predefined health outcomes, two options were given when calculating the health impact: to use WHO default values for BI and RR (95% CI), the level of scientific certainty of which is given according to the available epidemiological evidence, or to replace the WHO default values with estimates for BI and RR obtained from local

Table 1. Particle concentrations of PM_{10} and $PM_{2.5}$ in different seasons of the year

PM_{10} (µg m^{-3})						
Average			**Maximum**			**98th Percentile**
Annual	Summer	Winter	Annual	Summer	Winter	
79.6	84.37	74.86	395.95	395.95	261.57	237.39
$PM_{2.5}$ (µg m^{-3})						
Average			**Maximum**			**98th Percentile**
Annual	Summer	Winter	Annual	Summer	Winter	
33.01	34.95	31.07	180.41	180.41	85.32	94.88

epidemiological studies. In cases of the second option, the scientific uncertainty will be set to unknown by the program. In this research, the BI and RR values were selected based on similar studies (23,24).

Results

Table 1 shows a descriptive analysis of PM_{10} and $PM_{2.5}$ concentrations in the various seasons of 2015-2106. Table 2 shows the hourly average concentrations (µg m^{-3}) of PM_{10} and $PM_{2.5}$ at Bukan city from 2014 to 2015. Table 3 presents the RR with a 95% CI; this figure was used for the health effect estimates of PM_{10} and $PM_{2.5}$ particles. The correlation between PM_{10} and $PM_{2.5}$ concentrations and the percentage of estimated AP (attributed proportion, RR, and estimated number of excess cases [persons]) are shown in Table 4. Figure 3 shows the correlation between cumulative excess and PM_{10} concentration, including total mortality, cardiovascular mortality, respiratory mortality, hospital admissions (HA) for respiratory disease, and HA for cardiovascular disease.

Discussion

The average concentration of particulate matter was higher in summer than in winter. The concentrations of PM_{10} in summer and winter were 84.37 and 74.86 µg m^{-3}, respectively. The maximum concentration of PM_{10} was greater in summer (395.95 µg m^{-3}). The concentrations of $PM_{2.5}$ in summer and winter were 34.95 and 31.07 µg m^{-3}, respectively (Table 1). The maximum concentration of $PM_{2.5}$ was greater in summer (180.41 µg m^{-3}). The results reported in Table 1 show that neither the PM_{10} nor the $PM_{2.5}$ concentration changed significantly with seasonal variations; they were nearly constant. In recent years, dust storms have been the main causes of high PM_{10} and $PM_{2.5}$ concentrations in summer compared with other seasons (1). In Iran, dust storms have both internal and

Table 2. Hourly average concentrations (µg m-3) of PM_{10} and $PM_{2.5}$ particles in Bukan City from 2015 to 2016

		Maximum (µg m^{-3})	Minimum (µg m^{-3})	Mean (µg m^{-3})
January	PM_{10}	261.57	12.07	53.81
	$PM_{2.5}$	49.7	4.74	29.62
February	PM_{10}	230.72	19.92	75.33
	$PM_{2.5}$	66.52	16.61	27.66
March	PM_{10}	204.83	11.13	74.51
	$PM_{2.5}$	85.32	19.17	32.7
April	PM_{10}	179.11	19.31	62.48
	$PM_{2.5}$	54.18	6.75	19.55
May	PM_{10}	225.4	24.45	78.35
	$PM_{2.5}$	27.45	7.33	27.45
June	PM_{10}	395.95	6.92	97.5
	$PM_{2.5}$	164.98	7.71	40.08
July	PM_{10}	233.74	18.75	69.2
	$PM_{2.5}$	140	5.93	27.67
August	PM_{10}	144.99	17.05	62.55
	$PM_{2.5}$	180.41	1.83	38.85
September	PM_{10}	175.66	31.18	71.56
	$PM_{2.5}$	99.91	1.25	32.49
October	PM_{10}	248.99	3.16	75.05
	$PM_{2.5}$	81.44	1.55	32.76
November	PM_{10}	103.07	2.38	56.76
	$PM_{2.5}$	64.26	8.33	23.66
December	PM_{10}	116.62	3.02	49.54
	$PM_{2.5}$	51.43	0.87	35.26

external sources. The external sources of dust storms are the countries of Iraq, Jordan, and Saudi Arabia, and the internal sources are the provinces of Khuzestan, Kerman, and Sistan-Baluchistan. The reasons for the increase in dust storms in Iran include drought, lack of suitable vegetation, reduced rainfall and moisture in the air, destruction of forest and grasslands in Iraq, changes in air

Table 3. Relative risk with 95% confidence interval and corresponding reference

Health effects		Baseline Incidence	Relative risk per 10 µg m^{-3}		
			Low	Medium	High
Mortality	Total	543.5	1.004	1.006	1.008
	Cardiovascular	231	1.005	1.009	1.013
	Respiratory	48.8	1.005	1.020	1.013
Morbidity	HA Respiratory Disease	1260	1.005	1.008	1.011
	HA Cardiovascular Disease	436	1.006	1.009	1.013

Table 4. Health effects, relative risks, estimated AP, and estimated numbers of excess cases due to short-term exposure to PM10 levels above 10 μg m^{-3}

Health effects	RR (Medium)	Estimated AP (%)	Estimated number of excess cases (persons)
Total Mortality	Central	4.0332	49.3
	Lower	2.7254	33.3
	Upper	5.3062	64.9
Cardiovascular mortality	Central	5.9302	30.8
	Lower	3.3837	17.6
	Upper	8.3458	43.4
Respiratory mortality	Central	8.3458	9.2
	Lower	3.3837	3.7
	Upper	12.2876	13.5
HA respiratory disease	Central	5.3062	150.4
	Lower	3.2528	92.2
	Upper	7.2743	206.2
HA cardiovascular disease	Central	5.9302	58.2
	Lower	4.0332	39.6
	Upper	8.3458	81.9

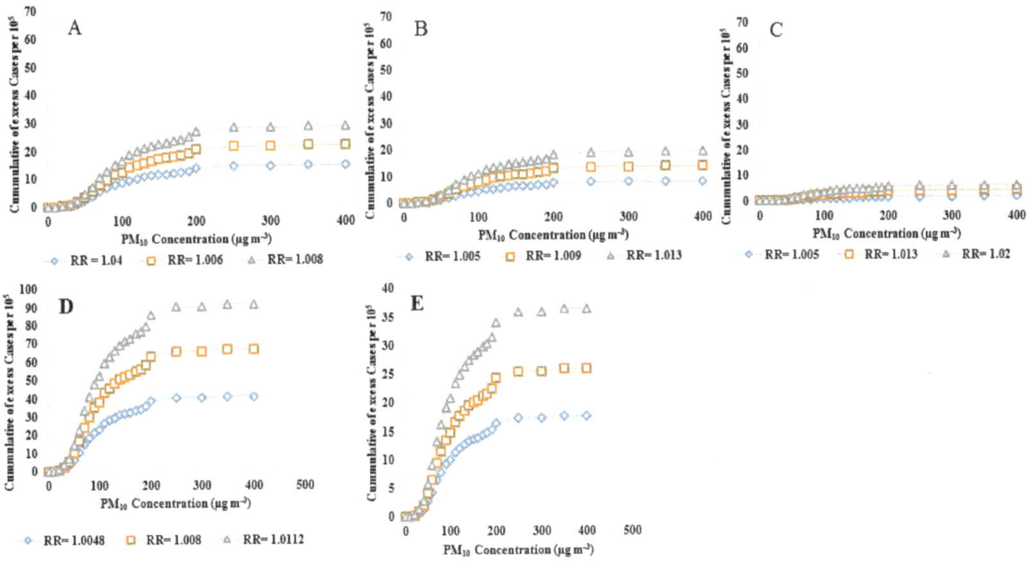

Figure 3. Cumulative excess of case related to PM$_{10}$ concentration: **A**: total mortality, **B**: cardiovascular mortality, **C**: respiratory mortality, **D**: HA for respiratory disease, **E**: HA for cardiovascular disease.

pressure, and strong winds from the deserts of Iraq and Saudi Arabia. The WHO guidelines for PM$_{10}$ and PM$_{2.5}$ particles are 50 and 25 μg m^{-3}, respectively (25). As shown in Table 2, the PM$_{10}$ and PM$_{2.5}$ concentrations measured in this study were higher than WHO guidelines in most months of the year.

The values shown in Table 3 were extracted from similar studies in Iran (24,26). Illustrated in Table 3 are the health effects of PM$_{10}$ particles that can be calculated in mortality, such as total mortality, cardiovascular mortality, respiratory mortality, and morbidity such as HA for respiratory disease and HA for cardiovascular disease. As illustrated in Table 4, the Air Q model predicted that the means of total mortality relative to PM$_{10}$ and PM$_{2.5}$ particles were 33.3 and 49.8 deaths, respectively. Figure 3, Part A shows the cumulative excess cases per 100 000 related to total mortality (lower, mean, and upper). In 2015-2016, there were 935 deaths, 57 of which were due to driving accidents. In other words, 878 people suffered a non-accidental death. As a result, 3.79% of total mortality was due to PM$_{10}$ particles. Similar studies have shown that the effects of PM$_{10}$ on total mortality were responsible for 2194 deaths in the city of Tehran in 2012 (24). Other studies have shown that the highest number of deaths caused by air pollution was related to PM$_{10}$ particles (100 deaths) (27). The Air Q model predicted that 17.6 deaths (mean), or 2.004% of total mortality in Bukan City were related to cardiovascular mortality. Figure 3, Part B shows the cumulative excess of cases per 100 000 related to cardiovascular mortality (lower, mean, and upper). Motalleby and colleagues' results showed that the effects of PM10 were responsible for 66 cardiovascular deaths in the city of Kashan in 2011 (27). The Air Q model predicted that 3.7 deaths from respiratory disease (mean) were related to the effects of PM_{10}. As a result, 0.42% of the total mortality in Bukan City was due to respiratory mortality. Figure 3, Part C shows the cumulative excess of cases per 100 000 related to cardiovascular mortality (lower, mean, and upper). The Air Q model predicted that 92.2 deaths (mean) were related to HA respiratory disease morbidity. Figure 3, Part D shows the cumulative excess of cases per 100 000 related to cardiovascular mortality (lower, mean, and upper). The Air Q model predicted that 39.6 deaths (mean) were related to HA cardiovascular disease. Figure 3, Part E shows the cumulative excess of cases per 100 000 related to cardiovascular mortality (lower, mean and upper). The continual evaluation of air quality data is necessary to investigate the effects of air pollution on human health.

Conclusion

This work used Air Quality software to assess the health risks of particulate matter. The health effects associated with particulate matter, such as total mortality, cardiovascular mortality, respiratory mortality, HA for respiratory disease morbidity, and HA for cardiovascular disease, were calculated.

This model can be useful in aiding data collection about the health effects of pollutants on exposed population.

Authors' contributions

All authors contributed equally and were involved in the study design, data collection, and article approval.

Competing interests

The authors of this article declare that they have no competing interests.

Acknowledgments

This study was supported by the Students Research Committee of Shahid Beheshti University of Medical Science, Iran (grant no. 2571).

References

1. Boloorani AD, Nabavi SO, Bahrami HA, Mirzapour F, Kavosi M, Abasi E, et al. Investigation of dust storms entering Western Iran using remotely sensed data and synoptic analysis. J Environ Health Sci Eng 2014; 12(1): 124. doi: 10.1186/s40201-014-0124-4.
2. Shahsavani A, Naddafi K, Jaafarzadeh Haghighifard N, Mesdaghinia A, Yunesian M, Nabizadeh R, et al. Characterization of ionic composition of TSP and PM_{10} during the Middle Eastern Dust (MED) storms in Ahvaz, Iran. Environ Monit Assess 2012; 184(11): 6683-92. doi: 10.1007/s10661-011-2451-6.
3. Sowlat MH, Naddafi K, Yunesian M, Jackson PL, Lotfi S, Shahsavani A. PM_{10} source apportionment in Ahvaz, Iran, using positive matrix factorization. CLEAN Soil Air Water 2013; 41(12): 1143-51. doi: 10.1002/clen.201200131.
4. Shao Y, Wyrwoll KH, Chappell A, Huang J, Lin Z, McTainsh GH, et al. Dust cycle: an emerging core theme in Earth system science. Aeolian Res 2011; 2(4): 181-204. doi:10.1016/j.aeolia.2011.02.001.
5. Seinfeld JH, Pandis SN. Atmospheric Chemistry and Physics. New York: John Wiley and Sons; 1998.
6. Anderson JO, Thundiyil JG, Stolbach A. Clearing the air: a review of the effects of particulate matter air pollution on human health. J Med Toxicol 2012; 8(2): 166-75. doi: 10.1007/s13181-011-0203-1.
7. Alizadeh Choobari O, Zawar-Reza P, Sturman A. The global distribution of mineral dust and its impacts on the climate system: a review. Atmospheric Research 2014; 138: 152-65.
8. Stedman JR, King K, Holland M, Walton H. Quantification of the health effects of air pollution in the UK for revised PM_{10} objective analysis. AEAT; 2002.
9. Xu LY, Yin H, Xie XD. Health risk assessment of inhalable particulate matter in Beijing based on the thermal environmentInt. J Environ Res Public Health 2014; 11(12): 12368-88. doi: 10.3390/ijerph111212368.
10. Sharafi K, Khosravi T, Moradi M, Pirsaheb M. Air quality and variations in PM_{10} pollutant concentration in western iran during a four –year period (2008-2011), kermanshah - a case study. Journal of Engineering Science and Technology 2015; 10(1): 47-56.
11. Kavousi A, Sefidkar R, Alavimajd H, Rashidi Y, Abolfazli Khonbi Z. Spatial analysis of CO and PM_{10} pollutants in Tehran city. Journal of Paramedical Sciences 2013; 4(3): 41-50.
12. Tiwary A, Colls J. Air Pollution: Measurement, Modelling & Mitigation. 3rd ed. London: Taylor and Francis Group; 2009.
13. Pengra B.The Drying of Iran's Lake Urmia and its Environmental Consequences. https://na.unep.net/geas/getUNEPPageWithArticleIDScript.php?article_id=79. Accessed Oct 2016.
14. Gilmour PS, Brown DM, Lindsay TG, Beswick PH, MacNee W, Donaldson K. Adverse health effects of PM10 particles: involvement of iron in generation of hydroxyl radical. Occup Environ Med 1996; 53(12): 817-22.
15. Nordenhäll C, Pourazar J, Ledin M, Levin JO, Sandström T, Ädelroth E. Diesel exhaust enhances airway responsiveness in asthmatic subjects. Eur Respir J 2001; 17(5): 909-15.
16. Chuang KJ, Chan CC, Su TC, Lee CT, Tang CS. The effect of urban air pollution on inflammation, oxidative stress, coagulation, and autonomic dysfunction in young adults. Am J Respir Crit Care Med 2007; 176(4): 370-6. doi: 10.1164/rccm.200611-1627OC.
17. Bell ML, HEI Health Review Committee. Assessment of the health impacts of particulate matter characteristics. Res Rep Health Eff Inst 2012; (161): 5-38.
18. Evans J, Donkelaar AV, Martin RV, Burnett R, Rainham DG, Birkett NJ, et al. Estimates of global mortality attributable to particulate air pollution using satellite imagery. Environ Res 2013; 120: 33-42. doi: 10.1016/j.envres.2012.08.005.
19. Kamarehie B, Ghaderpoori M, Jafari A, Karami M, Mohammadi A. Quantification of health effects related to SO2 and NO2 pollutants using air quality model. J

Adv Environ Health Res 2017; 5(1): 44-50. doi: 10.22103/JAEHR.2017.47757.
20. World Health Organization (WHO). Quantification of the Health Effects of Exposure to Air Pollution Report of a WHO Working Group. The Netherlands: WHO; 2000.
21. Karbassi A, Nabi Bidhendi G, Pejman A, Esmaeili Bidhendi M. Environmental impacts of desalination on the ecology of Lake Urmia. J Great Lakes Res 2010; 36(3): 419-424. doi: 10.1016/j.jglr.2010.06.004.
22. Jalili S, Kirchner I, Livingstone DM, Morid S. The influence of large-scale atmospheric circulation weather types on variations in the water level of Lake Urmia, Iran. Int J Climatol 2012; 32(13): 1990-96.
23. Ghanbari Ghozikali M, Mosaferi M, Nadafi K. Quantification of the health effects of exposure to ozone in tabriz by using airq model. Urmia Med J 2014; 25(6): 521-30. [In Persian].
24. Naddafi K, Hassanvand MS, Yunesian M, Momeniha F, Nabizadeh R, Faridi S, et al. Health impact assessment of air pollution in megacity of Tehran, Iran. Iranian J Environ Health Sci Eng 2012; 9(1): 28. doi: 10.1186/1735-2746-9-28.
25. WHO. Air quality guidelines: global update 2005: particulate matter, ozone, nitrogen dioxide, and sulfur dioxide. Geneva: World Health Organization; 2006.
26. Nourmoradi H, Goudarzi G, Daryanoosh SM, Omidi-Khaniabadi F, Jourvand M, Omidi-Khaniabadi Y. Health impacts of particulate matter in air by Air Q model in Khorramabad city, Iran. J Basic Res Med Sci 2015; 2(2): 44-52.
27. Motalleby M, Mazaheri A, Mosayebi M, Takhtfiroozeh SM. Assessing Health Impacts of Air Pollution in Kashan 2011. Arak Medical University Journal 2015; 18(5): 77-87. [In Persian].

Evaluation of cardiovascular and respiratory mortality attributed to atmospheric SO_2 and CO using AirQ model

Majid Kermani[1,2], Mohsen Dowlati[3,4], Sevda Fallah Jokandan[3], Mina Aghaei[5], Farshad Bahrami Asl[6], Sima Karimzadeh[7*]

[1]Associate Professor of Environmental Health Engineering, Research Center for Environmental Health Technology, School of Public Health, Iran University of Medical Sciences, Tehran, Iran
[2]Associate Professor of Environmental Health Engineering, Department of Environmental Health Engineering, School of Public Health, Iran University of Medical Sciences, Tehran, Iran
[3]MSc of Environmental Health Engineering, Department of Environmental Health Engineering, School of Public Health, Iran University of Medical Sciences, Tehran, Iran
[4]MSc of Environmental Health Engineering, Research Center for Environmental Health Technology, School of Public Health, Iran University of Medical Sciences, Tehran, Iran
[5]PhD Student of Environmental Health Engineering, Department of Environmental Health Engineering, School of Public Health, Tehran University of Medical Sciences, Tehran, Iran
[6]PhD Student of Environmental Health Engineering, Department of Environmental Health Engineering, School of Public Health, Hamadan University of Medical Sciences, Hamadan, Iran
[7]MSc of Environmental Health Engineering, Department of Environmental Health Engineering, School of Public Health, Urima University of Medical Sciences, Urima, Iran

Abstract
Background: Air pollutants have multiple adverse effects on human health. In this study, the health effects of exposure to carbon monoxide (CO) and SO_2 in the air of 6 Iranian metropolises in 2011-2012 were examined.
Methods: Raw data was collected from the Iranian Department of Environment and the Iran Meteorological Organization. After validation, the required statistical indices were calculated through programming and modifying temperature and pressure in Excel software. The output of Excel was given to the AirQ model, and the results were presented as the cases of death.
Results: The annual mean concentrations of SO_2 were 2.45, 1.55, 0.6, 0.55, 1.05, and 3.8 times higher than the guidelines of the World Health Organization (WHO) (20 μg/m^3) in Tehran, Mashhad, Isfahan, Shiraz, Tabriz, and Urmia, respectively. The concentrations of CO did not exceed the standard limit in any of the studied cities. The cumulative numbers of total deaths attributed to SO2 were 744, 122, 132, 44, 37, and 107 in Tehran, Mashhad, Isfahan, Shiraz, Tabriz, and Urmia, respectively. The highest mortality rate was found in Urmia at 2.9% followed by Tehran at 1.52%; the lowest rate of 0.46% was found in Tabriz.
Conclusion: The results show that of the 6 metropolises, the highest CO mortality rate of about 2.15% belonged to Isfahan followed by Arak with about 1.38%, and the lowest rate of 0.68% belonged to Mashhad. Because of the growing trend of air pollution and its mortality rate and adverse effects, practical solutions for the control and reduction of air pollution in Iranian metropolises are necessary.
Keywords: Air pollution, Software, Iran, Cities

***Correspondence to:**
Sima Karimzadeh
Email:
sima.karimzade@yahoo.com

Introduction

The increases in technology and industrialization without consideration given to sustainable development and environmental pollution, particularly the pollution of air which is an important factor of life, need to be given more attention (1-8). Based on the annual estimates of the World Health Organization (WHO), 800 000 premature deaths occur; of that number, about 1 500 000 of these deaths occur in South Asia (9). Annually, deaths caused by air pollution in the United States about 60 000 number. Nevertheless mortality attributable to pollution appears to be low; however, due to the large population that is exposed to air pollution and the existence of sensitive groups in society, the burden of disease attributable to pollution will increase (10,11). The effects of air pollution on human health can be categorized as chronic or acute. In determining acute effects, one examines important events that occurred in the 20th century in some cities of Europe and America, such as Meuse Valley, Belgium; London, England; and Donora, Pennsylvania in the United States (11-13). Over the past 2 decades, studies on the health effects of air pollution have determined and demonstrated that the rate of mortality attributable to air pollution is rising (12,13). Research has shown that the global burden of air pollution-related disease estimated by the WHO is 89% of total deaths caused by heart and respiratory disease (13). In the past few decades, many studies have demonstrated that the current levels of SO_2 and carbon monoxide (CO) are associated with cardiopulmonary respiratory deaths, hospitalizations, and respiratory symptoms (14-17). CO is a colorless, odorless, poisonous, and tasteless gas. It is often mixed with other gases that do have an odor, though it has no detectable odor itself. When carbon monoxide is in haled, it displaces oxygen in the blood and deprives the heart, brain, and other vital organs of oxygen. The six main symptoms of CO poisoning are headaches, vertigo, nausea, breathlessness, heart palpitations, and a loss of consciousness. Large amounts of CO can overcome a person in just a few minutes without prior warning, cause a loss of consciousness and eventually suffocation. Carbon monoxide is relatively stable in air and is one of the major pollutants related to the burning of natural gas and internal combustion engines. If the appliances burning fuel are properly kept and used, the amount of CO produced is not usually dangerous. About 85%-90% of CO comes from automobile exhaust (18-20). When fossil fuels which contain sulfur, like coal, are burned, sulfur dioxide is released. Generally, there are 2 reasons why SO_2 is hazardous to humans: first, it is in gaseous form, and second, it oxidizes to form sulfate. Aerosol SO_2, in comparison with other pollutants, is more soluble in water, and when it is combined with suspended solids and moisture, it creates harmful effects that are relayed by air pollution. Many studies have shown that the number of hospitalizations increase on days with high levels of SO_2 in the air. Asthmatics are generally considered the group most sensitive to high concentrations of SO_2. Another sensitive group comprises those who exercise regularly. This is due to the fact that SO_2 is highly reactive; consequently, the distribution of SO_2 along the conductive airways of the respiratory tract is non-uniform, depending on breathing volumes and types (21,22). Information on the effects of exposure for long periods (e.g., 24 hours) is obtained from epidemiological studies, which are indicative of the relationships among contaminants such as SO_2 and the health impacts on communities. To evaluate the evidence of effects on health related to SO_2 exposure for the New Zealand ambient air quality guideline values, Dennison et al studied the correlations between SO_2 and other contaminants in the air. They determined that it would be quite difficult to confidently attribute the impacts observed in epidemiological studies to SO_2 alone (23). Experimental studies were therefore applied to derive the dose-response relationships underpinning the ambient air quality guideline values for SO_2 in New Zealand (24). In a study during the years 1996-2000 in 15 cities of Italy, with increasing concentrations of CO and SO_2, the number of mortalities due to cardiovascular disease rose 0.93% and 1.11%, respectively (24). In the 8 Iranian metropolises studied in the current research, several pollutants are discharged from motor vehicles, industries, and commercial and domestic resources, and the concentrations of most of these pollutants rise above standards levels during different hours of the day. The situation has attracted the attention of a group of officials and people. Therefore, to reduce air pollution and aid decision-making in this regard, there is a significant need to quantify the health effects of pollution. The main purpose of this study was to quantify the short-term health effects of air pollution, specifically regarding the pollutants CO and SO_2, in 2011-2012 in 6 cities of Iran (Isfahan, Shiraz, Tabriz, Mashhad, Tehran, and Urmia). This study employed the software AirQ2.2.3.

Materials and Methods

Data related to air pollution were taken from the Environmental Protection Department of 6 large cities in Iran (Figure 1).

There are 21 valid, general monitoring stations for SO_2 and 25 valid, general monitoring stations for CO in the 6 Iranian cities investigated in this study. All stations monitor SO_2 and other gaseous pollutants (NO_2, PM_{10}, $PM_{2.5}$, O_3, and CO) hourly. The data related to pressure and temperature were obtained from the cities' metrological offices. Data regarding the cities' populations were obtained for use in statistical analysis. The population static over 65 years

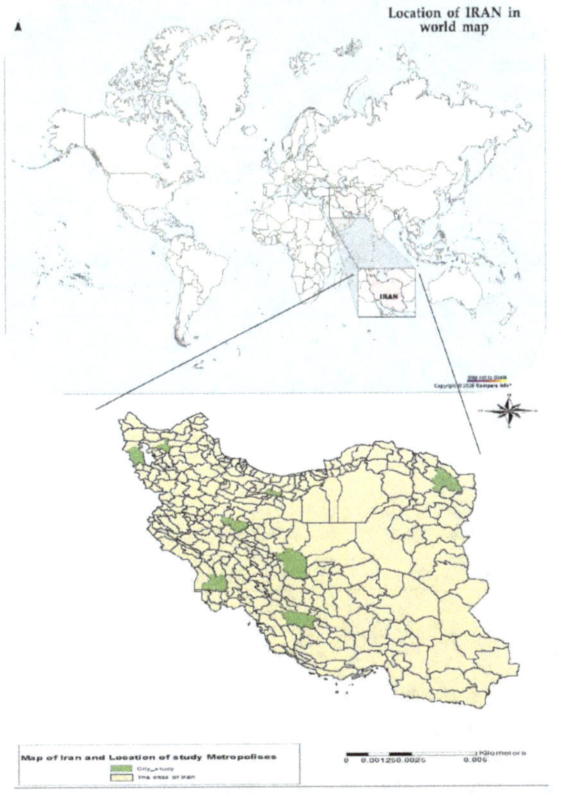

Figure 1. Map of Iran in world and location of study metropolises.

old were used for population that faced with CO. The data provided for consideration was volumetric base and needed to be gravimetric-based for entry into the selected software. Thus, by writing a program in Excel, new files were created with the model's required units. First, the raw data was changed based on temperature and measurement points. The following equation was used to correct the concentrations expressed in units.

$P_1V_1/T_1 = P_2V_2/T_2$

Then, the raw data was analyzed and valid data was selected based on WHO, European, and European Union (EU) criteria. Zero values meant that disturbances were removed from calculating average that conducted with moving average. Data on SO_2 and CO was placed on separate sheets, because the files for entry into the software for SO_2 were daily averages and that for CO was based on an hourly average. Initial and secondary filtering was done in Excel. In this part, the required statistical parameters were calculated and prepared for entry into AirQ software. For the quantification of both pollutants in the air, the software AirQ2.2.3 presented by the European Environment Office and the WHO was employed. It was also used to quantify the health effects of air pollution. Using this model, a kind of statistical and epidemiological method, the health outcomes were estimated using pollutant concentration and epidemiological parameters like baseline incidence, relative risk, and exposed population of the studied cities. The results were shown as attributable proportion (AP) and the number of excess cases of mortality. Finally, the results were presented as tables and charts of base line incidence (BI) and relative risk (RR) with 95% CI for estimated health endpoints attributable to SO_2 and CO in the present study (Table 1). The populations of the studied cities are shown in Table 2 (25,26).

Results

Table 1. Baseline incidence and relative risk with 95% CI for health endpoints

Health endpoint		Baseline Incidence (per 105 inhabitants)	RR (95% CI) per 10 μg/m³	
			SO_2	CO
	Total	543.5	1.004 (1.003-1.0048)	-
Mortality	Cardiovascular	231	1.008 (1.002-1.012)	BI:497; 1.007 (1.002-1.012)
	Respiratory	48.4	1.01 (1.006-1.014)	-

Abbreviations: BI, baseline incidence; RR, relative risk; CO, carbon monoxide.
Source: AirQ 2.2. 3 software

Table 2. Population of studied cities from the census reports on Iran

City	Exposed population	The population used in the software	Population over 65 years	Latitude	Longitude
Mashhad	2749374	2750 × 1000	200 × 1000	36.31	59.58
Tabriz	1494998	1495 × 1000	143 × 1000	38.08	46.28
Isfahan	1987168	1987 × 1000	135 × 1000	32.68	51.64
Shiraz	1549453	1540 × 1000	90 × 1000	29.62	52.52
Tehran	9000000	9000 × 1000	550 × 1000	35.34	51.25
Urmia	1615000	680 × 1000	40 × 1000	37.55	45.07

Table 3. Statistical parameters required for import into the program- CO (mg/m³) in 6 megacities

Parameter	Mashhad	Tabriz	Isfahan	Shiraz	Tehran	Urmia
Annual mean	2	2	2	2	2	2
Winter mean	2	3	2	2	2	2
Summer mean	2	2	2	2	2	2
Annual 98 Percentile (P_{98})	4	5	10	5	5	7
No. of station	8	6	4	2	10	1

Table 4. Statistical parameters required for import into the program- SO_2 (μg/m³) in six Megacities

Parameter	Mashhad	Tabriz	Isfahan	Shiraz	Tehran	Urmia
Annual mean	31	21	12	11	49	76
Winter mean	34	29	10	9	54	82
Summer mean	28	13	13	14	43	71
Annual 98 Percentile (P_{98})	48	66	19	25	94	159
Annual maximum	61	118	26	33	118	188
Winter maximum	61	18	26	34	118	176
Summer maximum	41	34	20	32	88	188
No. of station	7	5	4	2	9	1

Table 5. Comparison annual average concentration of SO_2 with the Iran national standard in 6 metropolis of Iran

City	The average annual concentration Iran national standard (μg/m³)	The ratio annual average concentration SO2 (μg/m³)
Mashhad	20	1.55
Tabriz	20	1.05
Isfahan	20	0.6
Shiraz	20	0.55
Tehran	20	2.45
Urmia	20	3.8

Based on the WHO's criteria, the data related to SO_2 and CO pollutants was studied. The required statistical parameters (annual and seasonal means and annual 98th percentiles) for CO and SO_2 were obtained from each city and are shown in Tables 3 and 4, respectively.

Table 3 shows the results that indicate the 1-hour average concentration of CO in 6 metropolitan cities was not higher than the standard level, and the highest annual concentration of CO was related to the (mg/m³) concentration of Tehran city. Table 4 shows that the annual mean concentrations of SO_2 were higher than the standard level (20 μg/m³) in Mashhad, Tehran, and Urmia with the highest annual SO_2 concentration being related to Urmia (76 μg/m³). The annual mean concentration of SO_2 was compared with Iran's national standard for average annual concentration in six metropolises of Iran, and the results are given in Table 5.

As indicated in Table 5, the annual mean concentrations of SO_2 were higher in Tehran and Urmia than in the other cities; their average ratios were 2.45 and 3.8 times greater than the average standard concentration. The province of West Azerbaijan is located in western Iran and is affected by wet weather from the Atlantic Ocean and Mediterranean Sea. In Urmia, the capital city of the province, there are approximately 300 vehicles for every 1000 people. That is about 1.5 times the average of the country. In Urmia, the number of vehicles and expansion grows with no regard to environmental issues, and this is the main factor threatening the quality of Urmia's air in view of the quickly increasing population. In most months of the year, Mashhad has a great number of pilgrims. Thus, air pollution in this city is caused by the heavy traffic and increasing use of necessary fuels. Table 6 shows the number of times the SO_2 concentration of each city exceeds standard level in a 24-hour period and the comparison of SO_2 levels in these cities with the standard level.

Based on the results presented in Table 6, the city experiencing largest number of 24-hour periods that the SO_2 concentration was higher than that recommended by the WHO is Mashhad, where levels were higher 365 days. According to the National Quality Standards of the EPA (Environmental Production Agency) and the National Standard of Clean Air of Iran, the standard assigned to CO for an 8-hour average is 9 ppm. CO concentrations did not exceed this standard level in any of the studied cities. Based on indicators of estimated relative risk shown in Table 7, the highest death rate is related to respiratory mortality due to contact with SO_2 in Urmia. According to the results, the total number of respiratory deaths compared to all deaths in the study period for the 6 studied cities was 365 out of 10 641 persons per year. Based on indicators of estimated relative risk shown in Table 8, the highest number of deaths is related to cardiovascular mortality due to contact with CO in Isfahan. According to the results, the estimated number of cardiovascular cases resulting in death compared to all deaths in the 6 studied cities during the study period was 64 out of 64 64 persons

Table 6. Comparison the average SO_2 concentration of 24 hours with guidelines and standards values in 6 metropolises

City	Guidelines and standards	Average 24-h	The No. of times that the SO_2 concentration of 24 h in each city is compared to a high standard
Mashhad	WHO Guidelines	20	365
	Iran national standard	100	0
	European standards	125	0
Tabriz	WHO Guidelines	20	128
	Iran national standard	100	1
	European standards	125	0
Isfahan	WHO Guidelines	20	267
	Iran national standard	100	17
	European standards	125	3
Shiraz	WHO Guidelines	20	153
	Iran national standard	100	0
	European standards	125	0
Tehran	WHO Guidelines	20	346
	Iran national standard	100	4
	European standards	125	0
Urmia	WHO Guidelines	20	351
	Iran national standard	100	109
	European standards	125	76

Table 7. Estimated attributable proportion expressed as percentage and number of excess cases in a year due to short-term exposure above 10 μg/m³ for SO_2

Health endpoints	Study city	AP (uncertainty range)*	No. of excess cases (uncertainty range)
Total mortality	Mashhad	0.81 (0.61-0.997)	122 (92-146)
	Tabriz	0.46 (0.34-0.55)	37 (28-45)
	Isfahan	1.21 (0.92-1.45)	132 (99-158)
	Shiraz	0.55 (0.41-0.66)	44 (33-53)
	Tehran	1.52 (1.14-1.81)	744 (560-890)
	Urmia	2.19 (2.90-3.46)	107 (81-128)
Cardiovascular mortality	Mashhad	1.61 (0.40-2.40)	103 (26-153)
	Tabriz	0.91 (0.23-1.37)	32 (8-47)
	Isfahan	2.4 (0.61-3.56)	111 (28-164)
	Shiraz	1.10 (0.28-1.65)	37 (9-55)
	Tehran	2.99 (0.76-4.42)	623 (159-920)
	Urmia	5.64 (1.47-8.23)	89 (23-129)
Respiratory mortality	Mashhad	2.01 (1.22-2.8)	27 (16-38)
	Tabriz	1.14 (0.69-1.6)	8 (5-12)
	Isfahan	2.99 (1.8-4.13)	29 (18-40)
	Shiraz	1.38 (0.83-1.92)	10 (6-14)
	Tehran	3.72 (2.26-5.12)	162 (99-223)
	Urmia	6.95 (4.29-9.47)	23 (14-31)

Table 8. Estimated attributable proportion expressed as percentage and number of excess cases in a year due to short-term exposure above 10 μg/m³ for CO

Health endpoints	Study city	AP (uncertainty range)	No. of excess cases (uncertainty range)
Cardiovascular mortality	Mashhad	0.68 (0.19-1.17)	9 (2-12)
	Tabriz	0.83 (0.24-1.42)	6 (2-10)
	Isfahan	2.15 (0.62-3.63)	14 (4-24)
	Shiraz	0.69 (0.19-1.17)	3 (1-5)
	Tehran	1.09 (0.31-1.86)	28 (8-48)
	Urmia	1.04 (0.3-1.77)	2 (1-4)

per year. According to the output charts obtained from the software, almost 50% of deaths attributed to contact with CO occurred in concentrations of less than 4 mg/m³. The results from the AirQ software are shown in graph form in Figure 2. These figures show the cumulative excess cases of cardiovascular mortality due to CO concentration in the 6 studied cities in Iran: *a*) Mashhad; *b*) Tabriz; *c*) Isfahan; *d*) Shiraz; *e*) Urmia; *f*) Tehran.

Discussion

The results shown in Tables 4 and 5 indicate that the 2011 concentrations of SO_2 were 49, 31, 12, 11, 21, and 76 in Tehran, Mashhad, Isfahan, Shiraz, Tabriz, and Urmia, respectively. Those figures are 2.45, 1.55, 0.6, 0.55, 1.05, and 3.8 times higher than those set out in the WHO guidelines (20 μg/m³). Therefore, the mean annual concentrations of SO_2 in Tehran, Mashhad, Tabriz, and Urmia were higher than the Iranian national standard and the EU standard, while it was reported as lower than the mentioned standards in Isfahan and Shiraz. As seen in Table 6, the mean annual concentration of SO_2 in Urmia was higher than the WHO standard for 96% of the days in a year. This rate was higher than the Iranian standard for 30% of days in a year (100 μg/m³) and higher than the EU standard on 20% of days in a year (125 μg/m³). In Tehran, the rates were 95% higher than the WHO standards, while it was only 2% higher than the Iranian standard and never exceeded the EU standard; this result indicates the deterioration of the situation of SO_2 in these cities. It should be noted that concentrations of SO_2 in Mashhad, Isfahan, Shiraz, and Tabriz were higher than the WHO standard on 100%, 73%, 42% and 35% of days in 2011, respectively. The results indicate that the status of SO_2 is critical in Urmia and Tehran. According to 2011 reports, there were about 300 cars for every 1000 individuals in Urmia; this rate is about 1.5 times the country's average (27). It seems that the high number of cars, the increased population, and the subsequent increased use of fossil fuels can be the causes for the increase in pollutants in the above-mentioned cities. On most days of the year in the studied cities, the distribution of the SO_2 concentration is in the range of 40-49 μg/m³ in the studied cities. As seen in Figure 2, the highest percentage of exposure to the pollutant occurred in Shiraz, Isfahan, and Tabriz with concentration intervals of 10-19 μg/m³, in Mashhad with 20-29 μg/m³, in Urmia with 30-39 μg/m³, and in Tehran with 40-49 μg/m³. Based on these figures, it becomes clear that the largest number of mortalities from cardiovascular

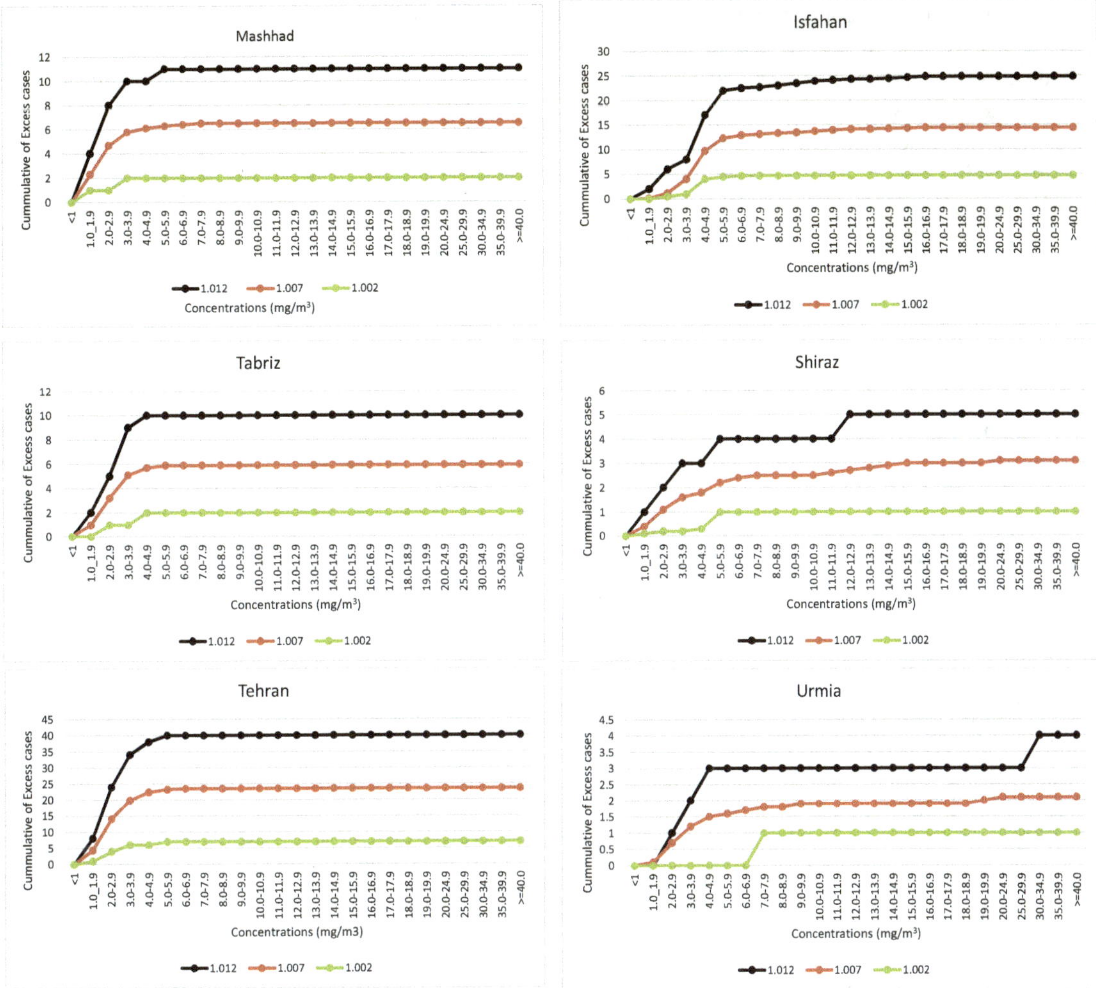

Figure 2. Cumulative of Excess cases for cardiovascular mortality of CO concentration in the six Iranian cities.

diseases have occurred at the same rate of concentration. In the case of CO, it was revealed that the concentration of the pollutant did not exceed the standard limits in any of the studied cities. According to Table 1 and considering RR and BI indices per 1000 population, the risk of cardiovascular deaths attributable to SO_2 and CO will increase 0.8% and 0.7% for each 10 μg/m³ concentration of SO_2 and 1 μg/m³ concentration of CO, respectively. Further more, it will increase the death rate 0.4% for each 10 μg/m³ increase in SO_2 concentration. In a study conducted in 8 cities of North America, it was found that per one unit of increase in concentration of carbon monoxide, a 2.79% increase in the number of cardiovascular patients was seen (28). As observed in Table 7, the cumulative total number of deaths attributed to SO_2 were 744, 122, 132, 44, 37, and 107 cases in Tehran, Mashhad, Isfahan, Shiraz, Tabriz, and Urmia, respectively. The results suggest that among the six studied metropolises, air pollution has caused the highest mortality rates in Urmia (about 2.19%) and Tehran (about 1.52%) and the lowest rate in Tabriz (0.46%). As is evident in Table 8, the cumulative numbers of cardiovascular deaths attributed to CO were 24, 7, 14, 3, 6, and 2 individuals in Tehran, Mashhad, Isfahan, Shiraz, Tabriz, and Urmia, respectively. The results suggest that among the six studied metropolises, air pollution caused the highest mortality rate in Isfahan (about 2.15%) and the lowest in Mashhad (0.68%). In a study examining 15 cities in Italy during the years 1996 to 2000, it was observed that the mortality rate caused by cardiovascular diseases increased with coefficients of 0.4%, 0.93%, 1.11%, and 0.54% in the concentration of NO_2, CO, SO_2 and PM_{10}, respectively (29). According to Figure 2, the largest and smallest cumulative numbers of deaths due to cardiovascular disease were 5.64% in Urmia and 0.9% in Tabriz for SO_2. For CO, the largest cumulative number was 2.15% in Isfahan. In a study carried out in Tucson (US) air pollutants, particles and carbon monoxide had significant and strong relationships with the referral rate of cardiovascular patients with coefficients of 2.75% and 2.79%, respectively, whereas other pollutants such as SO2, NO2, and O3 had weaker relationships with the referral rate of cardiovascular patients with coefficients of 0.14%, 0.69%, and 0.54%, respectively.

Conclusion

The current study, like other similar studies (30-41), showed that air pollution has a health effect on people. The results showed that in all calculated results attributed to SO_2, Tabriz had the lowest morality rate, while Tehran and Urmia had the highest mortality rates attributable to SO_2. Since the concentration of CO was not higher than the standard levels in the surveyed cities, the number of deaths from heart disease attributable to this pollutant was not high, while examination of the relationship between pollutant concentration and the number of deaths indicated that with increases in concentration, the number of deaths also increased. In general, statistics associated with the cumulative number of all deaths from cardiovascular disease extracted from the software clearly reflect the impacts of air pollution on human health. Thus, correct and effective planning is obviously required to control and reduce the harmful effects of air pollutants, especially SO_2 and CO. Thus, the adoption of effective methods to improve the quality of air and reduce the number of people exposed to air pollution should be considered by politicians.

Acknowledgments

The authors express their gratitude to the Environmental Protection Agency of all studied cities for their cooperation in data collection and to the Vice-Chancellery for Research of Iran University of Medical Sciences for its financial support of this study with grant No. 24221.

Competing interests

The authors hereby declare that in conducting this study, they had no competing interests.

Authors' contributions

All the authors contributed and participated equally in the collection, analysis, and interpretation of the data in this study. All authors critically reviewed, refined, and approved the manuscript.

References

1. Khorsandi H, Karimzade S, Aghaei M, KargarH, Mousavi Moghanjooghi S. Estimation and quantification of health effects attributed to NO2 pollutant in the air of Urmia, Iran. J Urmia Univ Med Sci 2016; 26(12): 1054-62. [In Persian].
2. Larsen B. Cost assessment of environmental degradation in the Middle East and North Africa region. The Economic Research Forum; 2011.
3. World Health Organization (WHO). Training pacage for the health sector. Outdoor air pollution. WHO; 2008.
4. Wong CM. Public health and air pollution in Asia (PAPA): coordinated studies of short term exposure to air pollution and dairy mortality in four cities. Boston: Health Effects Institute; 2010. p. 377-80.
5. Hirota K. Comparative studies on vehicle related policies for air pollution reduction in ten Asian countries. Sustainability 2010; 2(1): 145-62. doi: 10.3390/su2010145.
6. Bahrami Asl F, Kermani M, Aghaei M, Karimzadeh S, Salahshour Arian S, Shahsavani A, et al. Estimation of diseases and mortality attributed to NO_2 pollutant in five metropolises of Iran using AirQ model in 2011-2012. J Mazandaran Univ Med Sci 2015; 24(121): 239-49. [In Persian].
7. Arfaeinia H, Kermani M, Aghaei M, Bahrami Asl F, Karimzadeh S. Comparative investigation of health quality of air in Tehran, Isfahan and Shiraz metropolises in 2011-2012. Journal of Health in the Field 2014;1(4):36-44. [In Persian].
8. Kermani M, Bahrami Asl F, Aghaei M, Arfaeinia H, Karimzadeh S, Shahsavani A. Comparative investigation of air quality index (AQI) for six industrial cites of Iran. Urmia Med J 2014: 25(9): 810-9. [In Persian].
9. Cohen AJ, Ross Anderson H, Ostro B, Pandey KD, Krzyzanowski M, Künzli N, et al. The global burden of disease due to outdoor air pollution. J Toxicol Environ Health A 2005; 68(13-14): 1301-7. doi: 10.1080/15287390590936166.
10. Krzyzanowski M, Cohen A, Anderson R; WHO Working Group. Quantification of health effects of exposure to air pollution. Occup Environ Med 2002; 59(12): 791-3. doi: 10.1136/oem.59.12.791
11. Reed MD, Gigliotti AP, McDonald JD, Seagrave JC, Seilkop SK, Mauderly JL. Wealth effects of subchronic exposure to environment levels of diesel exhaust. Inhal Toxicol; 2004. 16(4): 93-177.
12. Samet JM1, Dominici F, Zeger SL, Schwartz J, Dockery DW. The national morbidity, mortality, and air pollution study. Part I: methods and methodologic issues. Res Rep Health Eff Inst 2000; (94 Pt 1): 5-14.
13. Ciocco A, Thompson DJ. A follow-up of Donora ten years after: methodology and findings. Am J Public Health Nations Health 1961; 51: 155-64.
14. Nemery B, Hoet PH, Nemmar A. The Meuse Valley fog of 1930: an air pollution disaster. Lancet 2001; 357(9257): 704-8. doi: 10.1016/S0140-6736(00)04135-0
15. Walters S, Phupinyokul M, Ayres J. Hospital admission rates for asthma and respiratory disease in the West Midlands: their relationship to air pollution levels. Thorax 1995; 50(9): 948-54.
16. Schwartz J. Short term fluctuations in air pollution and hospital admissions of the elderly for respiratory disease. Thorax 1995; 50(5): 531-8.
17. Lin H, An Q, Luo C, Pun VC, Chan CS, Tian L. Gaseous air pollution and acute myocardial infarction mortality in Hong Kong: a time-stratified case-crossover study. Atmos Environ 2013; 76: 68-73. doi: 10.1016/j.atmosenv.2012.08.043.
18. Health effects of outdoor air pollution. Committee of the Environmental and Occupational Health Assembly of the American Thoracic Society. Am J Respir Crit Care Med 1996; 153(1): 3-50. doi: 10.1164/ajrccm.153.1.8542133.
19. Shrestha K. An assessment of the contribution of micro scale activities to personal pollution exposure in commuting micro environments [dissertation].Canterbury: University of Canterbury; 2009.
20. Han X, Anther LP. A review of traffic-related air pollution exposure assessment studies in the developing world. Environ Int 2005; 32(1): 106-20. doi:10.1016/j.envint.2005.05.020.
21. Abdollahi M, Zadparvar L, Ayatollahi B, Baradaran M, Nikfar S, Hastaie P, et al. Hazard from carbon monoxide poisoning for bus drivers in Tehran, Iran. Bull Environ Contam Toxicol 1998; 61(2): 210-5.

22. WHO. Air Quality Guidelines: Global Update 2005: Particulate Matter, Ozone, Nitrogen Dioxide and Sulfur Dioxide. Geneva: World Health Organization; 2006.
23. Ministry for the Environment. Ambient Air Quality Guidelines. Wellington: Ministry for the Environment; 2002.
24. Scoggins A, Kjellstrom T, Fisher G, Connor J, Gimson N. Spatial analysis of annual air pollution exposure and mortality. Sci Total Environ 2004; 321(1-3): 71-85. doi: 10.1016/j.scitotenv.2003.09.020.
25. Buggeri A, Bellini O, Terracini B. Meta-analysis of the Italian studies on short-term effects of air pollution MISA 1996-2002. Epidemiol Prev 2004; 28(4-5 Suppl): 4-100. [In Italian].
26. Kermani M, Bahrami Asl F, Aghaei M, Karimzadeh S, Arfaeinia H, Godarzi G, et al. Quantification of health effects attributed to ozone in five metropolises of Iran using AirQ model. Journal of Health and Hygiene 2015; 6(3): 260-80. [In Persian].
27. Naddafi K, Hasanvand MS, Yunesian M, Momeniha F, Nabizade R, Faridi S, et al. Health impact assessment of air pollution in megacity of Tehran, Iran. Iran J Environ Health Sci Eng. 2012; 9(1). doi: 10.1186/1735-2746-9-28.
28. Khorsandi H, Amini Tapok F, Cargar H, Mousavi Moughanjogi S. Study of urmia city air quality according to the air quality index (AQI). Urmia Med J 2013; 23 (7): 767-75. [In Persian].
29. Burnett RT, Dales RE, Brook JR, Raizenne ME, Krewski D. Association between ambient carbon monoxide levels and hospitalization for congestive heart failure in the elderly in 10 Canadian cities.Epidemiology 1997; 8(2): 162-7.
30. Schwartz J. Air Pollution and hospital admissions for cardiovascular disease in Tucson. Epidemiology 1997; 8(4): 371-7.
31. Kermani M, Aghaei M, Gholami M, Bahrami Asl F. F, Karimzade S, Fallah Jokandan S, et al. Estimation of mortality attributed to PM2.5 and CO exposure in eight industrialized cities of Iran during 2011. Iran Occupational Health Journal 2016; 13(4): 49-61. [In Persian].
32. Motesaddi Zarandi S, Raei Shaktaie H, Yazdani Cheratee J, Hosseinzade F, Dowlati M. Evaluation of PM2.5 concentration and determinant parameters on its distribution in Tehran's metro system in 2012. Journal of Mazandaran University of Medical Sciences 2013; 22(2): 37-46. [In Persian].
33. Kermani M, Fallah Jokandan S, Aghaei M, Dolati M. Estimation the number of mortality due to cardiovascular and respiratory disease, attributed to pollutants O3, and NO2 in the air of Tehran. Journal of Health Research in Community 2016; 1(4):1-11. [In Persian].
34. Kermani M, Dowlati M, Jonidi Jafari A, Rezaei Kalantari R, Sadat Sakhaei F. Effect of air pollution on the emergency admissions of cardiovascular and respiratory patients, using the air quality model: a study in Tehran, 2005-2014. Health in Emergencies and Disasters Quarterly 2016; 1(3): 137-46. doi: 10.15412/J.HDQ.09010304.
35. Kermani M, Fallah Jokandan S, Aghaei M, Bahrami Asl F, Karimzadeh S, Dowlati M. Estimation of the number of excess hospitalizations attributed to sulfur dioxide in six major cities of Iran. Health Scope 2016; 5(4): e38736. doi: 10.17795/jhealthscope-38736
36. Kermani M, Aghaei M, Bahramiasl F, Gholami M, Fallah Jokandan S, Dolati M et al. Estimation of cardiovascular death, myocardial infarction and chronic obstructive pulmonary disease (COPD) attributed to SO2 exposure in six industrialized metropolises of Iran. Razi Journal of Medical Sciences 2016; 23(145): 12-21. [In Persian].
37. Kermani M, Dowlati M, Jonidi Jaffari A, Rezaei kalantari R. A Study on the Comparative Investigation of Air Quality Health Index (AQHI) and its application in Tehran as a Megacity since 2007 to 2014. Journal of Research in Environmental Health 2016; 1(4): 275-284. [In Persian].
38. Kermani M, Fallah Jokandan S, Aghaei M, Dowlati M. Estimation ofcardiovascular death, myocardial infarction and chronic obstructive pulmonarydisease (COPD) attributed to PM and SO2 in the air of Tehran metropolis. Journal of Research in Environmental Health 2016; 2(2): 116-126. [In Persian].
39. Kermani M, Dowlati M, Jonidi Jaffari A, Rezaei Kalantari R. A Study on the comparative investigation of air qualityin tehran metropolis over a five-year period using air quality index (AQI). Journal of Health Research in Community 2016; 2(1): 28-36. [In Persian].
40. Kermani M, Dowlati M, Jonidi Jafari A, Rezaei Kalantari R. Estimation of mortality, acute myocardial infarction and chronic obstructive pulmonary disease due to exposure to O3, NO2, and SO2 in ambient air in Tehran. Journal of Mazandaran University of Medical Sciences 2016; 26(138): 96-107. [In Persian].
41. Soleimani Z, Parhizgari N, Dehdari Rad H, Akhoond MR, Kermani M, Bagherian Marzouni M, et al. Normal and dusty days comparison of culturable indoor airborne bacteria in Ahvaz, Iran. Aerobiologia 2015; 31(2): 127-41. doi: 10.1007/s10453-014-9352-4.

21

Assessment of role of concrete factories in particulate matter emissions, 2015-2016, using the AQI index and zoning by GIS software (Case study: Nasr Kashan Concrete Factory)

Shahnaz Kushkbaghi[1], Mohammad Hassan Ehrampoush[2*], Seyed Abolghsem Mirhosseinidehabadi[3]

[1]MSc of Environmental Health Engineering, Department of Environment, School of Agriculture and Natural Resource, Yazd Branch, Islamic Azad University, Yazd, Iran

[2]Professor of Environmental Health Engineering, Research Center for Environmental Health Technology, Department of Environmental Health, School of Health, Shahid Sadoghi University of Medical Sciences, Yazd, Iran

[3]Associate Professor, Department of Environment, School of Agriculture and Natural Resource, Yazd Branch, Islamic Azad University, Yazd, Iran

Abstract

Background: Reducing the effects of climate change and air pollution is a global priority at present. To formulate effective policies for achieving such a reduction requires a good understanding of the underlying phenomena. This study assessed the role of Nasr Kashan Factory in the emissions of particulate matter (PM).

Methods: In this cross-sectional study, PM concentrations at 9 stations inside and around the Nasr Kashan Concrete Factory were determined at the unit's active and inactive times. The air quality index (AQI) was obtained and data was entered into ArcGIS 10.2 to obtain a zoning map of PM dispersion.

Results: The results showed that all AQI peaks were within the very healthy or the healthy range at the Factory's inactive times. When the factory was working, the AQIs ranged from 24.1 to 634 $\mu g/m^3$, which falls into the good and very hazardous categories. These results were dependent upon distance from the factory and were further affected by other produced factors of PM10.

Conclusion: The results of this paper showed that average PM emissions at the Nasr Kashan Concrete Factory were much lower during inactive times than during times of activity. Therefore, the Nasr Kashan Concrete Factory plays an important role in the emission of PM and in air pollution in the studied area. PM concentrations were higher near and inside the studied factory, and the AQI was in the hazardous category.

Keywords: Air pollution, Particulate matter 10, Software GIS, Air quality index, Kashan

***Correspondence to:**
Mohammad Hassan Ehrampoush
Email: m.ehrampush.ssu@gmail.com

Introduction

At present, reducing the effects of climate change and air pollution is a global priority. Therefore, devising effective policies is a challenge that requires a good understanding of the underlying phenomena of climate change and air pollution (1). Air pollution due to industrialization and urbanization is one of the major environmental issues of the current century, especially in developing countries. Air pollution is a mixture of different atmospheric pollutants such as particulate matter (PM), nitrogen dioxide (NO2), carbon monoxide, ozone, sulfur dioxide, etc. In recent decades, researchers have investigated short-term and long-term exposure to air pollutants and the outcome of such exposure on human health (2).

The chemical and physical properties of PM are of great importance in the area of environmental and health effects (3). Two groups of particles are particularly important: particles smaller than 10 microns (PM10) that enter the lower parts of the lung, and particles smaller than 2.5 microns (PM2.5) that are deposited in the alveoli and also enter the blood flow. Numerous studies conducted on the human body have shown that there is a significant relationship between upper and lower lung infections and increased concentrations of PM and sulfur dioxide in the air. On average, 35 $\mu g/m^3$ of PM10 cause 55 of each 100 000 deaths. The size of these particles is directly related to their ability to cause harm to human health. Particles with a diameter of 10 microns or less present a higher risk for

health (3).

To report air pollution through the mass media, indicators are used. First, the indicator of air pollution (PSI1) was used to report the severity and effects of air pollution. In 1999, the US Environmental Protection Agency (EPA) introduced the air quality index (AQI), which emphasized smaller particles (PM2.5). The AQI shows the effects of polluted air on health. This indicator is calculated using a formula and the concentration of pollutants (carbon monoxide, ozone in the Earth's surface, PM, sulfur dioxide, and NO2). After calculating, the range 0-500 is divided into different zones and each zone shows the amount of air pollution (4).

In general, the AQI of a region enables people to determine the qualitative status of the weather as it regards health and hygiene. In addition, managers and officials use the AQI to prescribe precautions required for each of the items of air quality.

The most important sources of PM in the air of large cities include particles worn from vehicle brake pads, asphalt streets, and metal compounds from industrial processes such as lead, cadmium, sulfates, pollen, microorganisms, particles, and soot (5).

An important and effective measure for finding suitable methods for removing the risks and damages of air particles is to determine the actual amount of particulate matter emissions, compare the air quality with standards, and give simple notification to the public when air quality and pollution go beyond standard levels (6,7).

This study assessed the particulate matter emissions of Nasr Kashan Concrete Factory using the AQI and zoning with GIS software.

Studies in other cities have shown that high PM_{10} levels affect increases in morbidity and mortality rates (8). Studies have indicated that common concentrations of PM_{10} adversely impact health in many urban areas. These impacts include aggravation of existing respiratory disease and decline in lung function (9).

The study by Hosseini et al on the city of Sanandaj showed that the average PM_{10} concentration was 160.63 µg/m, and the lowest and highest concentrations of particulate matters occurred in the months of May and June, respectively. Average concentrations of PM_{10} on non-dusty days was 96.88 (µg/m), which is 4.8 times higher than on dusty days. On dusty days, the dominant elements in PM_{10} were Na, Ca, Mg, Al, and Fe contributing to 95.72% of total measured metals. Concentrations of PM_{10} during dusty days were considerably higher than that during non-dusty days. The WHO ranked Sanandaj as the third most polluted city in the world in terms of PM_{10} (10).

The WHO ranked Sanandaj as the third most polluted city in the world in terms of PM_{10} (11).

Materials and Methods

Study area

The Nasr Kashan Concrete plant is located in northeastern Kashan at the intersection of Nosh Abad and Mohammad Abad roads. The latitude and longitude of this area is 51° 26′ 30″ East and 34° 1′ 38″ North, and its altitude is 920 meters above sea level (Figure 1).

There are seven truck mixers and three concrete transfer pump machines in this plant. The daily production rate is about 480 tons of concrete and includes all two sand tissues, gravel and pebble sand for different uses. In addition, there are 5 cement silos at this plant. The plant has an area of about 2300 m², and the height of the wall is about 230 cm.

Sampling

To measure the amount of pollution created by the plant in terms of PM in the air, 9 stations in areas surrounding the plant were identified. Because of the heterogeneous nature of the environment around the plant (vacant lands, other factories, gardens, etc), sampling was done mainly on vacant lands along roadways; pollution caused by the plant and noise pollution caused by traffic on the roads were also taken into consideration. Figure 2 and Table 1 show the position of sampling stations.

Sampling was performed with 12 reps at each station, based on the National Institute for Occupational Safety and Health (protocol 0500) (9). This method was used to determine the concentration of suspended particles that

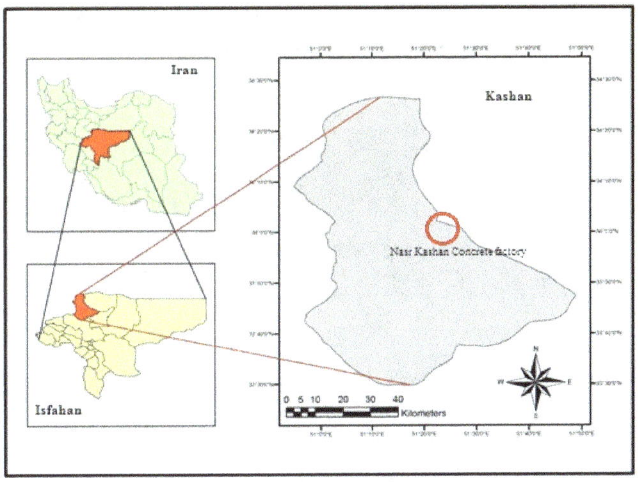

Figure 1. Location of Kashan city and Nasr Kashan Concrete factory.

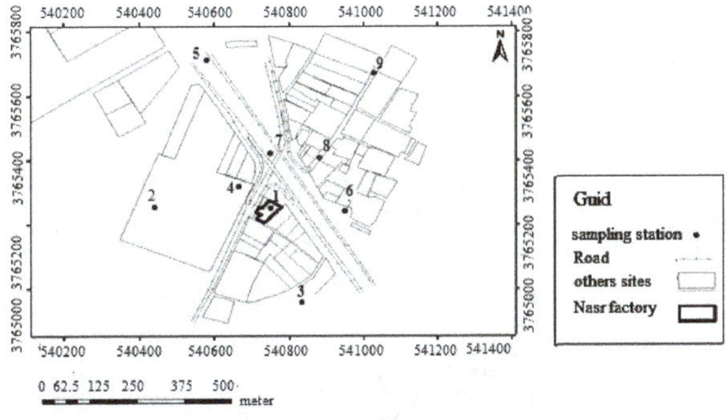

Figure 2. Sampling stations in studied area.

Table 1. Location of sampling stations in studied area

Station	Coordinate (m)		Distance of the factory (m)	Location
1	540750/5	3765252/55	0	Inside of the studied factory
2	540439/6	3765255/57	310.88	Empty land in the West of the
3	540835/7	3764960/03	304.68	Empty area out of structures in the south of Nasr factory
4	540667/1	3765320/02	107.3	Empty land in the West of the studied factory
5	540581/5	3765713/03	490.5	Between Mohammad Abad road in north of Nasr factory
6	540951/1	3765242/16	200.8	East Road of Nasr factory on the edge of the road and private places
7	540749/2	3765423/58	171	Crossing the road of Noushabad and Mohammad Abad in the north of Nasr factory
8	540883/7	3765408/76	205.3	Inside of sub alley in the North East of Nasr factory
9	541028	3765670/6	501.8	Sub northeastern end of the sub alley in the North East of Nasr factory

affect people working in the plant. However, because the weather outside the factory was calm and without much air flow, the same method was used to measure pollutants. PVC filters with a diameter of 37 mm and 5 mm mesh and an SKC pump with an input capacity of 2 L/m were used in sampling. About 75 L of air was passed per filter station. Before sampling, filters were coded under laboratory conditions and then placed in special cassettes in sampling place was connected to the pump. After sampling, the cassettes were transferred directly to the laboratory and weighed with weighing scales (accurate to the milligram). Since the idle time in the factory was like the empty sampling time (Blank), the weight difference created in the filter was considered as the weight of PM. The concentration of particles in units of milligrams per cubic meter was obtained using the following equation:

$$C = \frac{(W_2 - W_1)}{V} \times 10^3 \qquad (1)$$

where *W1* and *W2* are weights of the filter before and after sampling (unit = mg), and *V* is the volume of air (75 mL).

Air quality index

Since the filters have 5-micron pores, the pollutant was PM10, the main pollution caused by factories producing materials.

The AQI was calculated for ground level ozone, particle pollution, carbon monoxide, and sulfur dioxide (the four major air pollutants regulated by the Clean Air Act). The EPA has established national air quality standards for each of these pollutants to protect public health (9,10). The AQI is divided into six levels of health concerns shown in Table 2.

Equation 2 is used by the EPA to calculate the AQI in terms of PM10 pollution intensity:

$$I = \frac{I_{high} - I_{low}}{C_{high} - C_{low}}(C + C_{low}) + I_{low} \qquad (2)$$

Where I_{high} and I_{low} are the upper and lower air quality indices for air quality, C_{high} and C_{low} are the upper and lower limit emissions (PM10) in the group of air quality, and C is pollutant concentration (11).

After determining the amount of pollution and the status of air quality, an air quality zoning map was generated using ArcGIS 10.2 software, and the measurements were taken at times of activity and inactivity at the factory.

Results

The average, maximum, and minimum PM concentrations and the zoning map of the PM concentrations taken from Nasr factory at both active and inactive times in the studied area are illustrated in Table 3 and Figures 3-5. Figures 6 and 7 show the zoning maps of the PM concentrations ($\mu g/m^3$) in the area.

Table 2. AQI and Health Implications (9,10)

AQI	Level of air pollution	Implications of health
0–50	Excellent	No health implications.
51–100	Good	Few hypersensitive individuals should reduce outdoor exercise.
101–150	Lightly Polluted	Slight irritations may occur, individuals with breathing or heart problems should reduce outdoor exercise.
151–200	Moderately Polluted (Unhealthy)	Slight irritations may occur, individuals with breathing or heart problems should reduce outdoor exercise.
201–300	Heavily Polluted (Very Unhealthy)	Healthy people will be noticeably affected. People with breathing or heart problems will experience reduced endurance in activities. These individuals and the elderly should remain indoors and restrict activities.
300+	Severely Polluted (Hazardous)	Healthy people will experience reduced endurance in activities. There may be strong irritations and symptoms and other illnesses may be triggered. The elderly and the sick should remain indoors and avoid exercise. Healthy individuals should avoid outdoor activities.

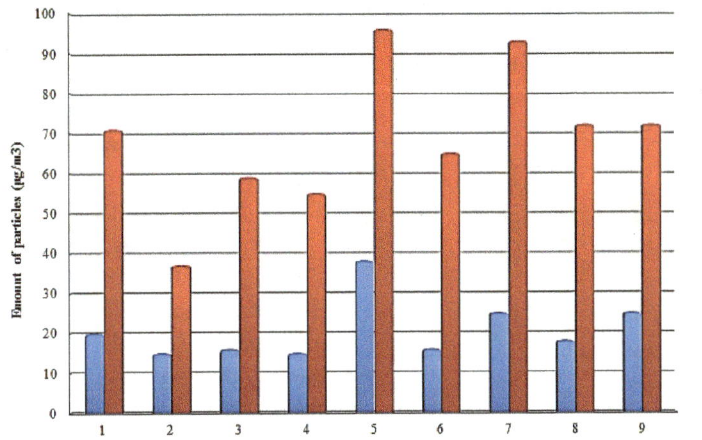

	1	2	3	4	5	6	7	8	9
the lowest of PM	20	15	16	15	38	16	25	18	25
the highest of PM	71	37	59	55	96	65	93	72	72

Figure 3. Maximum and minimum particulate matter concentrations at the time of inactivity of the factory in the studied area (µg/m³).

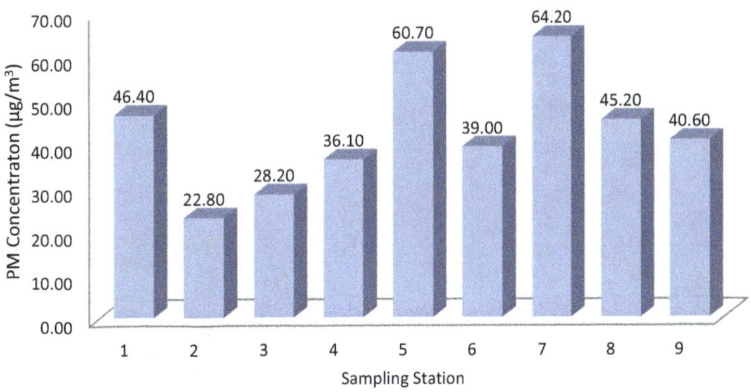

Figure 4. Mean concentrations of PM (µg/m³) at the time of inactivity of factory in the studied area.

The results showed that during inactive times, the PM air pollution around the factory is low. It became clear that the two stations on the periphery of the factory (Stations 5 and 7) had the highest amounts of PM, but levels were at a healthy level. The remaining stations were also low. Measurements showed that contamination was minimal in places where the land area was small and surrounded by walls.

Table 3 shows the standard deviation (SD) of PM at active and inactive times of the Nasr Kashan Concrete factory.

When the factory was active, the PM concentrations showed that pollution was highest at 738 µg/m³ in Station 1 inside the factory and lowest at 26 µg/m³ in Station 2. Moreover, there were significant increases in PM concentration at Stations 4, 6, and 8 (Table 1). PM dispersion measurements showed that significant pollution was created inside the studied factory and reached a distance of 100 to 200 m around it.

The results showed that the average amount of PM at the time of inactivity of Nasr factory was lower than the value recommended by the EPA (150 µg/m³) and WHO guidelines (50 µg/m³), except at stations 5 and 7; however, at the active times of the Nasr factory, the average PM concentration was higher than the value recommended by WHO guidelines, except at stations 9, 5, and 2, and lower than the EPA standard at all stations except Stations 4 and 2.

PM zoning maps for active times of the factory showed that the factory causes significant pollution, such that the PM10 concentration inside the factory was more than 500 µg/m³. As distance from the factory increased, air quality improved; PM concentrations were balanced at a distance of about 200 m from the factory (Figure 6).

Air quality index

The average, maximum, and minimum estimated AQIs taken from the Nasr factory at active and inactive times are compared in Table 4, and zoning maps for the AQI of PM are shown in Figures 8 and 9.

The calculated AQI at the time of inactivity showed that when the factory was inactive, the lowest AQIs (less than 30 µg/m³) were estimated at Stations 2 and 3. Zoning maps

Table 3. Standard deviation (SD) of PM at active and inactive times of Nasr factory

Station	SD of data at time activity	SD of data at time inactivity
1	119.49	14.42
2	8.85	6.78
3	20.68	13.11
4	73.59	13.01
5	11.70	14.85
6	57.29	16.67
7	45.66	20.88
8	75.79	19.00
9	14.52	13.54

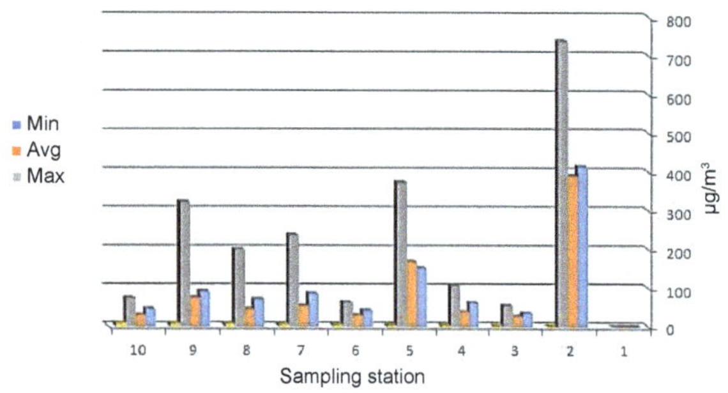

Figure 5. Concentration of particulate matter (µg/m^3) at the time of activity in the studied area.

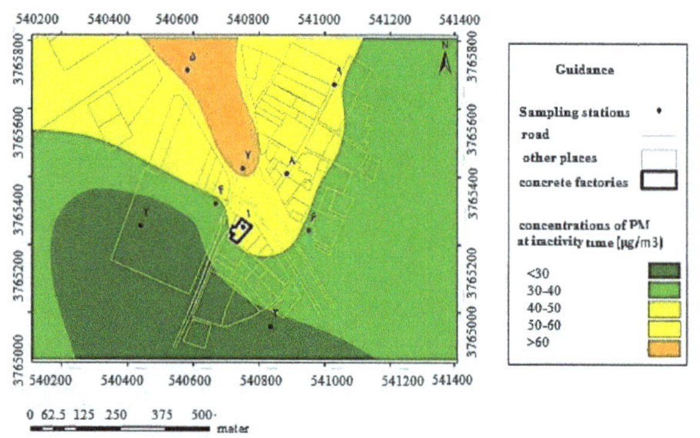

Figure 6. Zoning map of particulate matter concentrations (µg/m^3) at the time of inactivity of the factory in the studied area.

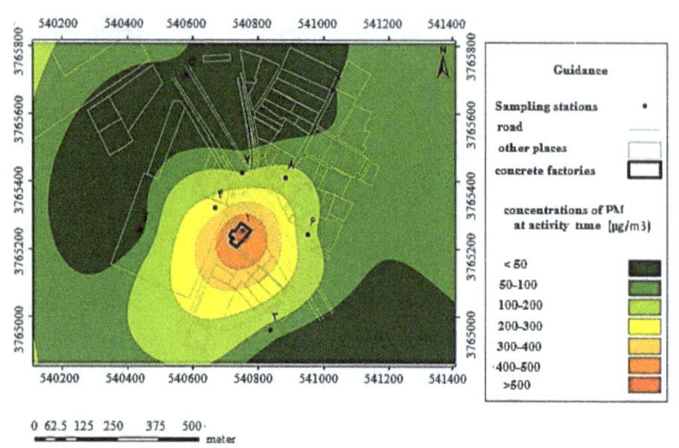

Figure 7. Zoning map of particulate matter concentrations (µg/m^3) at the time of activity of Nasr Kashan Concrete factory in the studied area.

at inactive factory times showed the highest amounts of pollution were found at Stations 5 and 7; the weather was reasonably clean and the AQI was in the range of very healthy (0-50) to healthy (51-100).

When the factory was inactive, the average AQI in the higher level was estimated to be 413.6 µg/m^3 and the air pollution level was hazardous. The lowest AQI (less than 50 µg/m^3) was estimated at Stations 2, 5, and 9 (Table 4). Maximum AQIs were estimated at Stations 4, 6, 7, and 8 and were equal to 225.4, 141.6, 123.3, and 184.2 µg/m^3, respectively.

The AQI zoning map showed that the air quality was very healthy at Stations 2, 5, and 9 (outside the factory) and unhealthy and very hazardous at Stations 4 (60 to 80 m from the factory) and 1, respectively, at active factory times (Figure 8); therefore, the air quality was improved at greater distances from the factory. Finally, at a distance of 100 to 200 m, the air quality returned to normal levels.

Discussion

The results of this paper showed that the average PM concentration was much lower at inactive times than at active times of the Nasr factory; hence, Nasr Kashan Concrete Factory played an important role in the emissions

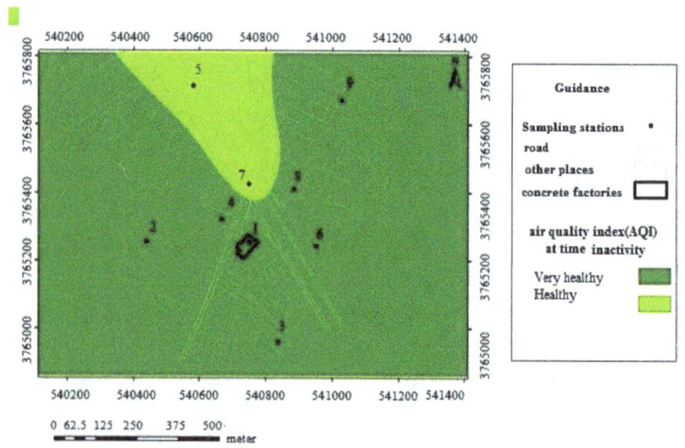

Figure 8. Zoning map of AQI of PM at inactive times of the Nasr factory in the studied area

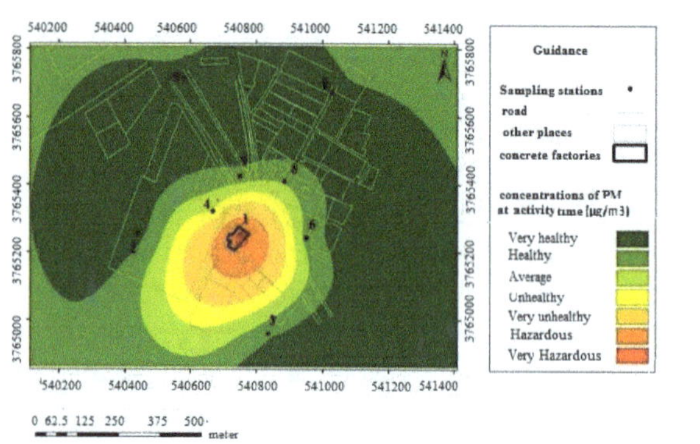

Figure 9. Zoning map of air quality index of particulate matter at active times of the Nasr factory in the studied area.

Table 4. Comparison of air quality indexes at active and inactive factory times (μg/m³)

Station	AQI at time activity			AQI at time inactivity		
	Maximum	Minimum	Average	Maximum	Minimum	Average
1	634	249.8	413.6	59.3	18.5	43
2	51	24.1	34.4	34.3	13.9	21.1
3	76.2	35.2	61.4	53.5	14.8	26.1
4	225.4	107.4	151.8	51.5	13.9	33.4
5	55.4	26.9	41.6	71.6	35.2	53.8
6	141.6	51	86.5	56.4	14.8	36.1
7	123.3	41.7	71.3	70.1	23.1	55.5
8	184.2	61.3	91.6	59.8	16.7	41.8
9	60.8	26.9	45.4	59.8	23.1	37.6

of particulate matters and air pollution in the studied area, such that the particulate matter concentration increased near and inside the studied factory, and the AQI reached the hazardous level. This pollution can pose a serious threat to workers and experts working in the factory. Particulate matter is the main factor of many respiratory diseases occurring among citizens in their places of residence and work. A study conducted in 51 countries found that when the air pollution index increases up to 60 ppm, incidence of coronary heart disease also increases up to 10% (12). Particulate matter 2.5 (PM2.5) are well-known criteria pollutants that pose a risk to public health (9-11). Studies have shown that ambient air pollution is associated with increased risk of respiratory disease and cardiovascular disease (CVD) mortality (13).

In addition, increasing concentrations of particulate matters and secondary hydrocarbons and ozone cause significant increases in rates of ventricular heart and blood pressure and complications in older people (14,15). Long-term increases in these pollutants with ozone cause heart attack and fatal cardiovascular disease (16,17). Increase in the amount of particulate matter (10 micrograms per cubic meter) increases these attacks by 2% percent (7).

In this study, the average concentration of particulate matter at inactive times of Nasr factory (22/8-64/2 μg/m³) was lower than the recommended EPA standard (155-254 μg/m³), but at times of activity of Nasr factory, the average concentration of PM was higher than the value recommended by WHO guidelines (5,18). In the same study by Jafarzadeh Haghighi et al (19) on the national Iranian steel industry, the average TSP concentration in sampled air was higher than the standard value and the standard of Iran (EPA = 250 μm/m³). The annual average of the samples was 649 micrograms per cubic meter. So this study showed that environmental factors affect the dispersion and distribution of air pollution. Hence, the height of the Nasr Kashan Concrete factory wall may be an important factor in reducing the dispersion of pollution. The emission height of PM10 (mixing tank cement, sand, and water) is 3 m when the factory is active, but the height of the factory wall is 230 cm. Therefore, raising the height of the factory walls to higher than 3 m will make a significant reduction in the amount of particles dispersed. An important subject is that concrete companies are easy to move and settle; therefore, when large civil projects are in progress in an area, concrete companies are easily established and increase PM pollution in that area, especially in large cities. Thus, it is recommended that concrete factories be established outside residential areas and the establishment of this type of factory in city centers and crowded places be prevented, especially at the time of the large construction operations.

Muindi et al (20) stated that outside sources have an impact on inside sources and levels, especially in areas closest to the studied area. Since the Nasr factory is located at the intersection of two major highways, it seems the transit of vehicles causes dust and dispersion of particulate matter in the streets and increases the volume of PM in the studied area, such as Stations 4, 6, and 7.

Conclusion

In this study, the AQI zoning map showed that the activity of the factory increased the PM10 concentration in the studied area with the highest levels found at stations inside the factory; however, PM10 levels decreased at distances of 200 m from the factory. It can be concluded that the Nasr Kashan Concrete factory causes PM pollution in the studied area.

The results showed that all peaks of the AQI were less than 60, falling into the good and very good categories of air quality at the inactive times of the factory. Thus, the AQI was in the range of very healthy (0-50) to healthy (51-100). When the factory was active, AQIs were in the range of 24.1 to 634 μm/m³, falling into the good and very hazardous categories. It seems that the index values were related to the distance of the stations from the factory. Based on the results of this study, it is recommended that the factory walls be raised as high as possible and fast-growing trees be cultivated near the factory. Furthermore, materials must be wet before production is started. Since lowlands are the best places for factories, it is proposed that the concrete plant be established outside of residential areas where people are most exposed to the greatest amounts of pollution caused by these activities.

Summary of recommendations:

- Transfer concrete factory to outside the city to reduce emissions of PM from the factory;
- Minimize particulate emissions to surrounding areas by growing plants and trees such as spruce and constructing walls as high as possible around the concrete plant to act as windbreaks;
- Conduct further studies in seasons other than autumn, when this research was conducted.

Acknowledgments

This research is derived from a Master's thesis. The authors express their appreciation to Iran's Environmental Protection Organization and the Nasr Beton factory for their cooperation in providing data.

Competing interests

The authors have no competing interests to declare.

Authors' contributions

All authors participated in data acquisition, analysis, and interpretation. All authors critically reviewed, refined, and approved the manuscript.

References

1. Mitran G, Ilie S. Study of particulate matters pollution related with meteorological factors for a city from South-Central of Romania. European Journal of Sustainable Development 2014; 3(4): 17-28. doi: 10.14207/ejsd.2014.v3n4p17.
2. Omidi Y, Goudarzi G, Heidari AM, Daryanoosh SM. Health impact assessment of short-term exposure to NO_2 in Kermanshah, Iran using Air Q model. Environmental Health Engineering and Management Journal 2016; 3(2): 91-7. doi: 10.15171/ehemj.2016.06.
3. Ali K, Budhavant KB, Safai PD, Rao PS. Seasonal factors influencing in chemical composition of total suspended particles at Pune, India. Sci Total Environ 2012; 414: 257-67. doi: 10.1016/j.scitotenv.2011.09.011.
4. Colls J. Air Pollution (Clays Library of Health & the Environment). 2nd ed. London: Spon Press; 2002.
5. EPA. Air Quality Index (AQI): Office of Air Quality Planning and Standards (OAQPS). USEPA, USA: 2006. http://www.epa.gov/airs/criteria.html.
6. Sharma M, Maloo, S. Assessment of ambient air PM_{10} and $PM_{2.5}$ and characterization of PM_{10} in the city of Kanpur: India. Atmos Environ (1994) 2005; 39(33): 6015-26. doi: 10.1016/j.atmosenv.2005.04.041.
7. Naddafi K. Nabizadeh R, Nazmara SH, Nurmordadi HA, Mohamadi Moghadam F. Investigation of TSP and PM10 and describing the air quality based on AQI index in the air of central areas in Tehran in 2007-2006. Health System Researches 2009; 6 (4): 657-65. [In Persian].
8. Naddafi K, Ehrampoush M, JafariV, Nabizadeh R, Younesian M. Investigation of total particulate matters and compounds of its constituent materials in the central region of Yazd. J Shahisadoghi University of Medical Sciences and Health Services of Yazd 2007; 6(4): 21-5. [In Persian].
9. NIOSH. NIOSH Health Hazard Evaluation Report No. 93-0775. http://www.cdc.gov/niosh/hhe/reports/pdfs/1993-0775-2398.pdf.
10. Hoseini G, Teymouri P, Shahmoradi B, Maleki A. Determination of the concentration and composition of PM10 during the Middle Eastern dust storms in Sanandaj, Iran. J Res Health Sci. 2015; 15(3): 182-188.
11. US EPA. Air Quality Index (AQI) - A Guide to Air Quality and Your Health. EPA; 2011. http://www.airnow.gov/index.cfm?action=aqibasics.aqi.
12. Ahmadi H, Ahmadi T, Shahmoradi B, MohammadiSh, Kohzadi Sh. The effect of climatic parameters on air pollution in Sanandaj, Iran. Journal of Advances in Environmental Health Research 2015; 3: 49-61.
13. Balluz L, Wen XJ, Town M, Shire JD, Qualter J, Mokdad A. Ischemic heart disease and ambient air pollution of particulate matter 2.5 in 51 counties in the U.S. Public Health Rep 2007; 122(5): 626-33. doi: 10.1177/003335490712200510.
14. Dockery DW, Schwartz J, Spengler JD. Air pollution and daily mortality: associations with particulates and acid aerosols. Environ Res 1992; 59(2): 362-73. doi: 10.1016/S0013-9351(05)80042-8
15. Thurston GD, Ito K, Kinney PL, Lippmann M. A multi-year study of air pollution and respiratory hospital admissions in three New York state metropolitan areas: result for 1988 to 1989 summers. J Expo Anal Environ Epidemiol 1992; 2(4): 429-50.
16. Prioleau WH. Fine particulate air pollution and cardiovascular disease. J S C Med Assoc 2009; 105(6): 202-3.
17. Chen LH, Knutsen SF, Shavlik D, Beeson WL, Petersen F, Ghamsary M, et al. The association between fatal coronary heart disease and ambient particulate air pollution: Are females at greater risk? Environ Health Perspect 2005; 113(12): 1723-9. doi: 10.1289/ehp.8190.
18. EPA. Air Quality Index Air Quality Index [A Guide to Your Health Air and Radiation]. EPA; 2003. http://www.epa.gov.
19. Rafiei M, Gadgil AS, Ghole VS, Jaafarzadeh N, Gore SD, Aberomand M, et al. Investigation of respirable particulate matter pollutants on air-breathing zone workers in the Beam Rolling Mills Factory (Iran National Steel Industrial Group), Ahvaz, Iran. Indian J Occup Environ Med 2008; 12(2): 71-5. doi: 10.4103/0019-5278.43264.
20. Muindi K, Kimani-Murage E, Egondi T, Rocklov J, Ng N. Household air pollution: sources and exposure levels to fine particulate matter in Nairobi slums. Toxics 2016; 4(3): 12. doi: 10.3390/toxics4030012.

Regeneration and treatment of sulfidic spent caustic using analytic hierarchy process

Asadollah Karimi[1], Esmaeil Fatehifar[2*], Reza Alizadeh[3], Iraj Ahadzadeh[4]

[1]Ph.D. Student, Environmental Engineering Research Center, Faculty of Chemical Engineering, Sahand University of Technology, Tabriz, Iran
[2]Professor, Environmental Engineering Research Center, Faculty of Chemical Engineering, Sahand University of Technology, Tabriz, Iran
[3]Associate Professor, Environmental Engineering Research Center, Faculty of Chemical Engineering, Sahand University of Technology, Tabriz, Iran
[4]Assiatant Professor, Faculty of Chemistry, Tabriz University, Tabriz, Iran

Abstract
Background: Sulfur compounds must be removed from petroleum because they contribute to environmental pollution. A strong alkaline solution such as caustic soda is used to remove these compounds. This spent caustic has high values for chemical oxygen demand (COD) concentration, pH and total sulfur. In this study, the regeneration and treatment methodology of sulfidic spent caustic was investigated by applying the analytic hierarchy process (AHP).
Methods: The evaluation index system developed was based on group decision-improved AHP. Expert Choice software was used to simplify decision-making when choosing a practical method and prioritizing treatment of spent caustic. Cost, environmental considerations, availability and scale-up were chosen as criteria and wet air oxidation and biological and catalytic methods were selected as alternative methods. The treatment and regeneration of spent caustic was carried out in a batch bubble column reactor loaded with IVKAZ catalyst and the effluent was treated in a precipitation-stirred tank reactor.
Results: Evaluation indicated that cost ranked first among criteria at 40.9%. The results showed that the proposed process produced about 13% (wt) of caustic, 50 g/L of COD and 36 g/L of S^{2-}.
Conclusion: The results indicate that the catalytic method was more effective (0.45) than wet air oxidation and the biological method. This process regenerated more than 85% of initial caustic and the economy of the process improved by the recycling of the stream of caustic.
Keywords: Catalytic oxidation, Wastewater treatment, Recovery, Expert Choice

***Correspondence to:**
Esmaeil Fatehifar
Email: fatehifar@sut.ac.ir

Introduction

Industrial wastewater is a major source of pollution in the environment and has negative consequences for human life. Refineries create deleterious waste that must be treated. Caustic scrubbing solutions are commonly used in liquefied petroleum gas units to eliminate impurities and acid constituents such as mercaptans, H_2S and CO_2. Spent caustic in wastewater is strictly handled and disposed of because it contains high amounts of contaminants. Spent caustic is a hazardous waste that can be classified reactive and highly corrosive because it contains sulfide and has a high pH value, respectively. Highly odorous spent caustic, usually sulphitics, may contain high levels of sulfide, mercaptan and phenol (1-3). The US Environmental Protection Agency (EPA) under the Resource Conservation and Recovery Act defines spent caustic as hazardous waste (2) and it is a major effluent from oil refineries (4). Table 1 lists the characteristics of spent caustic from liquified petroleum gas.

Conventional disposal methods such as dumping into deep wells or in the ocean are not acceptable solutions to this problem (3,5); this effluent must be treated and handled properly. Treatment of spent caustic can be carried out by either biological, chemical or thermal processes, each of which can be divided into subcategories (1). Treatment methods such as advanced oxygen process, wet air oxyidation (WAO), incineration, and biological or catalytic pathways which can be used separately or in combination are suggested for treatment of organic compounds (such as spent caustic waste) and refractory substances (6-8). Incineration is suitable for handling of effluent having more than 100 g/L of chemical oxygen

Table 1. Charactricties of spent caustic produced from liquefied petroleum gas

Item	Value
COD	100-200 g/L
S^{2-}	80-90 g/L
Mercaptans	0-30 g/L
pH	12-13.5
Phenols	0.002-0.3 g/L
Specific gravity	1.1
NaOH	4-5 wt%

demand (COD), but this treatment is expensive and produces more hazardous compounds (9). WAO is generally applied under strict operating conditions (10) using either low, medium or high temperature systems (11). The biological method is generally employed after pretreatment and cannot be applied directly or alone (12-14). The catalytic treatment is applied to research and industrial waste (15) and can reduced the COD 50% under mild operating conditions. The main oxidation reactions of spent caustic are (16,17):

$$NaOH + \frac{1}{2}\,Na_2S_2O_3 + O \rightarrow Na_2SO_4 + \frac{1}{2}\,H_2O \quad (1)$$
$$NaSH + 2O_2 + NaOH \rightarrow Na_2SO_4 + H_2O \quad (2)$$
$$NaSH + 2O_2 \rightarrow \frac{1}{2}\,Na_2S_2O_3 + \frac{1}{2}\,H_2O \quad (3)$$
$$2RSNa + \frac{1}{2}\,O_2 + H_2O \rightarrow RSSR + 2NaOH \quad (4)$$

In this study, analytic hierarchy process (AHP) was applied to simplify decision-making when choosing the most practical method from among WAO, biological and catalytic methods. AHP was also used to prioritize treatment and regeneration of spent caustic. Expert Choice software was chosen for evaluation of the three methods and was applied to predict the optimal methods of regeneration and treatment of spent caustic. The regeneration and treatment of spent caustic was developed at bench pilot plant scale. In this system, the spent caustic was oxidized in a heterogeneous batch reactor. The effluent of the first reactor was then precipitated with hydrated lime in the stirred mixed reactor. All experiments were carried out at the Environmental Engineering Research Center of Sahand University of Technology in October 2015. Figure 1 shows a schematic of the steps required.

Methods

Software preparation

The focus of this study was on spent caustic regeneration. The purpose was to specify the criteria for the intermediate levels and the decision alternatives (18). AHP addresses the influencing criteria and factors that require manual calculation or the use of software. Expert Choice software is easy to use for collaborative decision-making (18) and is the best choice for analyzing data having many variables to fulfill research objectives and limited resources.

The first step in AHP and the software is to develop a hierarchy by breaking the problem down into its components. The main criteria are developed in accordance with the spent caustic regeneration and treatment process. The four criteria selected are cost, environmental impact, availability and scale-up and the three methods selected were WAO, biological and catalyst methods. Figure 2 shows the hierarchy for this analysis. The basic design consists of pairwise criteria and alternatives.

Experimental procedure

Catalytic oxidation was used to treat and regenerate spent caustic from waste solution provided by a refinery in Iran. Figure 3 is a schematic of the two 500 mL batch reactors. The oxidation reactor is a bubble column with 40 µm pore size. The precipitation stirred tank reactor is a cylindrical glass column with an agitator (Figure 3). The cobalt phthalocyanine catalyst (JSC) was employed to treat and regenerate waste in the first reactor.

The temperature was determined using a 500 mL (shof-balloon of DW2) in the first reactor. A thermocouple was applied to detect the reactor temperature. The second reactor operated at ambient temperature. The system was operated at a constant stirring rate of 50 rpm for 60 minutes. Both reactors operated at atmospheric pressure. Catalytic oxidation reactions (1)-(4) were carried out in the first reactor. All solutions were made with deionized water. Standard thiosulfate titrant, standard iodine titrant, HCl and indicator were purchased from Merck for titration (S^{2-} and alkalinity). H_2SO_4, Ag_2SO_4, and $HgSO_4$ were purchased from Merck for COD determination. $CaCO_3$ was obtained from Carlo Erba for the lime solution. The alkalinity, pH, COD and S^{2-} of the effluent were analyzed using standard methods for the examination of water and wastewater (19). The COD concentration was measured by the dichromate method with a UV-Vis spectrophotometer (Jenway 6705). A pH analyzer (Metrohm) was applied for pH measurement. Temperature, reaction time and air flow were selected as the independent variables because these parameters contribute to completion of the reaction in the bubble column reactor. Experiments were also carried out

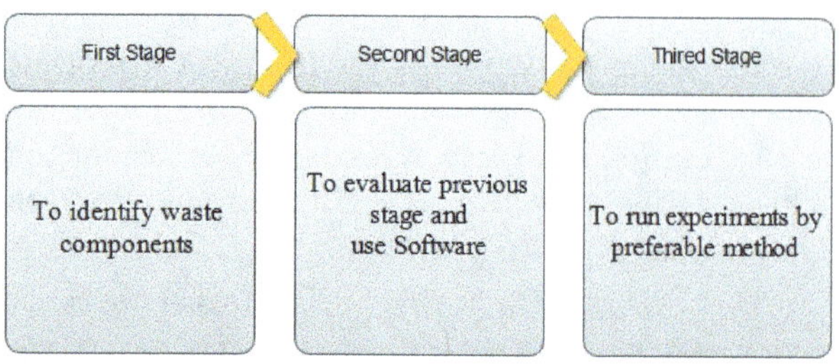

Figure 1. Study steps.

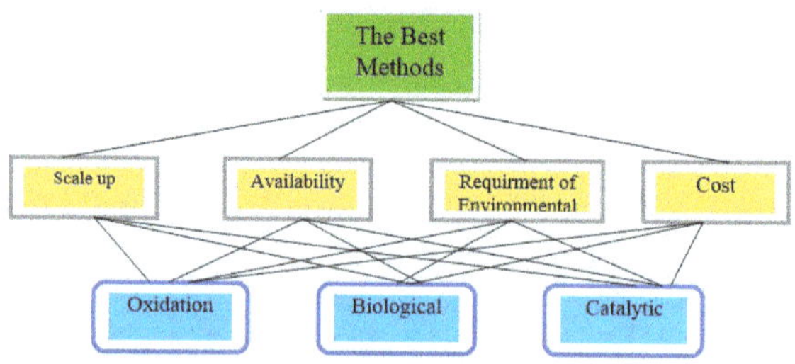

Figure 2. Hierarchy view of criteria and alternatives.

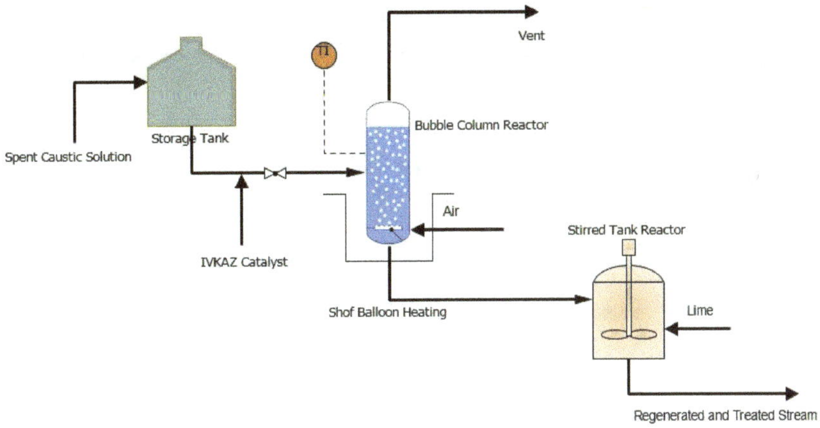

Figure 3. Schematic of bench scale pilot.

to assess temperature, reaction time and air flow. Table 2 lists the independent variables.

Results

Software results

A pairwise comparison was done based on the results for alternatives and criteria. The questionnaire design used a numerical scale ranging from 1 to 9 as shown in Table 3. The priority and importance of the alternatives and criteria were compared pairwise. Table 4 shows the pairwise comparison matrix of the main criteria.

The results of pairwise comparison are shown in Figure 4. The greatest preference was for cost at 40.9% and environmental impact ranked a strong seond (about 28%) after cost. Figure 5 shows that the overall inconsistency of these methods as rated by Expert Choice was 5%.

Experimental results

NaOH regeneration is shown in Figure 6 at 80 and 90°C for different reaction times at 7 and 10 L/min of air flow. Reaction time and temperature influenced the treatment efficiency of catalytic oxidation as evidenced by the improvements seen.

Figure 7 shows the S^{2-} concentration under the same conditions as in Figure 6. An increase in reaction time and temperature allowed reactions 1-4 to be completed, causing the S^{2-} concentration to decrease. Figure 8 shows that a decrease in S^{2-} decreased the COD concentration. COD concentration also decreased as the air flow increased at 80 and 90°C for 20-30 minutes of reaction time.

Table 2. The independent test variables

Independent variables	Value
Temperature (°c)	80-90
Reaction time (min)	20-30
Air flow (L/min)	7-10

Table 3. Preference qualitative for pair wise comparison method (20)

Value	Preferences
9	Extremely preferred
7	Very strongly preferred
5	Strongly preferred
3	Moderately preferred
1	Equally preferred
8, 6, 4, 2	-

Table 4. Pairwise comparsion matrix

	Cost	Requirement of environmental	Availability	Scale up
Cost	1	1	4	3
Requirement of environmental		1	3	1
Availability			1	4
Scale up				1

Inconsistency: 0.06

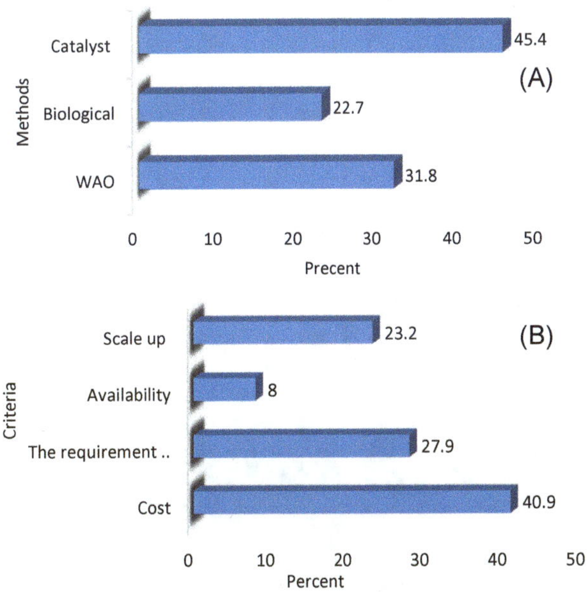

Figure 4. The result of pairwise comparison in expert choice software (A) Alternatives of regeneration (B) Criteria factor.

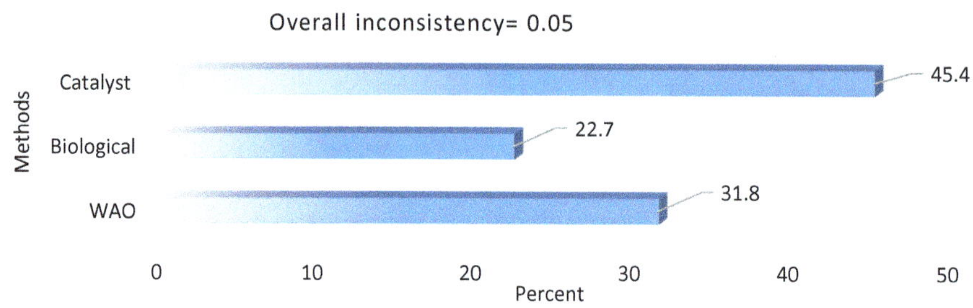

Figure 5. Overall inconsistency result in expert choice software.

Discussion

Software

The energy consumption of the WAO method was very high, so this process had a high fixed cost in comparison with the catalytic and biological methods. WAO is generally used as a pretreatment (8,9); therefore, the present method should be used as an auxiliary treatment. Although WAO cannot satisfy environmental requirements alone, it is one way to help alleviate pollutants such as COD and S^{2-}.

The performance of the biological method relates to COD concentration, phenolic components and pH. This method is restricted and could not be applied directly because a high level of COD and phenolic components can cause loss of microorganisms and treatment would cease (10,20). This means that the biological method must be employed through means such as WAO, which increases the total cost of processing.

The catalytic method decreased the COD concentration by 50% (15) and the operating condition were mild and employed separately. The investment and operational costs of the catalytic method was lower than the other methods. Note that catalytic oxidation scales up easily and can be employed without pretreatment (15); thus, it has top priority as an alternative method.

Overall inconsistency is a major area of evaluation of the AHP method. An inconsistency ratio of about 10% or less is usually considered "acceptable," but particular circumstances may warrant the acceptance of a higher value.

Experimental

Figure 6 shows that the impact of reaction time was more perceptible. An increase in temperature aided completion of reaction 4, increasing the percentage of caustic to 13.4% (wt). Temperature was the most remarkable variable, so the focus was on this factor. The LPG unit used 15% (wt) caustic for desulfurization of hydrocarbon and 13.4% (wt) of the caustic could be recycled back to the unit. The recycled stream helped reduce processing costs, which

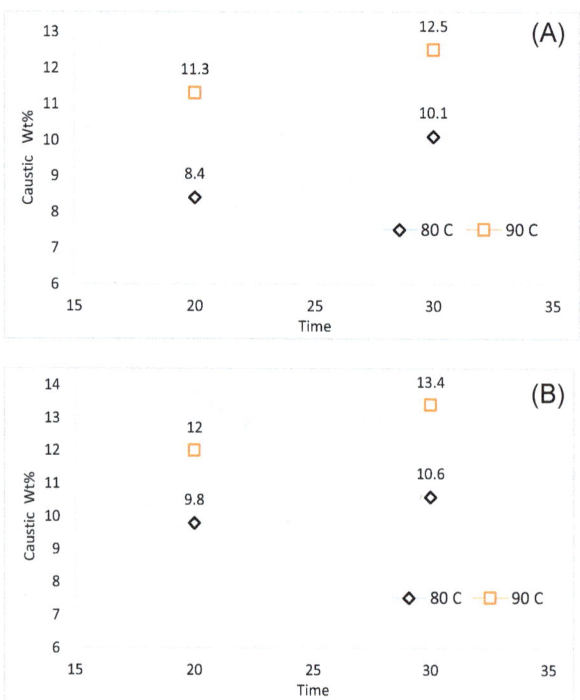

Figure 6. Amount of caustic after regeneration (A) 7 L/min and (B) 10 L/min.

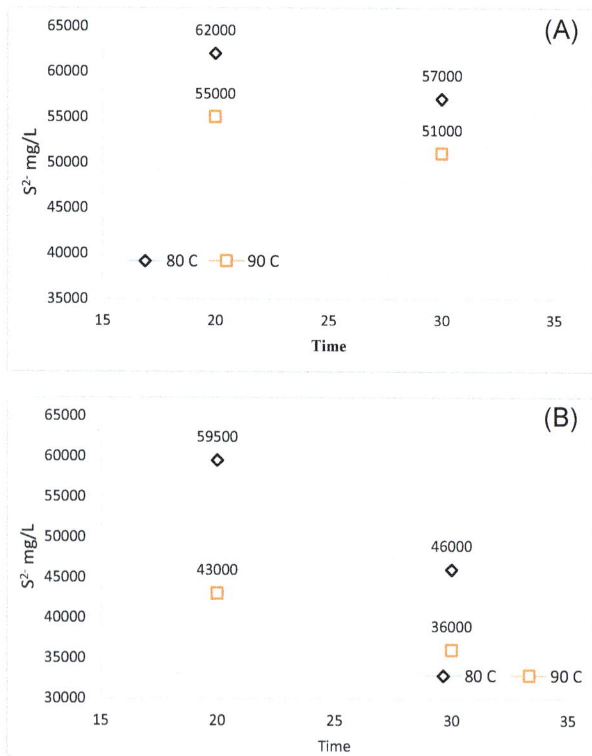

Figure 7. S^{2-} concentration value (A) 7 L/min and (B) 10 L/min.

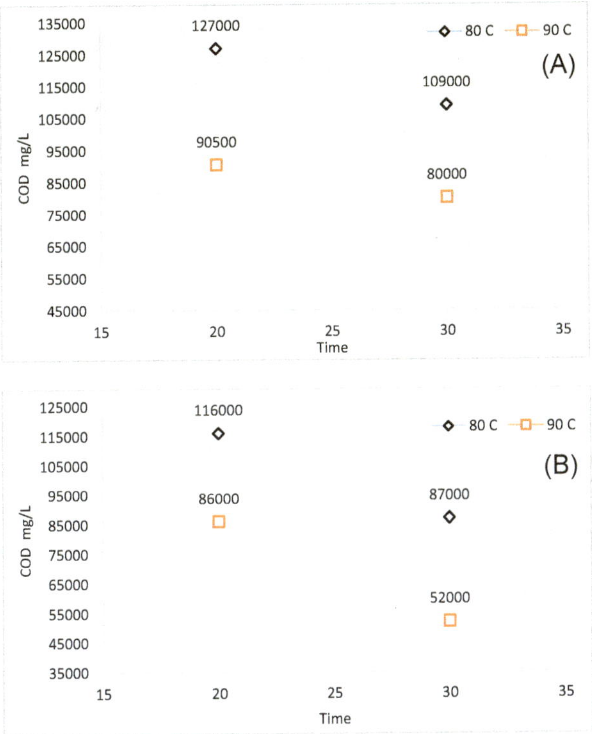

Figure 8. COD concentration value (A) 7 L/min and (B) 10 L/min.

were high. The reaction time was not long and was more favorable than for the WAO, advanced oxidation and biological methods (2,10,14,22).

Figure 7 demonstrated that efficient air flow decreasaed the S^{2-} concentration because the reactions reach completion in the bubble column reactor. Thiosulfate in alkaline media is a product of the chemical oxidation of sulfide (23-25). As the temperature increased, catalytic oxidation causedmore sulfides to be converted to sulfate and thiosulfate. The sulfate generated in the oxidation reactor occurs according to the precipitation reaction shown in Eq. (5) in the stirred tank reactor with lime.

$$Na_2SO_4 + Ca(OH)_2 \rightarrow CaSO_4 (s) \downarrow + 2 NaOH \quad (5)$$

The customary method of eliminating sulfate from wastewater is by the addition of hydrated lime. The precipitation reactor was designed to carry the reaction to completion; thus, sulfate and thiosulfate were generated in the bubble column reactor and reacted with $Ca(OH)_2$. Increased deposition of calcium sulfate occurred in the second reactor, decreasing the S^{2-} concentration.

Figure 6 shows a decrease in NaOH recovery from the spent caustic stream were the result of increased production of disulfides. As a result of catalytic oxidation (reactions 1 and 2), COD decreased because the sulfate was completely oxidized. The decline in generation of tiosulfide and sulfate increased the amount of S^{2-} and COD in Figures 7 and 8, respectively. It was found that increasing the air flow assisted in completion of the reactions. Figures 6-8 show that an increase in oxygen shifted the reaction to the right by eliminating the sulfide ions easily during reactions 20 and 3.

Conclusion

This study was divided into 2 parts: the AHP followed by a batch pilot plant study. The goal of AHP was to determine the optimum method for treating spent caustic waste. The preferred method was the catalytic method at 45.4% and this was selected as the proposed method. After selecting the best method for spent caustic regeneration and treatment, experiments were conducted using catalytic air oxidation in a batch bubble column and a mixed precipitation reactor. The best value for recovery of NaOH was 13.4% (wt) for an initial weight of 4% (wt), which could then be recycled. Reusing this stream improved the system by decreasing the cost of materials and reducing wastewater effluent. The temperature and pressure conditions were mild in this process. The S^{2-} of the effluent decreased from 81 to 36 g/L under the optimal conditions. This decreased the amount of S^{2-} by 45%. This decrease in S^{2-} decreased the COD in wastewater from 160 to 52 g/L.

Acknowledgments

The authors would like to thank the Environmental Engineering Research Center for their cooperation.

Competing interests

The authors declare that no competing interests exist.

Author contributions

All authors contributed equally and all authors participated in the data acquisition, analysis, and interpretation.

References

1. Hawari A, Ramadan H, Abu-Reesh I, Ouederni M. A comparative study of the treatment of ethylene plant spent caustic by neutralization and classical and advanced oxidation. J Environ Manage 2015; 151: 105-12. doi: 10.1016/j.jenvman.2014.12.038.
2. Sheu SH, Weng HS. Treatment of olefin plant spent caustic by combination of neutralization and Fenton reaction. Water Res 2001; 35(8): 2017-21. doi: 10.1016/S0043-1354(00)00466-8.
3. Ahmad W. Neutralization of Spent Caustic from LPG Plant at Preem AB Goteborg [dissertation]. Goteborg, Sweden: Chalmers University of Technology; 2010.
4. Munirasu S, Haija MA, Banat F. Use of membrane technology for oil field and refinery produced water treatment—A review. Process Saf Environ Prot 2016; 100: 183-202. doi: 10.1016/j.psep.2016.01.010.
5. Grover R, Gomaa HM. Proven technologies manage Olefin plant spent caustic. Hydrocarbon Processing 1993; 72(9): 61-70.
6. Yadav A, Teja AK, Verma N. Removal of phenol from water by catalytic wet air oxidation using carbon bead – supported iron nanoparticle containing carbon nanofibers

in an especially configured reactor. J Environ Chem Eng 2016; 4(2): 1504-13. doi: 10.1016/j.jece.2016.02.021.

7. Golmohammadi S, Ahmadpour M, Mohammadi A, Alinejad A, Mirzaei N, Ghaderpoori M, et al. Removal of blue cat 41 dye from aqueous solutions with ZnO nanoparticles in combination with US and US-H_2O_2 advanced oxidation processes. Environmental Health Engineering and Management Journal 2016; 3(2): 107-13. doi: 10.15171/EHEM.2016.08.
8. Jaafarzadeh Haghighi Fard NA, Jorfi S, Ahmadi M, Mirali S, Kujlu R. Treatment of mature landfill leachate by chemical precipitation and Fenton advanced oxidation process. Environmental Health Engineering and Management Journal 2016; 3(1): 35-40.
9. Debellefontaine H, Chakchouk M, Foussard JN, Tissot D, Striolo P. Treatment of organic aqueous wastes: wet air oxidation and wet peroxide oxidation. Environ Pollut 1996; 92(2): 155-64. doi: 10.1016/0269 7491(95)00100-X.
10. AlNaizy R. Economic analysis for wet oxidation processes for the treatment of mixed refinery spent caustic. Environ Prog Sustain Energy 2008; 27(3): 295-301. doi: 10.1002/ep.10261.
11. Zhu W, Bin Y, Li Z, Jiang Z, Yin T. Application of catalytic wet air oxidation for the treatment of H-acid manufacturing process wastewater. Water Res 2002; 36(8): 1947-54. doi: 10.1016/S0043-1354(01)00419-5.
12. Conner JA, Beitle RR, Duncan K, Kolhatkar R, Sublette KL. Biotreatment of refinery spent-sulfidic caustic using an enrichment culture immobilized in a novel support matrix. Appl Biochem Biotechnol 2000; 84-86: 707-19.
13. de Graaff M, Bijmans MF, Abbas B, Euverink GJ, Muyzer G, Janssen AJ. Biological treatment of refinery spent caustics under halo-alkaline conditions. Bioresour Technol 2011; 102(15): 7257-64. doi: 10.1016/j.biortech.2011.04.095.
14. Oh SY, Shin DS. Removal of total dissolved solids in spent caustic using biochar: pretreatment for subsequent biological treatment. Clean Soil Air Water 2015; 43(1): 92-5. doi: 10.1002/clen.201300784.
15. UOP LLC. http://www.uop.com. Accessed August 1, 2007.
16. Mohammadbeigi K, Tajerian M. Demercaptanization of Distillate (DMD). Petroleum & Coal 2004; 46(1): 17-22.
17. Matthews R. Performance update: low pressure wet air oxidation unit at Grangemouth, Scotland. Environ Prog Sustain Energy 1997; 16(1): 9-12. doi: 10.1002/ep.3300160113.
18. Ramanathan, R. A note on the use of the analytic hierarchy process for environmental impact assessment. J Environ Manage 2001; 63(1): 27-35. doi: 10.1006/jema.2001.0455.
19. Eaton AD, Clesceri LS, Rice EW. Standard Methods for the Examination of Water and Wastewater. 21st ed. Washington DC: American Public Health Association; 2005.
20. Ghodsipur SH. Multiple objective decision making (MODM). Tehran: Amirkabir University Press; 2006. [In Persian].
21. Najaf Poor AA, Dousti S, Joneidi Jafari A, Hosseinzadeh A. Efficiency in phenol removal from aqueous solutions of pomegranate peel ash as a natural adsorbent. Environmental Health Engineering and Management Journal 2016; 3(1): 41-6.
22. Czimer B, Kovács A, Petró J. Treatment of Spent Merox Caustic Waste in Industrial Ecology Frames. Period Polytech Chem Eng 2015; 59(3): 215-20. doi: 10.3311/PPch.7601.
23. Millano EF, Sorber CA. Treatment of thiosulfate-containing wastewater in activated sludge systems. J Water Pollut Control Fed 1986; 58(9): 917-923.
24. Karimi A, Fatehifar E, Alizadeh R, Ahadzadeh I. Regeneration of Spent Caustic of Olefin Unit in a Bubble Column Reactor: Treatment and Recovery Optimization. Environ Prog Sustain Energy 2016. doi: 10.1002/ep.12433.
25. Rolia E, Chakrabarti CL. Kinetics of decomposition of tetrathionate, trithionate, and thiosulfate in alkaline media. Environ Sci Technol 1982; 16(2): 852-7. doi: 10.1021/es00106a006.

23

Modeling of CO and NO_x produced by vehicles in Mashhad, 2012

Ali Asghar Najafpoor[1], Ahmad Hosseinzadeh[2,3], Somaye Allahyari[2,3*], Allah Bakhsh Javid[4], Habibollah Esmaily[5]

[1]Associate Professor, Health Sciences Research Center, Department of Environmental Health Engineering, School of Health, Mashhad University of Medical Sciences, Mashhad, Iran
[2]MSc Student, Health Sciences Research Center, Department of Environmental Health Engineering, School of Health, Mashhad University of Medical Sciences, Mashhad, Iran
[3]Student Research Committee, Mashhad University of Medical Sciences, Mashhad, Iran
[4] Assistant Professor, Department of Environmental Health Engineering, School of Health, Tehran University of Medical Sciences, Tehran, Iran
[5]Associate Professor, Health Sciences Research Center, Department of Biostatistics, School of Health, Mashhad University of Medical Sciences, Mashhad, Iran

Abstract
Background: In large cities, the share of vehicles in air pollutants emissions is nearly 70% that is mainly due to use of fossil fuels. Environmental simulation has many advantages such as accuracy and speed of modeling. Present study was conducted to create a model of air pollution [Carbon Monoxide (CO) and Nitrogen Oxides (NO_x)] from vehicles in fifty following years, in Mashhad.
Methods: According to the collected data from license plate, traffic and transportation organizations, modeling of CO and NO_x was performed by STELLA software. Hence, five strategies, including reduction in the number of imported vehicles and the proportion of distance traveled by vehicles, increase in the number of junked vehicles, application of Euro 4 standards instead of Euro 3 and a combination of their application, were applied in the model.
Results: In the current condition, CO and NO_x concentrations are 27,894 and 2,121, and after 50 years they would be 26,227,930 and 2,070,011 ton/year, respectively. Applying the aforementioned strategies, their concentrations were declined approximately (35% and 35%), (50% and 50%), (16% and 16%), (7% and 47%) and (75% and 85%), correspondingly.
Conclusion: Developed model showed that if the present condition remains stable, air quality will be more and more undesirable in the 50 following years. However, application of the second method, reduction of the distance traveled, was the most effective strategy in reducing the amounts of ones, so it will be better that this strategy is considered in the administrative policies. Nevertheless, as far as possible all of them ought to be taken advantage of.
Keywords: Modeling, Air pollution, CO, NO_x, Mashhad

***Correspondence to:**
Somaye Allahyari
Email: allahyaris891@gmail.com

Introduction

Air pollution is a notable environmental threat for human health, and its impacts on economic activities carry on to be a global anxiety. Air pollution is the presence of one or more pollutants or the blend of them in atmosphere for a certain period of time (1). Air pollution is composed of industrial progression, cities enlargement, population accumulation, increasing motorist vehicles, increasing the use of oil production, and in some cases, regional and topography circumstances (2). Although technology improvement plays an important role to decline vehicles emissions, decrease of air pollution will remain as a challenge owing to increase transportation demand (3). Numerous pollutants, such as CO, NO_x, SO_x, O_3, and dust the combination of which forms photochemical smog are produced in cities (4). Based on conducted studies, the share of vehicles in air pollutants emissions is nearly 70% in metropolises that is mainly due to use of fossil fuels, also CO and NO_x were known as the most common pollutants produced in vehicles (5). Since pollutants have a destructive effect on human health, animals, plants, and buildings, they cause types of cancers, optical diseases, breath disorders, genetic mutation, and also environmental problems such as acid rain and ozone layer depletion. Determination of the real concentrations of the pollutants and description of air quality in comparison with standards are effective ways to control air quality (6). Nowadays, modeling in many scientific fields, especially environmental science is vastly used among which air pollution modeling is also placed (7). Modeling is transformation of statistical concepts to mathematical relations which is necessary for perception of a process. In fact, cause and effect relations among variables can obviously be evaluated by a model. Development of mathematical model requires skill, talent, experience, creativity, and innovation. Mathematical models can be used in research, development, design, and engineering economics. Mathematical modeling often requires numerous assumptions that are reasonable as possible. Most complicated models that have minimal assumptions for their development require a lot of time in order to simulate. When evaluating the results of the model, limitations imposed by assumptions should be considered (8). In many countries as well as Iran, plenty of studies have been conducted about modeling of air pollution. Modeling and prediction of carcinogenic polycyclic aromatic compounds and ozone concentration have been performed in Tehran and Mashhad, respectively (9,10). In a study in Greece and Finland, multiple regression model was used for prediction of NO_x and PM_{10} concentrations, which were compared with those of artificial neural network model (11). Modeling the spread of pollutants can show the effects of different parameters changes in production and emission of pollutants. Environmental simulation in the form of environmental models, particularly done by modern computers, has many advantages such as modeling accuracy and speed. A model can simulate the effects of new programs and ideas without spending time in the real world. Mashhad city is located in the northeast of Iran and between Binalood and Hezar Masjed mountain ranges. It is the capital of Khorasan Razavi province with 204 square kilometer area and attitude of 985 meters above the sea level. According to the 2011 census, its population was nearly 3,070,000 (12). The most important factor of air pollution in Mashhad, like all other Iranian metropolises, is transportation, so management of this problem requires a special attention. Present study was conducted to create a model of air pollution (CO and NO_x) from vehicles in fifty following years, in Mashhad.

Methods

This cross-sectional study was carried out for modeling the concentration of CO and NO_x produced by vehicles except diesel vehicles, buses, and minibuses in the next 50 years, using STELLA 8 software in Mashhad city. Data of vehicles were collected from license plate, Traffic and transportation organizations. STELLA software was used as a tool for dynamic simulation. To design dynamic systems model, in design page of the software, the figures of systems can easily be drawn using specific toolbars. After you draw figures, the software makes a convert of drawn figures to mathematical equations. To draw the general plane of system, the related icon was selected from the top of page and transferred into design page. In order to achieve desired system, these icons are displaced to achieve desired system. After drawing the general plane of system and determination of its equations in window environment, the simulation results can be shown as figures or tables. After completing the model, it can be implemented by referring to Stella table of contents and selecting Run or pressing on Ctrl-R keys. Also, with selection of Time space from Run, during the time period which has been considered for implementation of model, a change can be made in the calculations. First to run this model, the entire considered vehicles of Mashhad (514183) were classified into four groups by age, including up to 5, 5-10, 10-15, and over 15 years. For each one of the groups, a stock and a converter coefficient with regard to the number of junked vehicles including 0.002, 0.004, 0.007 and 0.013, respectively, were considered. It is necessary to mention that 18,000, the number of imported vehicles in that year, were added to the first stock. In this way, a system diagram was created on canvas and then transformed into mathematical relationships by STELLA. At the end of modeling, concentrations of the aforementioned pollutants were predicted in the following fifty years. Then to improve the future air quality, five strategies, including decreasing the number of imported vehicles and amount of distance traveled by vehicles, increasing the number of junked vehicles, applying Euro 4 standards instead of Euro 3, and combined application of these strategies, were applied in the software and influence of each was evaluated. The illustrative features of the developed model in the present study are exposed in Figure 1.

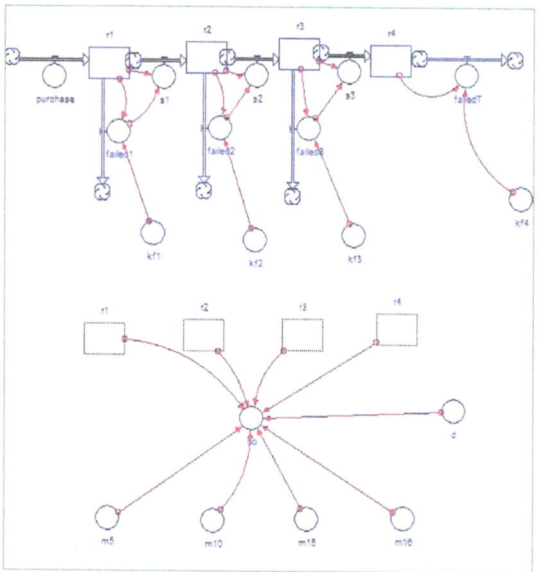

Figure 1. Dynamic model of air pollution for simulating the concentrations of CO and NO_x produced by vehicles using STELLA

Results

The results of STELLA software prediction for CO and NO_x, which were obtained based on aforementioned strategies over following fifty years have been presented in Tables 1 and 2, correspondingly.

In the first strategy, the is reduction of imported vehicles, if the number of bought vehicles decreases to half of its initial number (from 18,000 to 9,000), the amounts of CO and NO_x will be based on third columns of Tables 1 and 2, respectively. With application of this strategy, the amounts of CO and NO_x will be declined to nearly 9 million tons (from 26 to 17) and approximately 0.7 million tons (from 2 to 1.3), in that order.

In the second strategy, that is increasing the number of junked vehicles, with a double increase of convert coefficients from 0.002, 0.004, 0.007 and 0.013 to 0.004, 0.008, 0.014 and 0.026, junking rate can be augmented in the software. In this way, the amounts of CO and NO_x will be based on the forth column of Tables 1 and 2, correspondingly, and decrease of pollutants concentrations can be clearly observed; that is, the proportions of CO and NOx will be declined to almost 4 million tons (from 26 to 22) and 0.3 million tons (from 2 to 1.7), respectively.

In the third strategy, which is reduction of distance traveled by vehicles, if the amount of annual distance traveled by vehicles plummet to half of its initial proportion (from 20,000 to 10,000 km), as they have been presented in the fifth columns of Tables 1 and 2, the amount of CO and NOx will be plunged to half (from 26 and 2 to 13 and 1.03 million tons), correspondingly, in the next fifty years.

In the forth strategy, application of Euro 4 standards instead of Euro 3, if Euro 4 standards the application of which is necessary for cars since 2012 are replaced instead of Euro 3 in m5, m10, m15 and m16 converters, the amount of CO and NOx will be decreased approximately to 2 and 1 million tons, in that order, as it has been shown in the sixth columns of Tables 1 and 2. The Euro 4 and Euro 3 standards are displayed in Table 3.

In the fifth strategy, combined application of aforementioned strategies, if the number of imported vehicles along with annual distance traveled by vehicles are decreased, the number of junked vehicles is augmented, and Euro 4 standards are replaced instead of Euro 3, the amount of CO and NO_x will be fallen back based on the seventh columns of Tables 1 and 2, respectively. As it is observed, 74.74% and 85.5% decline can be the effects of this strategy in decreasing these two pollutants, in that order.

Discussion

According to the obtained model, if conditions of this present study do not change, life will be impossible in the future years owing to the increasing proportion of pollutants. In this study, the sensible result of each considered

Table 1. Amounts of CO in different conditions up to 50 next years (ton/year)

1	2	3	4	5	6	7
Year	Amount of CO with current conditions (2012)	Amount of CO with decline of imported vehicles	Amount of CO with increase of junked vehicles	Amount of CO with decrease of distance traveled	Amount of CO with application of Euro 4 standards instead of Euro 3	Amount of CO with combination of these four strategies
2012	27894	27894	27894	13947	23010	11505
2022	657353	570763	633867	328677	604292	253018
2032	2879861	2227775	2681220	1439931	2666909	956868
2042	7458985	5339300	6716488	3729493	6920845	2216682
2052	15053702	10197139	13123998	7526851	13978827	4094289
2062	26227930	17048996	22155481	13113965	24365203	6625708

Table 2. Amounts of NO_x in different conditions up to 50 next years (ton/year)

1	2	3	4	5	6	7
Year	Amount of NO_x with current conditions (2012)	Amount of NO_x with decline of imported vehicles	Amount of NO_x with increase of junked vehicles	Amount of NO_x with decrease of distance traveled	Amount of NO_x with application of Euro 4 standards instead of Euro 3	Amount of NO_x with combination of these four strategies
2012	2121	2121	2121	1060	1131	566
2022	51704	44924	49852	25852	27575	11531
2032	227056	175687	211381	113528	121097	43431
2042	588459	421282	529855	294230	313845	100506
2052	1187938	804744	1035615	593969	633567	185555
2062	2070011	1345629	1748534	1035006	1104006	300210

Table 3. Euro 4 and 3 standards for vehicles emissions (g/km)

		Euro 4 standards	Euro 3 standards	Convertor
CO	For vehicles up to 5 years old	1	2.3	m_5
	For vehicles over 5 years old	2.65	2.85	m_{10}
NO_x	For vehicles up to 5 years old	0.08	0.15	m_{15}
	For vehicles over 5 years old	0.12	0.225	m_{16}

2.85 and 0.225 have been calculated from the ratio between American and Euro 3 standards.

2.65 and 0.12 have been calculated from the ratio between American and Euro 4 standards.

strategy is shown by the obtained model. As the five proposed approaches were applied to the model in this study, the best strategy that had the lowest pollutants produced was the reduction of distance traveled by vehicles. In the following studies, modeling has been used for predicting future air quality as well. In a study by Saide *et al* (13), PM_{10} and $PM_{2.5}$ pollutions have been predicated by WRF-chem CO tracer in overnight steady-state conditions. The forecasting system has been based on precisely-simulating CO as a $PM_{10}/PM_{2.5}$ surrogate, since there is a strong correlation (over 0.95) amongst these pollutants. Therefore, the PM has been estimated by particular forecasting CO. Eventually, with regard to the simulations, forecasts which can be achieved by the system are proposed here. In fact, this is the largest merit of the presented systems (13). In another study by Banerjee *et al* (14), NO_2 concentration in Pantnagar (India) was determined by two mathematical models including Gaussian and combined models that are used for linear and industrial resources, respectively. These models illustrated that contribution of NO_2 produced in industries and vehicles is nearly 45-70% and 9-39%, correspondingly, and in air quality control, annual average of NO_2 is 32.6 μg/m^3. Thus, with statistical analysis, the accuracy of the model was obtained 61.9% (14). In the same study by Voukantsis *et al* (15), principle component analysis and artificial neural networks were used for the comparison of air pollution patterns of Thessaloniki and Helsinki and control of data in these regions. Then air quality forecast models were developed in the mentioned regions. Also forecasting model of PM_{10} and $PM_{2.5}$ concentrations was used for the following day predictions and the agreement index of daily data was measured. According to the model, the average of PM_{10} was between 0.8 and 0.85 that has been improved in comparison with prior studies prediction of quality parameters. In other words, performance of the model was evaluated by comparison of the obtained results from this model and the real condition, that indicates the results are pleased. In the present study, forecasting of CO and NO_x concentrations was performed by condition in 2012 (15).

Conclusion

To sum up, the amounts of the pollutants will decrease by applying each of the four main strategies listed above. Since the obtained results from the present study have proven that the greatest decline (nearly 50% in the quantity of CO and NO_x) was achieved by applying the third approach which is the reduction of the distance traveled by vehicles, so it will be better that this strategy is considered in the administrative policies. However, it needs to be mentioned that the highest reduce was obtained in the last strategy that is combination of first four method. Therefore, as far as possible, all the approaches mentioned above should be applied to implement the pollution reduction.

Acknowledgements

The authors would like to express their gratitude to the authorities of license plate, Traffic and Transportation organizations for their cooperation in this study. This study was financially supported by Mashhad University of Medical Sciences (MUMS).

Competing interests

The authors declare that they have no competing interests.

Authors' contributions

All authors participated equally in data acquisition, analysis and interpretation. All authors reviewed and approved the manuscript.

References

1. Alidadi H, Shakeri MT, Hoseinzadeh A, Noorani A. Relation between Mortality Rate and air pollutant concentrations in Mashhad, 2007-2009. Iranian Journal of Health Sciences 2013; 1(2): 68-74. [In Persian]
2. Khorasani N, Cheraghali M, Nadafi K, Karami M. Survey and comparison of Tehran and Isfahan air quality in 1378 and represntation of improvement methods. Iranian J Natural Res 2003; 55(4): 559-67. [In Persian]
3. Potoglou D, Kanaroglou PS. Carbon monoxide emissions from passenger vehicles: predictive mapping with an application to Hamilton, Canada.

Transportation Research Part D: Transport and Environment 2005; 10(2): 97-109.
4. Rowshan GR, Khosh Akhlagh F, Negahban S, Mirkatouly J. Impact of pollution on climate fluctuations in Tehran city. Environmental Sciences 2009; 7(1) 173- 92. [In Persian]
5. Emamzade A, Ghadamian H, Etabi F, Chehrazi S. Analyze and evaluate effects of turbocharge systems on fuel consumption and pollutants emmiss ions, "Tehran Bus" Company. JEST 2006; 8(2): 7-24. [In Persian]
6. Golbaz S, Jonidi Jafari A. A comparative study of health quality of air in Tehran and Isfahan; 2008-2009. Razi Journal of Medical Sciences 2011; 18(84): 38-46. [In Persian]
7. Nagendra SM, Khare M. Line source emission modelling. Atmospheric Environment 2002; 36(13): 2083-98.
8. Peiravi Minaee R, Alidadi H, Najafpoor A. Modeling of drought effects on variation of chemical water quality in the rural wells of Kashaf Rood area in Mashhad plain, 2006-2010 [Master dissertation]. Mashhad: Mashhad University of Medical Sciences; 2013. [In Persian]
9. Halk F. Determination of carcinogenic polyaromatic compounds in air by using dispersion modeling GIS. Environmental Studies 2008; 34(47): 37-42. [In Persian]
10. Seghatoleslami N, Moussavi M, ALAMI M. Modeling and forecasting of ozone in air of Mashhad city' using neural networks. Chemical Engineering of Iran 2013; 12(66): 12-20. [In Persian]
11. Vlachogianni A, Kassomenos P, Karppinen A, Karakitsios S, Kukkonen J. Evaluation of a multiple regression model for the forecasting of the concentrations of NOx and PM10 in Athens and Helsinki. Sci Total Environ 2011; 409(8): 1559-71.
12. Khosaran Razavi portal [home page on the internet]. Available from: http://www.khorasan.ir/tabid/60/Default.aspx
13. Saide PE, Carmichael GR, Spak SN, Gallardo L, Osses AE, Mena-Carrasco MA, *et al.* Forecasting urban PM10 and PM2.5 pollution episodes in very stable nocturnal conditions and complex terrain using WRF-Chem CO tracer model. Atmospheric Environment 2011; 45(16): 2769-80.
14. Banerjee T, Barman SC, Srivastava RK. Application of air pollution dispersion modeling for source-contribution assessment and model performance evaluation at integrated industrial estate-Pantnagar. Environ Pollut 2011; 159(4): 865-75
15. Voukantsis D, Karatzas K, Kukkonen J, Räsänen T, Karppinen A, Kolehmainen M. Intercomparison of air quality data using principal component analysis, and forecasting of PM10 and PM2.5 concentrations using artificial neural networks, in Thessaloniki and Helsinki. Sci Total Environ 2011; 409(7): 1266-76.

Evaluation and analysis of gaseous emission in landfill area and estimation of its pollutants dispersion

Amirreza Talaiekhozani[1*], Somaye Bahrami[2], Seyed Mohammad Javad Hashemi[3], Sahand Jorfi[4,5]

[1]Assistant Professor, Department of Civil Engineering, Jami Institute of Technology, Isfahan, Iran
[2]PhD Student of Environmental Engineering, School of Post Graduate, Islamic Azad University Branch of Bushehr, Bushehr, Iran
[3]M.Sc, Department of Civil Engineering, Jami Institute of Technology, Isfahan, Iran
[4]Assistant Professor, Environmental Technologies Research Center, Ahvaz Jundishapur University of Medical Sciences, Ahvaz, Iran
[5]Assistant Professor, Department of Environmental Health Engineering, School of Health, Ahvaz Jundishapur University of Medical Sciences, Ahvaz, Iran

Abstract
Background: The biogases are the mixture of gases produced through the microbial decomposition of organic waste which are amply observed in the landfills. The main purpose of this study was to estimate the emission rates of landfill gases such as carbon dioxide, methane and non-methane organic compounds (NMOCs) in the solid waste landfill of Rodan city in Hormozgan province.
Methods: All the necessary information such as population, geographic and climate of Rodan city were collected. Solid waste analysis was then conducted. Afterward, the LandGEM software is used in this study for the purpose of estimation of total biogas, methane, carbon dioxide and NMOCs emission from Rodan's landfill.
Results: The analysis of results showed that only 24.18% of the produced waste in this city is perishable. The calculations indicate that the peak of biogas production which is equal to 420 tons per year would be achieved in the year 2019. The production rates of carbon dioxide and methane in the same year would be equal to 308 and 112 tons per year respectively. The pollutants transmittance calculations in the vicinity of the landfill revealed that the maximum pollutant concentration is within the maximum distance of 200 m.
Conclusion: The results obtained in this study could be used for the purpose of design and installation of extraction or incineration equipment in the landfill of Rodan.
Keywords: Solid waste, Landfill, Biogas, Rodan city, LandGEM

***Correspondence to:**
Amirreza Talaiekhozani
Email: atalaie@jami.ac.ir

Introduction

In today's world, the waste compounds are addressed as environmental pollutants which would result in severe problems if not properly disposed. With this in mind, the waste disposal areas would play a vital role in the waste disposal networks which is the pivotal aspect of the general waste management strategy. The gas extraction equipment and energy consumption are presently the most significant component of the landfill areas (1,2). The disposed waste in landfill areas would be subjected to a variety of biochemical and physical reaction which could lead to the production and emission of substantial amount of gaseous components and liquids. Among these gasses, carbon dioxide and methane have significant importance due to their greenhouse properties (3). The installation of necessary equipment for the extraction of these gasses is essential in order to prevent their release into the atmosphere (4).

Biogas is the mixture of gases produced through microbial decomposition of organic compounds in anaerobic conditions. Generally, the biogases are dominantly composed of 40%-75% methane and 15%-50% carbon dioxide in addition to little amounts of water vapor (5%-10%), hydrogen sulfide (0.005%-2%), less than 6% halogenic hydrocarbon, less than 1% ammonium, less than 0.6% carbon monoxide, 0%-2% nitrogen and minimal amounts of non-methane organic compounds (NMOCs) (5,6). Usually, for every ton of waste, about 250 kg of biogas is produced which can be consumed through extraction and treatment (7). Hajbagheri et al (5) introduced the LandGEM software and its applications in the calculation of the biogases production rates such as carbon dioxide, methane and NMOCs. Their evaluations revealed that the LandGEM software is a reliable and appropriate tool for the purpose of estimating a wide range of gaseous compounds. They have also investigated the effects of the waste composition on the estimation accuracy of LandGEM software (5). Results indicated that 60% of the produced biogas in landfills of Shiraz was methane which would be financially beneficial if extracted. Omrani et al (8) have also conducted another study by using the LandGEM software which illustrated that the emission rates of methane and carbon dioxide from the landfills of Shiraz are equal to 24 and 60 m^3/y respectively (8). Safari et al have also employed the LandGEM software to investigate the gases produced in the landfills of Mashhad. After the initial estimations, two disposal options which were incineration and energy production were investigated. The study results revealed that the environmental benefits would be significant despite high initial costs of energy production from methane (7). Zoghi and Ghavidel (4) estimated the rate of methane production in the municipal landfills by utilizing artificial neural networks. These researchers provided an estimation model for produced gases by considering parameters such as latex circulation and landfill properties. Mahvi and Rodbari (9) calculated the rate of produced biogases in the landfills of Shahrod using LandGEM software. The study results indicated that 488 m^3 methane and 46 m^3 carbon dioxide are released into the atmosphere from this landfill annually. Mahdipour et al (10) have also modeled the produced gasses in the landfills of Ahvaz, Abadan and Dezfol. They have concluded that these landfills possess high potentials for producing substantial amounts of methane. The main purpose of this study was to estimate the gas emission rates in the landfill including carbon dioxide, methane and NMOCs in the municipal waste landfill of Rodan city located in Hormozgan province. In the first step, the required information such as waste composition and production rates were investigated. Then LandGEM software, developed by the United States Environmental Protection Agency (USEPA), was employed to estimate the emission rates of the produced gases. Lastly, the Screen View software was used in modeling the biogas emission. The results obtained in this study are applicable for the purpose of design and installation of gas extraction systems in the landfill. The study results have also illustrated the pollutant range of motion in the atmosphere and their concentrations within various seasons.

Methods

Future population estimation

The population of Rodan city was calculated between years 2016 and 2019 by considering the present population of the city and the population growth coefficient using Eq.1:

$$P_n = P_0 (1 + r)^n \tag{1}$$

where, P_n is the population in year n, P_0 is the population in the origin year, r is the average population growth rate and n is the number of years.

Geographic and climatic characteristics of Rodan

This study is conducted on the landfill of Rodan, Hormozgan province. Based on the capitation conducted in 2011, the city comprised a population of 118 547 individuals. The landfill is situated 5 km away from the city. Based on the reports of Iranian climatology agency, the average precipitation within the course of 10 years in 2003 to 2013 is 208.12 mL per year and the average maximum temperature of the city is 39.3°C within the course of 10 years. Based on Talaiekhozani's report (11), the selection of existing coefficients and parameters in LandGems software including the methane production rate (k) and methane production potential capacity (Lo) is dependent on the climate of the area under study.

The climate of an area is indicated by the aridity index. The aridity index is used as an indicator to determine the level of dryness of the climate at a specific area. Although there are several aridity indices, but majority of them are not applicable for Iranian climate. De Martonne method (Eq. 2) was selected as the most compatible aridity index for Iran climate among the different methods used to determine the aridity index (Eq. 2) (11).

$$I = \frac{P}{(T+1)} \tag{2}$$

where I is the De Martonne dryness parameter, T is the average annual temperature in °C and P is the average annual precipitation in mm. The results obtained from Eq.2 are compared with Table 1 in order to determine the climate type.

Waste analysis method

All analysis was conducted by the municipal recycling agency of Rodan city in year 2012. The municipal authorities have attempted to obtain a set of samples from the city waste. Four waste transport trucks, with predetermined load capacity were selected for this purpose. These trucks dispose four loads of municipal wastes on a daily basis. The density of disposed waste is then determined in respect to its volume and weight. This process was repeated every month for a year. It is worth mentioning that no samples were obtained before and after holidays to insure the minimum possible error in sampling. A composite sample was also obtained in order to determine the quality and quantity of the solid waste including the percentage of perishable and non-perishable compounds, the percentage of organic and volatile organic matters and humidity which was based on standard methods (2).

Table 1. De Martonne dryness coefficient range and related climate type

Climate types	*I*
Dry	Smaller than 10
Semi dry	10 to 19.9
Mediterranean	20 to 23.4
Semi humid	24 to 27.9
Humid	28 to 34.9
Intense humidity	Higher than 35

Source: Reference 12.

Evaluation of gas emission rate

The gas emission rate of the landfill was evaluated using LandGEM software. The LandGEM software is developed by the USEPA. LandGEM is an automated tool used in estimating total biogas, methane, carbon dioxide and NMOCs from municipal solid waste landfills (11). This software is utilized for estimation of gases emission based on either site-specific data or default parameters. LandGEM has two groups of default parameters known as specifically inventory defaults and Clean Air Act (CAA) defaults. The CAA defaults have been developed based on federal regulations for municipal solid waste landfills. The CAA defaults are utilized to determine if a specific landfill requires the control of gases emission or not. The inventory defaults have been developed based on emission factors in environmental protection agency (11). A first-degree equation is provided by the software in order to estimate the rate of the produced gases Eq. 3.

$$Q_{CH4} = \sum_{i=1}^{n} \sum_{j=0.1}^{1} KL_0 \left[\frac{M_i}{10} \right] e^{-Kt_{ij}} \quad (3)$$

Where Q_{CH4} is the produced methane in the calculated year (cubic meter per year, i is the step index in year, n is the year of origin-first year of operation, j is equal to 0.1 time increment in year, K is reverse of years of methane productions, L_0 is the methane production potential in cubic meter per ton, M_i is the disposed waste mass in year i in ton, and t_{ij} is the age of the j portion of the waste in the year i within the operation year. The characteristics of the Rodan landfill were then fitted into the model according to Table 2.

Results

Climate of Rodan

The Rodan's landfill is located in a plain area with hills and vegetation such as mesquite, lotus and sorrel. Registered statistics of synoptic station in the course of 10 years from 2003 to 2013 were analyzed in order to determine the precipitation quantity of this region. Table 3 presents the average precipitation rates during various seasons of the year. The average annual precipitation was equal to 208.12 mm. The average temperature of Rodan was 39.3°C. Based on the De Martonne coefficient of 5, the climate classification is said to belong to a dry climate type. Wind statistics in the course of 2003 to 2013 was utilized to determine and analyze the wind speed. The average wind speed was 3.4 m/s in July and the minimum speed was 2.5 m/s in September. The average wind speed throughout the year was 2.95 m/s. The location of Rodan's solid waste landfill is shown in Figure 1.

Waste qualitative analysis

The percentage of the waste compositions are variable based on the region, economic and social conditions of the people, the geographic location, climate, seasons, and the waste recovery rate (legal or illegal) (2). Therefore, in order to achieve an accurate evaluation, a separate analysis of the solid waste in every region is needed throughout the course of the various seasons. The important fact is that the solid waste produced in various regions of a city

Table 2. The characteristics of the Rodan landfill

Parameter	Value	Unit
Year of the operation start	2009	Year
Year of the operation shutdown	2019	Year
Calculate the operation shutdown model?	No	-
Methane production rate (K)	0.05	$Year^{-1}$
Methane production potential (L_0)	170	Ton per cubic meter
Concentration of NMOCs	4000	ppmv as hexane
Methane components	50	% by volume

Table 3. The average precipitation in the range of 2003 to 2013

Title	Month											
	March	April	May	June	July	August	September	October	November	December	January	February
The average of total precipitation(mm)	15	1	0.5	0.5	2.2	0.02	0	3.1	6.4	3.4	54	7.3

Source: Reference 13.

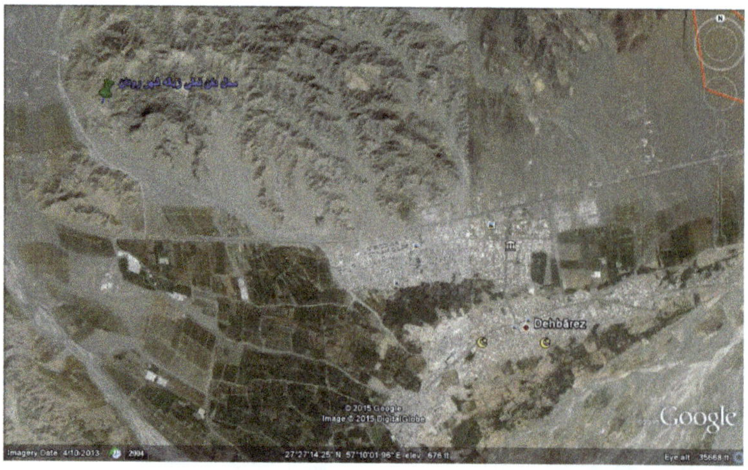

Figure 1. A satellite picture of Rodan's solid waste landfill.

could have significant differences in respects to their composed material. Table 4 illustrates the average percentage weight of different fraction of the wastes in Rodan. As it is presented, the perishable organic components account for 24.18% of the entire wastes in the city. Plastic and rubber constitute 28.07% of this city wastes. Paper and glass constitute 8.26% and 6.05% of the wastes, respectively. Hence, the application of the recycling process in this city could result in the recovery of a large portion of plastic, rubber, paper, cardboard, metal and glass. The humidity of the waste has also been estimated to be 16.53%.

The waste production quantity

The Rodan's landfill was established in 2009 and is still under operation until 2019. After the closure, a new site will be selected based on the general waste plan studies. Studies reveal that the annual waste production rate in Rodan is 402 g/capita/day. The annual waste production rate is illustrated in Table 5. Based on Table 5, 54 824 tons of waste is disposed in this landfill in the course of 10 years of operation.

The production of biogas

Biogas is a mixture of carbon dioxide, methane and NMOCs. The rate of the produced biogas is dependent on the volume of the disposed waste in the landfill. LandGEM software has been introduced as an appropriate model to estimate the rates of biogases production such as carbon dioxide, methane and NMOCs. Hajbagheri et al (5) showed that the LandGEM software is a reliable and appropriate tool for the purpose of estimating a wide range of gaseous compounds (5). As it is shown in Figure 2, the produced biogas is increased through the rise of the disposed waste mass. After the landfill closure in 2019, the waste production would be decreased but not ceased. Based on our calculation, the biogas production would continue for 150 years after the operation shutdown until 2169. The maximum biogas production in the landfill after the closure is achieved in 2020 which is equal to 420 tons per year. It is necessary to prevent the emission of NMOCs into the atmosphere because biogases contain little amounts of these gases which are toxic and carcinogenic (2). Presently, the Rodan landfill lacks any biogas extraction equipment. Thus, it is essential to design such

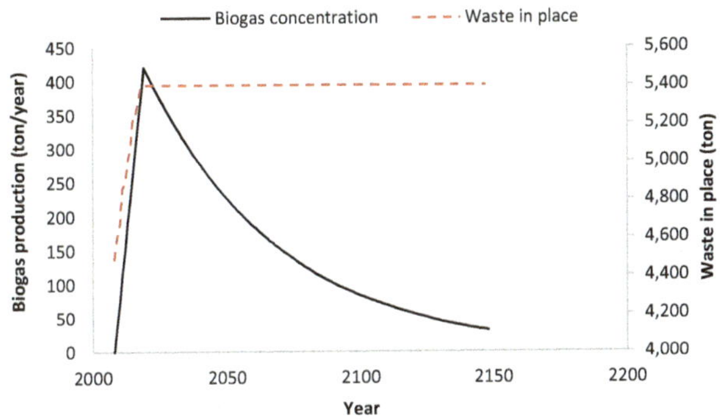

Figure 2. Amount of biogas production in Rodan's landfill between 2009 and 2169.

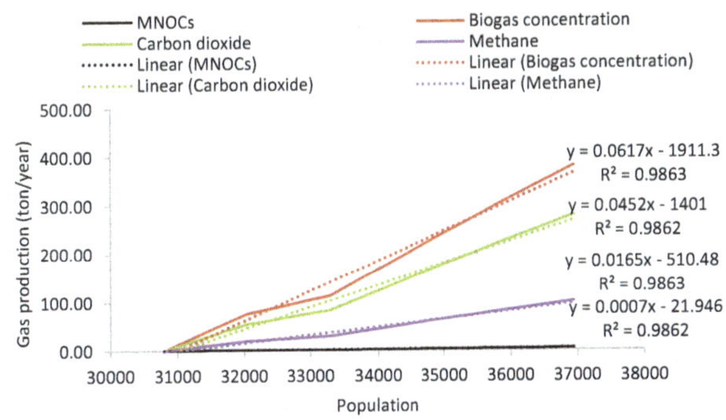

Figure 3. The relationship between population and gas production rate in the Rodan's landfill.

Table 4. The average weight percentage of the waste components in Rodan

Type	Percentage of the components
Perishable organic compounds	24.18
Paper, cardboard and box file	8.26
Plastic and rubber	28.07
Glass	6.05
Metal	3.85
Bones	1.65
Textile	13.76
Wood	8.81
Apartment waste	4.95
Others	0.42

Table 5. The population of Rodan and the waste production rate during 2009 to 2019

Year	Population	Weight of the produced waste (ton/day)	Weight of the produced waste (ton/year)	Waste production rate (g/capita/day)
2009	30 789	12.3	4490	399
2010	31 404	12.6	4599	401
2011	32 032	12.8	4672	399
2012	33 285	13.3	4855	399
2013	33 784	13.4	4891	396
2014	34 291	13.7	5000	398
2015	34 805	13.9	5074	400
2016	35 327	14.4	5256	407
2017	35 857	14.4	5256	401
2018	36 395	14.6	5329	401
2019	36 941	14.8	5402	400

system.

Figure 3 presents the relationship between the population and the total biogas, carbon dioxide, methane and NMOCs production rates. The presented relation could be utilized in estimating the produced gases in the landfill.

Carbon dioxide and methane production

Carbon dioxide and methane are among the important greenhouse gasses. Carbon dioxide is a colorless and odorless gas which plays a vital role in sustaining life on earth. The average concentration of carbon dioxide in the atmosphere is approximately 0.00756 g/m^3. Volcanoes and hot water springs are the natural sources of carbon dioxide. Although in comparison to manmade sources, their capacity is very limited. Microorganisms are capable of producing carbon dioxide through anaerobic and aerobic processes (Eqs. 4 and 5). However methane is only produced through anaerobic processes of organic matter decomposition by microorganisms.

$$Organic\,compounds + O_2 \xrightarrow{\text{Aerobic microorganisms}} CO_2 + H_2O \qquad (4)$$

$$Organic\,compounds \xrightarrow{\text{Aerobic microorganisms}} CO_2 + CH_4 + H_2O \qquad (5)$$

This study revealed that high levels of methane and carbon dioxide are released into the atmosphere from the Rodan's landfill (Figure 4). Omrani et al (8) illustrated that 60% of the produced biogas in the landfills of Shiraz was methane which would be financially beneficial if extracted. They have also carried out a study by using the LandGEM software which illustrated that the emission rate of methane from the landfills of Shiraz is equal to 24 m^3/y (8). The emission rate of carbon dioxide of Rodan's landfill from 2009 to 2169 is presented in Figure 3. As it is shown, the production and emission rate of carbon dioxide and methane is increased with the increase of the disposed waste in the landfill which would reach its maximum in 2020, a year after shutdown. In 2020, the carbon dioxide and methane production rates will be equal to 308 and 112 tons respectively. Although, it is often suggested to convert the produced carbon dioxide into biomass by algae and utilize it as raw material for biodiesel, however none of the proposed methods are financially cost effective (14). Based on our calculations, after 11 years of operation, the Rodan's landfill would emit 1537 tons of carbon dioxide and 560 tons of methane into the atmosphere. Presently, the cost of every ton of liquid carbon dioxide is 12 dollars. Thus revenue of 18 444 is achievable after 11 years of operation by selling the carbon dioxide. It is worth mentioning that the initial costs for equipment and purification must also be considered in decision making. However due to the existence of ample impurities in the produced biogas, the cost of purification will appear to be very high.

Methane accommodates more utilization methods when compared to carbon dioxide. One of these is energy production. Approximately 0.00165 MW of energy is achievable per every cubic meter of methane. It is estimated that throughout the years of operation, the Rodan's landfill would produce only 1 MW of energy. No energy recycling approach is proposed for this landfill since the electric charge produced in this landfill is significantly low. It is proposed to burn the produced methane in order to inhibit the emission.

The Production of NMOCs

The NMOCs are the collection of chemical compounds with different chemical structure but with similar behavior in the atmosphere. NMOCs are produced and emitted from wide range sources such as burning, solvents, anaerobic decomposition of organic compounds and production stages (11,13). NMOCs could also result in the formation of tropospheric ozone which poses much health risks for humans. Several other NMOCs including benzene or 1.3 Butadiene are also highly dangerous for humans (14,15). Large portions of the NMOCs are among the volatile organic compounds (VOCs) which are highly dangerous. The production rate of NMOCs within the years of 2009 and 2169 are presented in Figure 5. As shown in Figure 5, the levels of NMOCs are increased with the increase in the disposal rate of waste in the landfill of Rodan. However, after 1 year of landfill closure, the production rate of NMOCs would significantly decline. The climax of NMOCs production rate is observed in the year 2020 which is one year after the shutdown and 4.82 tons of these compounds are released into the atmosphere. Although the levels of NMOCs in the atmosphere are very small, its inhibition is highly essential due to its high toxicity.

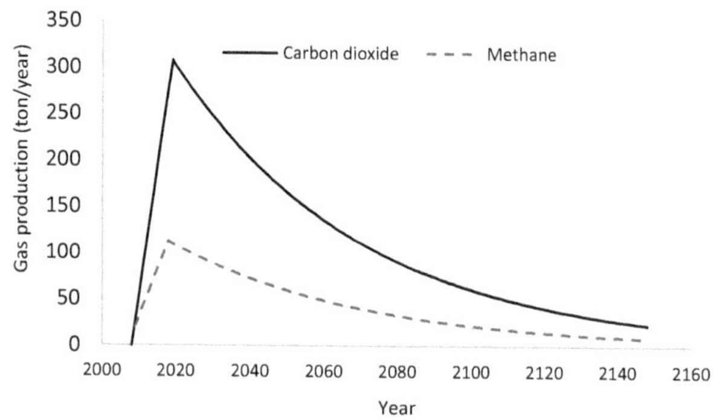

Figure 4. The carbon dioxide and methane production rates in 2009 to 2169

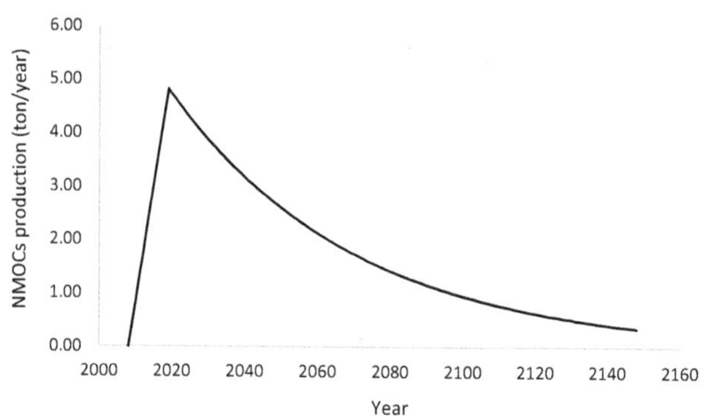

Figure 5. The NMOCs production rate within the years of 1387 to 1527.

Table 6. The emission rate of NMOCs in 2016 in the landfill of Rodan

Gas/Pollutant	Emission rate (ton/year)	Gas/Pollutant	Emission rate (ton/year)
Total landfill gas	266.8	Dichlorobenzene - (HAP for para isomer/VOC)	0.000274
Methane	71.2	Dichlorodifluoromethane	0.017190
Carbon dioxide	195.5	Dichlorofluoromethane – VOC	0.002378
NMOCs	3.063	Dichloromethane (methylene chloride) – HAP	0.010570
1,1,1-Trichloroethane (methyl chloroform) - HAP	0.000569	Dimethyl sulfide (methyl sulfide) – VOC	0.004306
1,1,2,2-Tetrachloroethane - HAP/VOC	0.001641	Ethane	0.237800
1,1-Dichloroethane (ethylidene dichloride) - HAP/VOC	0.002111	Ethanol - VOC	0.011060
1,1-Dichloroethene (vinylidene chloride) - HAP/VOC	0.000172	Ethyl mercaptan (ethanethiol) - VOC	0.001270
1,2-Dichloroethane (ethylene dichloride) - HAP/VOC	0.000361	Ethylbenzene - HAP/VOC	0.004340
1,2-Dichloropropane (propylene dichloride) - HAP/VOC	0.000181	Ethylene dibromide - HAP/VOC	0.000002
2-Propanol (isopropyl alcohol) - VOC	0.026710	Fluorotrichloromethane - VOC	0.000928
Acetone	0.003613	Hexane - HAP/VOC	0.005054
Acrylonitrile - HAP/VOC	0.002971	Hydrogen sulfide	0.010900
Benzene - No or Unknown Co-disposal - HAP/VOC	0.001319	Mercury (total) - HAP	0.000001
Benzene - Co-disposal - HAP/VOC	0.007635	Methyl ethyl ketone - HAP/VOC	0.004550
Bromodichloromethane – VOC	0.004513	Methyl isobutyl ketone - HAP/VOC	0.001691
Butane – VOC	0.002582	Methyl mercaptan – VOC	0.001069
Carbon disulfide - HAP/VOC	0.000392	Pentane - VOC	0.002116
Carbon monoxide	0.034850	Perchloroethylene (tetrachloroethylene) – HAP	0.005452
Carbon tetrachloride - HAP/VOC	0.000005	Propane - VOC	0.004310
Carbonyl sulfide - HAP/VOC	0.000262	t-1,2-Dichloroethene – VOC	0.002412
Chlorobenzene - HAP/VOC	0.000250	Toluene - No or Unknown Co-disposal - HAP/VOC	0.031930
Chlorodifluoromethane	0.000999	Toluene - Co-disposal - HAP/VOC	0.139200
Chloroethane (ethyl chloride) - HAP/VOC	0.000745	Trichloroethylene (trichloroethene) - HAP/VOC	0.003269
Chloroform - HAP/VOC	0.000032	Vinyl chloride - HAP/VOC	0.004054
Chloromethane – VOC	0.000538	Xylenes - HAP/VOC	0.011320

The LandGEM software is capable of calculating the emission rate of 48 chemical compounds in NMOCs collection. The calculation results are presented in Table 6. Based on this table, the emission rate of compounds such as vinyl chloride and benzene in the atmosphere are estimated to be 0.004 and 0.011 tons respectively in 2016. Aspiration of high concentrations of vinyl chloride in low intervals would result in negative effects on the central nervous system which is followed by symptoms such as vertigo, insomnia and headache. Low levels of vinyl chloride can dissolve in surface and underground water sources which could enter the human digestion system. Prolonged contact with low concentration of vinyl chloride by aspiration or digestion could damage the liver. The aspiration of vinyl chloride would increase the risk of liver cancer. Thus, the USEPA has classified vinyl chloride as carcinogenic compounds. Reports of the destructive effects of vinyl chlorides on the human reproduction system have also been provided (16). Although, various epidemiological studies have confirmed the relation of vinyl chloride with birth defects, however several other studies found no such connection (17). Several other studies have also confirmed that men who were in contact with vinyl chloride at works have faced abortion (16). However, various other studies have denied such connection. Studies report a reduction in fertility in mouse that was exposed to low quantities of vinyl chloride in the course of 12 months (16). The half-life of vinyl chloride in the atmosphere is only a few hours, however, in the case of wind blow; this harmful substance can be transmitted across the nearby areas which could pose threat for the residents of those areas. The contact of vinyl chloride with the human body would demand a concentration of 1.3 mg/m^3. Otherwise it could pose serious threat to human health as it was mentioned that the compounds such as vinyl chloride have serious consequences for human body. Thus the inhibition and control of this substance is highly significant in Rodan's landfill. Majority of the compounds in Table 6 are members of VOCs and hazardous air pollutants (PAH) which are indicated in the table.

The modeling of the pollutants emission in the atmosphere

In this section, the total biogas transmittance of carbon dioxide, methane and NMOCs in the atmosphere is modeled in the direction of the wind using Screen View software. Figure 6 presents the total concentration of biogases in the nearby atmosphere of the Rodan's landfill. As it is shown, the concentrations of both pollutants would reach their maximum within the distance of 200 m. The concentration of the total biogas and carbon dioxide within the distance of 200 m of the landfill is equal to 202580 and 10430 μg/m^3. The total concentration of the biogas and carbon dioxide would decrease by taking the distance from the landfill in such a way in which it would reach 3507 and 2534 μg/m^3 respectively within the distance of 100 m. Since the average concentration of carbon dioxide in the atmosphere is 7560 μg/m^3 (14), the produced car-

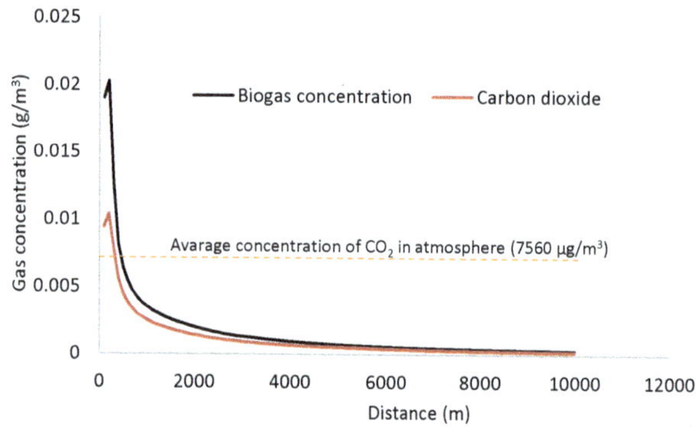

Figure 6. Total biogas emission and carbon dioxide in the vicinity of the landfill of Rodan in the direction of the wind.

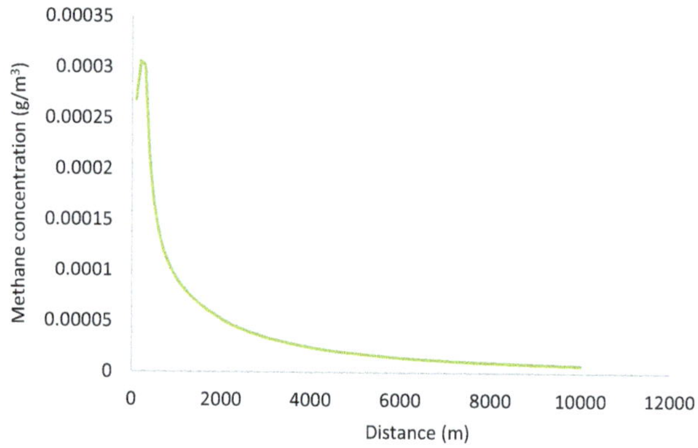

Figure 7. The transmittance of methane around the landfill of Rodan in the direction of the wind.

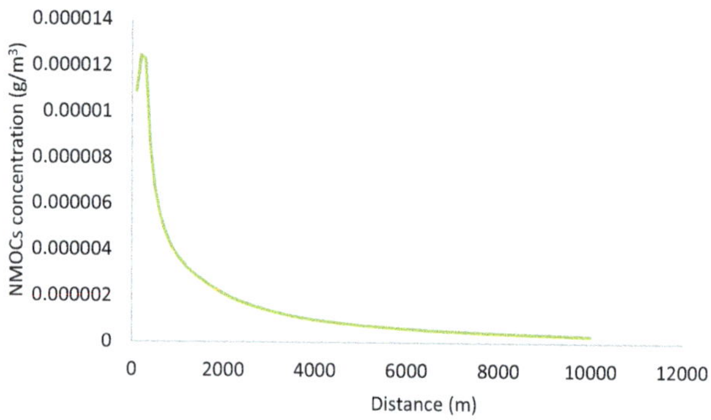

Figure 8. The concentration of NMOCs within various distances from the landfill in the direction of the wind.

bon dioxide in the landfill could reach 17 990 and 10 097 μg/m³ respectively within the distance of 200 and 1000 m. This implies that within the distance of 200 m of the landfill, the concentration of the carbon dioxide which is 2.3 and is within its normal levels, would reach the concentration of 1.3 within the distance of 1000 m.

The emitted methane from the landfill has similar conditions to carbon dioxide. The maximum concentration of gas which is equal to 306 μg/m³ is reached within the distance of 200 m. The concentration of methane would reach 94.41 μg/m³ when the distance is increased over 1000 m and within the distance of 10 000 m, it would be reduced to 7.92 μg/m³. Methane is considered as a gas with greenhouse properties. The heating capacity of methane is 25 times stronger than carbon dioxide thus the inhibition of this gas is of significant importance. Generally, the effects of methane on human health are through the replacement of oxygen and lowering of its concentration (19,20). Headaches, vertigo and nausea are the symptoms of high concentration of methane in the breathing air. However based on the conducted calculations, the concentration of methane around the landfill of Rodan is not high enough to pose any threats for human health (Figure 7).

The NMOCs include dangerous substances such as vinyl chloride. Thus determining their concentrations in the vicinity of the landfill is of great importance. As it is presented in Figure 8, the highest level of concentration which is equal to 12.46 μg/m³ is observed in the distance of 200 m from the landfill. By taking the distance from the landfill, the concentration of NMOCs would decrease, which would reach a concentration of 3.75 μg/m³ in the distance of 1000 m. The concentration of NMOCs in the distance of 10 000 m from the landfill would be equal to only 0.32 μg/m³.

Conclusion

In this study, we investigated the production and emission of carbon dioxide, methane and 48 NMOCs in the landfill of Rodan by using the LandGEM software. We have also modeled the transmittance of the produced pollutants in the nearby areas of the landfill by using the Screen View software. The results suggested that the maximum gas production in the landfill would be achieved one year after the operation shutdown which is in the year 1398. In this year, the production rate of carbon dioxide, methane and NMOCs would be equal to 308, 112 and 4.82 ton per year respectively. The results have also suggested that this landfill would only have the capacity for 1 MW of energy production due to the triviality of the methane production in the course of 11 years of operation. Thus it is suggested to incinerate the produced gas in order to protect the environment and inhibit the greenhouse property. Based on our calculations, the concentration of carbon dioxide, methane and NMOCs would be equal to 94.41, 10 097 and 3.75 mg/m³ respectively within the distance of 1000 m from the landfill. The concentration of carbon dioxide within the distance of 1000 m is 1.3 which is equal to the universal standard. The results obtained in this study could be used for the purpose of design and installation of extraction or incineration equipment in the landfill of Rodan.

Competing interests

The authors declare that there is no conflict of interest that would prejudice the impartiality of this scientific work.

Authors' contribution

All authors of this study have a complete contribution for data collection, data analyses and manuscript writing.

References

1. Porahmad A, Habibi K, Zahraee S, Nazariadli M. Using phase algorithm for relocating of municipal equipment (case study: Babolsar landfill). Environment Journal 2008; 42: 31-42. [In Persian].
2. Jonidi Jafari A, Talaiekhozani A. Introduction to Solid Waste Material. 1st ed. Tehran: Ebadifar; 2011. [In Persian].
3. Poralaghebandan H, Shahsavari A, Hamsizadeh A, Sami S. Municipal Solid Waste Engineering. 1st ed. Tehran: Press the municipalities and the village administrations of Iran; 2010. [In Persian].
4. Zoghi M, Ghavidel A. Prediction of methane percentage in landfills by using artificial neural networks. Iranian Journal of Health and Environment 2009; 2(2): 140-9. [In Persian].
5. Hajbagheri H, Safari A, Yavri A. Introducing of LandGEM model for estimation of emitted biogas from landfill and its effective parameters. The First Conference of New Clean Energy; Hamedan, Iran.
6. Talaiekhozani A, Bagheri M, Rostami Najafabadi N, Borna E. Effect of nearly one hundred percent of municipal solid waste recycling in Najafabad city on improving of its air quality. Journal of Air Pollution and Health 2016; 1(2): 111-22.
7. Safari E, Asadollahfardi GR, Joghtaee F. Evaluation of reducing possibility of produced methane pollution in municipal landfill based on sustainable development mechanism in Rasht city. Forth National Congress on Waste Management; Mashhad; 2010.
8. Omrani GA, Mohseni N, Haghighat K, Javid AH. Technical and sanitary assessment of methane extraction from Shiraz landfill. Journal of Environmental Science and Technology 2009; 10(4): 175-82. [In Persian].
9. Mahvi A, Rodbari A. Calculation of methane emission from Shahrod landfill by using LandGEM software. Fifth Conferences of Solid Waste Management; April 22-23, 2010; Mashhad, Iran.
10. Mahdipour A, Sekhavatjo M, Neisi A, Takdastan A. Estimation of gas production from municipal solid waste landfills by using LandGEM software (case study of Ahwaz, Dezfol, Abadan and Khoramshahr). The fifith National Conference and Exhibition on Environmental Engineering; Tehran; November 11-14, 2011. [In Persian].
11. Talaiekhozani A. Landfill Gas Emissions Model (LandGEM) Version 3.02 User's Guide (internet); 2015 (cited 2016 January 8) Available from Netlibrary: http://www.researchgate.net/publication/282943665___3.02___. doi: 10.13140/RG.2.1.4758.3442.
12. Maliva R, Missimer T. Aridity and drought. In: Maliva R, Missimer T, eds. Arid lands Water Evaluation and Management. Berlin Heidelberg: Springer; 2012. p. 21-39.
13. Talaiekhozani A, Bagheri M, Goli A, Talaei Khozani MR. An overview of principles of odor production, emission, and control methods in wastewater collection and treatment systems. J Environ Manage 2016; 170: 186-206. doi: 10.1016/j.jenvman.2016.01.021.
14. Roshan A, Talaiekhozani A, Roodpeyma Sh. A Review on Removal of Pollutants from Air Using Biological Methods. The 5th Conference on Application of Chemistry in Novel Technology. Isfahan. Iran. December 17, 2015. doi: 10.13140/RG.2.1.4239.1288.
15. Alaee S, Talaiekhozani A, Ziaee GR, Lohrasbi P. Evaluation of Iranian college students' awareness about infertility risk factors. Jundishapur J Health Sci 2016; 8(2): e34172. doi: 10.17795/jjhs-34172.
16. Alaee S, Talaiekhozani A, Rezaei S, Alaee K, Yousefian E. Cadmium and male infertility. Journal of Infertility and Reproductive Biology 2014; 2(2): 62-9.
17. Agency for Toxic Substances and Disease Registry (ATSDR). Toxicological Profile for Vinyl Chloride (Update). Atlanta, GA: Public Health Service, U.S. Department of Health and Human Services; 1997.
18. Agency for Toxic Substances and Disease Registry (ATSDR). Case Studies in Environmental Medicine. Vinyl Chloride Toxicity. Atlanta, GA: Public Health Service, U.S. Department of Health and Human Services; 1990.
19. Talaiekhozani A, Masomi B, Hashemi SMJ. Evaluation of Gaseous Pollutants Emission Rate from Marvdasht Landfills. Journal of Advanced Medical Sciences and Applied Technologies 2016; 2(1): 162-75.
20. I.R. OF Iran Meteorological Organization. Weather Station Rudan; 2016 [cited 2016 Jan 10]. Available from: http://www.irimo.ir/eng/wd/701-Weather-Forcast-Rudan.html?id=132.

25

An assessment on dispersion of carbon monoxide from a cement factory

Gholamreza Goudarzi[1], Rajab Rashidi[2], Fariba Keishams[3], Mahsa Moradi[4], Shahram Sadeghi[5], Fereydoun Masihpour[6], Mojtaba Shegerd[6], Ehsan Abouee Mehrizi[7], Mohammad Veysi Shikhrobat[8], Yusef Omidi Khaniabadi[4,9*]

[1]Associate Professor of Environmental Health, Air Pollution and Respiratory Diseases Research Center, Ahvaz Jundishapur University of Medical Sciences, Ahvaz, Iran
[2]Assistant Professor of Occupational Health, Department of Occupational Health, Nutrition Health Research Center, School of Health, Lorestan University of Medical Sciences, Khorramabad, Iran
[3]MSc Student of Environmental Health, Department of Environmental Health, School of Health, Isfahan University of Medical Sciences, Isfahan, Iran
[4]MSc of Environmental Health, Air Pollution and Respiratory Diseases Research Center, Ahvaz Jundishapur University of Medical Sciences, Ahvaz, Iran
[5]MSc of Environmental Health, Environmental Health Research Center, Kurdistan University of Medical Sciences, Sanandaj, Iran
[6]BSc of Occupational Health, Health Center of East, Ahvaz Jundishapur University of Medical Sciences, Ahvaz, Iran
[7]PhD Student of Environmental Health, Department of Environmental Health Engineering, School of Public Health, North Khorasan University of Medical Sciences, Bojnurd, Iran
[8]BSc of Health Services Administration, Health Center of East, Ahvaz Jundishapur University of Medical Sciences, Ahvaz, Iran
[9]MSc of Environmental Health, Health Care System of Karoon, Ahvaz Jundishapur University of Medical Sciences, Ahvaz, Iran

Abstract

Background: Modeling the dispersion of pollutants from factory stacks addresses the problem of matching emissions of a cement plant with the capacity of the environment to avoid affecting the environment and society. The main objective of this study was to simulate the dispersion of carbon monoxide (CO) from the main stack of a cement plant in Doroud, Iran using SCREEN3 software developed by the US Environmental Protection Agency (US EPA).

Methods: Four samplings were conducted to measure the concentration of CO in the three-stack flow of a cement factory. The input parameters were those affecting gas dispersion and included CO rate, meteorological parameters, factors associated with the stack, and various factors related to the receptor. All factors were incorporated in the model, and dispersion was modeled by SCREEN3.

Results: Southwesterly winds have been dominant in the past 5 years. According to the results of this study, the highest and the lowest CO levels were estimated by the model in spring and autumn as having maximum amounts of 842.06 and 88.31 $\mu g/m^3$, respectively, within distances of 526 and 960 m from the cement plant, respectively, at a downwind southwesterly direction from the plant.

Conclusion: Although the maximum predicted CO levels in each of the four seasons were lower than the NAAQS criteria, the simulation results can be used as a base for reducing CO emissions to prevent the potentially significant health and environmental impacts imposed by long-term contact to such emissions.

Keywords: Modeling, Carbon monoxide, SCREEN3, Cement plant.

***Correspondence to:**
Yusef Omidi Khaniabadi
Email: yusef_omidi@yahoo.com

Introduction

Air pollution attributable to the growth of industries is known as one of the environmental problems in the world, especially in Iran, a country that faces Middle Eastern Dust (MED) storms (1-5). Development in urban areas, increasing consumption of energy, and population growth are some of the most important factors that threaten health and environment (6-10). Combined cycle processes are the major sources of air pollutants in terms of quality and quantity of fuel combustion (11). When the fuels are burned, they emit toxins and global warming emissions, the most important of which are oxides of monoxide, oxides of sulfur, and dioxide, that are being discharged into the atmosphere (12-18).

The city of Doroud in Loresan province of western Iran is enclosed on three sides by the Zagros Mountains. Air pollutants, especially those from the Doroud Cement Plant and other industries associated with ruck extraction activities, have affected this city. The Doroud Cement Plant is located near the city center. Carbon monoxide (CO) emissions from the defective combustion of fuel-burning process of this plant have caused inhabitants of the city to encounter large amounts of CO. The kiln fuel of this factory is natural gas through the first six months of the year; during autumn and winter, mazut is used.

Global concerns about CO emissions prompted the US Environmental Protection Agency (EPA) to establish primary and secondary standards for the concentration of CO in the air.

To diminish these concerns, it is important to identify how an air pollutant is dispersed in the troposphere (13,19,20). Various parameters affect gas dispersion, including wind speed and direction, ground conditions, and atmospheric stability (19,21-23). Software tools based on Gaussian distribution are commonly used to estimate the concentrations of various pollutants (24). The application of atmospheric models provides information useful to atmospheric pollution control programs. The Gaussian model combines source linked factors and meteorological parameters from a source to assess a pollutant concentration. The model assumes that the pollutant does not undergo any chemical reaction and is not eliminated through other processes such as dry or wet deposition.

The basic equation for determining ground level concentrations using the Gaussian model (25) is presented in Eq. (1) and (2).

$$X = \frac{Q}{2\pi u_s \delta_y \delta_z}\left\{\exp\left[-0.5\left(\frac{z_r - h_e}{\delta_z^2}\right)^2\right] + \exp\left[-0.5\left(\frac{z_r + h_e}{\delta_z^2}\right)^2\right] + A\right\} \quad (1)$$

$$A = \sum_{N=1}^{K}\left[\exp\left(\frac{-0.5(z_r - h_e - 2Nz_i)}{\delta_z}\right)^2 + \exp\left(\frac{-0.5(z_r + h_e - 2Nz_i)}{\delta_z}\right)^2 + \exp\left(\frac{-0.5(z_r - h_e + 2Nz_i)}{\delta_z}\right)^2 + \exp\left(\frac{-0.5(z_r + h_e + 2Nz_i)}{\delta_z}\right)^2\right] \quad (2)$$

where X is downwind concentration (μg/m^3), Q is emission rate (g/s), u_s is wind speed at stack height (m/s), δ_y and δ_z are standard deviations of lateral and vertical dispersion (m), respectively, z_r and z_i are the receptors height above ground level and mixing high (m), respectively, and h_e is central plume height (m).

The main objective of this study was to model CO emissions from the main stack of Doroud Cement Plant using SCREEN3 software.

Methods

Study area

Doroud Cement Plant (33°29'MN, 49°4'ME) is one of the productive industries in the city of Doroud, Lorestan province, located in southwestern Iran (Figure 1). This factory started up in 1959 with a manufacturing capacity of 300 tons per day. Doroud Cement Plant is located in the vicinity of residential areas (26). Several atmospheric contaminants (such as CO) emitted from this factory can be harmful to the health of people living downwind of the cement factory.

Measurement

Conducted in 2014, this study performed sampling in four periods (May, August, November, and February) to measure the amount of CO emitted from the flow of three stacks. The CO samples were taken from the gas flow based on ASTMD5522-EPACTM-030 standard using Testo (XL350), which is a portable emissions analyzer designed for short-term industrial stack gas monitoring. This analyzer was calibrated by Behrooz measurement tools. It has an internal calibration with measurement accuracy of ± 2 mg and response time of about one minute. To assess CO dispersion, the SCREEN3 model was used. Table 1 shows the results of measured data and CO concentrations.

SCREEN3

SCREEN3 (Likes Environmental Software, Waterloo, Ontario, Canada), developed by the US EPA, is software that predicts pollutant concentrations away from the source. In this study, SCREEN3 was used to simulate CO dispersion from the stack of a cement plant. This EPA-approved air dispersion model is a screening version of the Industrial Source Complex Dispersion Models (ISC3) and is used to analyze single-source release scenarios over simple or complex terrain. To estimate concentration, SCREEN3 incorporates different factors related to the source of the emission and meteorological parameters based on the Gaussian model (15,27). SCREEN3 can be used for dispersion modeling at distances less than 100 km from the source (28). The data required to run the software includes source type, emission rate (g/s), source stack height (m), stack inner diameter (m), stack exit velocity (m/s), temperature of exit gas (°K), air temperature (°K), height of receptor from ground level (m), wind direction, and urban or rural option. CO samples obtained from three stacks of the cement plant, including Electro filters 1 and 2 and Kiln (unit 3), and their averages were applied for the explication of the model during four seasons. Table

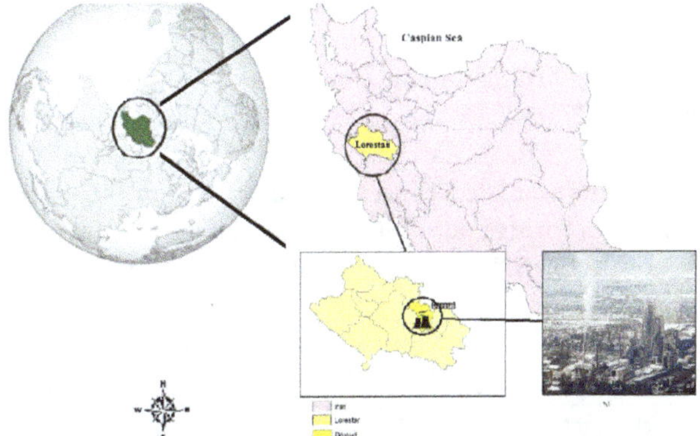

Figure 1. Doroud Cement Plant, the study area.

Table 1. Data related to the cement factory stacks

Number of stack		Unit 1	Unit 2	Unit 3
Q (m^3/s)		97.2	144.4	222.2
Spring	Velocity of gas (m/s)	7.8 ±1.3	10.9 ± 2	12.7 ±1.6
	Temperature of gas (°C)	160.22 ± 22	112 ± 25	71 ± 12
	CO (PPM)	271±13.2	252±12.08	2378±76
Summer	Velocity of gas (m/s)	182 ± 8	18.8 ± 3.6	11.6 ± 0.5
	Temperature of gas (°C)	33.22 ± 5.4	135 ± 3.5	80.3 ± 9
	CO (PPM)	58±5.3	220±7	260±36
Autumn	Velocity of gas (m/s)	176 ± 13	14.6 ± 6.7	14.6 ± 6.7
	Temperature of gas (°C)	36.1 ± 2.1	142 ± 10	142 ± 10
	CO (PPM)	85±12	141±16.9	221±25.8
Winter	Velocity of gas (m/s)	8.5 ± 0.6	14.8 (2.6)	9.1 ± 5
	Temperature of gas (°C)	166 ± 26	134 ±11	89 ± 4.9
	CO (PPM)	719±26.9	426±16.9	630±53.04

2 illustrates the physical factors related to units 1, 2, and 3 of the cement factory.

Meteorological data

The meteorological data required for this modeling effort was obtained from surface weather observatory stations located near the cement factory. Surface wind speeds and wind directions at 10 m above ground level were used in the meteorological analysis to evaluate the environmental impact (HIA) of CO emissions. The 5-year results of wind speeds and direction were obtained from the meteorological stations and then used to draw the wind rose plot using WRPLOT View software. For short time periods, a constant representative atmospheric stability was assumed.

Results

Figure 2 shows a five-year wind rose plot of wind speeds and directions based on the data recorded daily by the meteorological station in Doroud. Southwesterly winds dominated during these 5 years. The maximum percentage of time that wind blew from the dominant direction was 40%.

The percentage of calm winds was zero. Wind speed ranged 17-21 knots per second.

The plots of different concentrations of CO predicted by the SCREEN3 at X downwind direction are illustrated in Figures 3 to 6. As can be seen in these figures, the maximum predicted concentrations of CO in the warm seasons of spring and summer were 842.06 and 119.19 µg/m^3, respectively. Figures 4 and 5 also show the plots of CO levels at different distances away from the plant during the autumn and winter seasons. As seen, the maximum estimated CO concentrations were 88.31 and 429.88 µg/m^3, respectively.

Table 2. Physical factors related to cement factory stacks

Parameters associated with stack	Unit 1	Unit 2	Unit 3
Stack height (m)	54	70	90
Stack diameter (m)	2.8	2.85	4

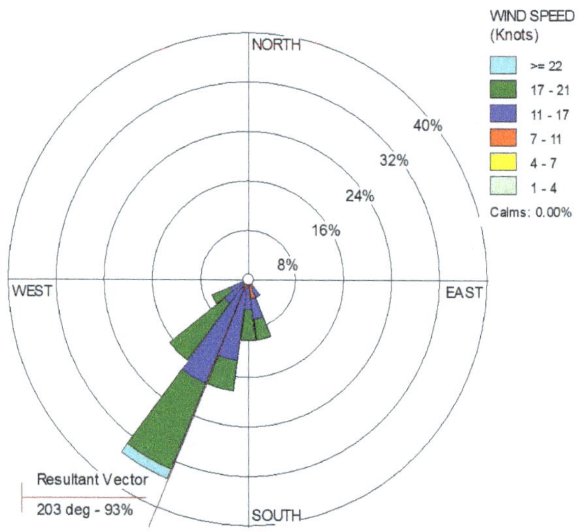

Figure 2. Five-year wind rose of wind speed and direction.

The figures also show that, for distances close to the source, the pollutant concentration was lower. At distances up to 526, 584, 960, and 2647 m from the source, CO levels rapidly increased at ground level, and after drifting downward to a distance of 4000 m, they were found to be 89.91, 11.04, 32.94, and 425.52 µg/m^3, respectively. Thus, the pollutants in the study area do not exceed the NAAQS standard. The worst atmospheric condition was noted in spring.

Discussion

In recent decades, air pollution has been considered a serious threat for the environment, the quality of human

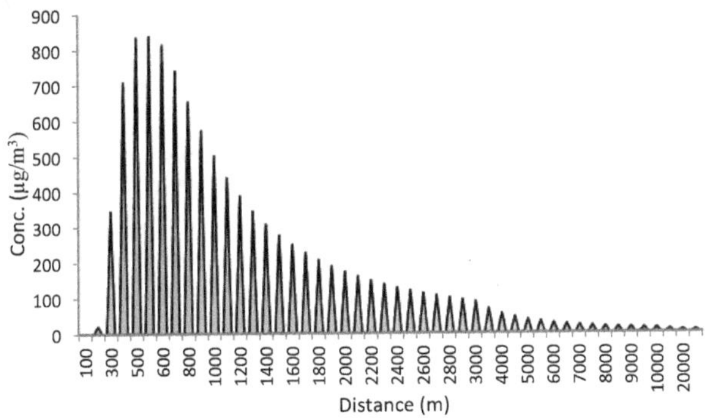

Figure 3. The concentration distribution of CO during spring.

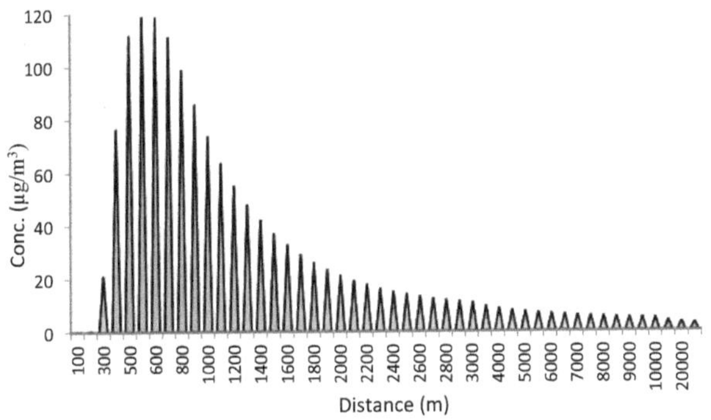

Figure 4. Concentration distribution of CO during summer.

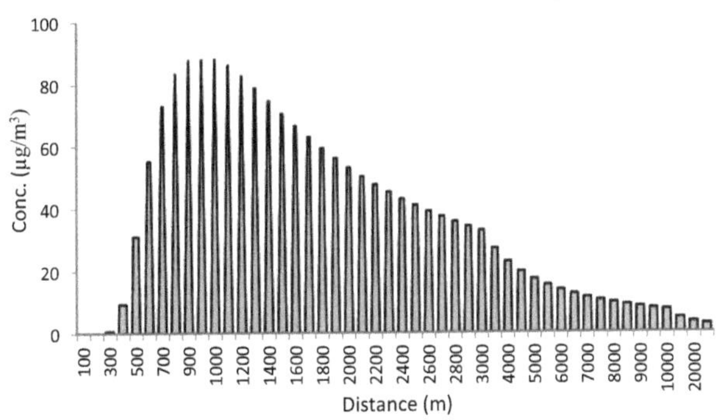

Figure 5. Concentration distribution of CO during autumn.

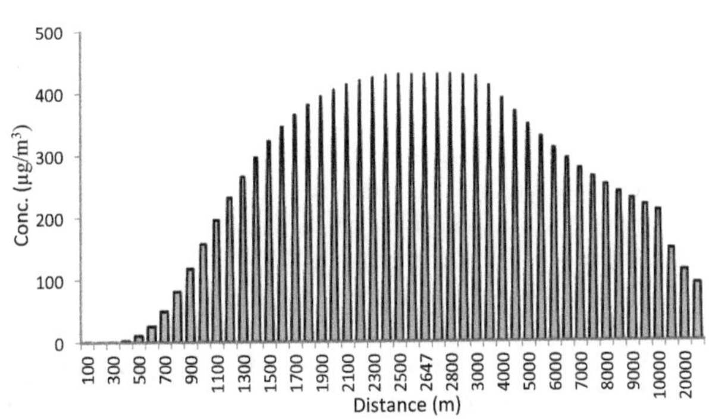

Figure 6. Concentration distribution of CO during winter.

life, and human health around the world. The current study assessed the distribution of CO from the stacks of a cement plant in Doroud, Lorestan, Iran the SCREEN3 model. Southeasterly winds were dominant during this 5-year analysis of wind speeds and directions. Seangkiatiyuth et al showed that winds were below the instrument detection limit 6.9%, 17.7%, and 47.8% of the one year (19). Abril et al reported stronger winds coming from a southerly direction, and these winds were more frequent than the others (29). These findings are consistent with the results of the current study. Maximum CO concentrations for the four seasons were estimated to be 842.06, 119.19, 88.31, and 429.88 μg/m^3 in spring, summer, autumn, and winter, respectively. The worst condition occurred in spring in an unstable condition in which the maximum concentration of pollutant measured near the cement plant was at a higher level than in the other seasons. Doroud is well known for the extraction and manufacture of rock materials as well as the existence of a large cement plant located in the vicinity of the city center which affects the quality of the air in nearby communities.

Major sources of CO that increase the risks from anthropogenic sources of air pollution are road traffic, defective combustion, and industrial processes. This can be seen in studies conducted in other industries with a wide range of basic conditions, such as population, climate, economic and social conditions, and pollutant concentrations. Few studies have investigated modeling CO exited from cement plant stacks. Sari et al showed the modeling of pollutants from the stacks of a palm oil mill using SCREEN3 software. The highest concentration of CO on the west and east was found to be 49.6 μg/m^3 at an X downwind distance of 1403 m from the source (15). Maximum CO levels in spring, summer, autumn, and winter occurred within distances of 526, 584, 960, and 2647 m from the cement plant, respectively.

Abdulkareem et al illustrated that the simulated results are in good agreement with the dispersion pattern and that continuous gas flaring irrespective of the quantity will, in the long run, lead to changes in the quality of the physical atmosphere (30). Visscher showed that SCREEN3 is a good model for forecasting the distribution of air pollutants (31).

Abu-Allaban and Abu-Qudais predicted the concentration of CO gas emitted from a cement plant in Jordan using the AERMOD model. In their study, the maximum 1-hour predicted concentration of CO was estimated at 0.086 ppm at a distance of 2000 m from the source in a west-east direction (32); this is lower than the findings of the current study. Kahforoshan et al demonstrated that the maximum CO level in a stack in Nigeria was 14640 μg/m^3 at a distance of 20 m from the stack at ground level (33). Maximum CO concentrations were lower than the US National Ambient Air Quality Standard (NAAQS) with an average value of 40 000 μg/m^3. This condition had no significant impact on the health of nearby communities settled in an X downwind from the south and east direction.

Otaru et al reported that, due to fugitive emissions from cement plants, a simulated distance of 7000 meter from the source is recommended for safe human settlement and activities (34). Schuhmacher et al indicated that exited pollutants from a cement plant stack are not considered causal predictors of mortality, but they increase by about 0.2% the risk of asthma visits (35).

Momeni et al modeled the spread of air pollution using SCREEN3 and meteorological information. Their measurements indicated that CO levels were lower than the standard (36), and this finding is consistent with the results of the present study.

Conclusion

The results of this study showed that the SCREEN3 software is one of the most effective models for estimating air pollutant distribution. The dominant direction of CO dispersion was from the southwest. The highest and lowest concentrations were predicted in spring and autumn, respectively. Maximum CO concentrations in different seasons were not higher than the NAAQS recommendations. Thus, it can be concluded that CO emissions from the cement plant have no impact on health in nearby communities. It is important to emphasize the fact that applying atmospheric dispersion models can be useful when they are applied together and with measured data in order to permit more robust and improved predictive atmospheric studies. In addition, to decrease emissions from fuel combustion, fuel type must be selected with attention to reducing CO concentrations. Although the maximum CO concentrations in four seasons predicted by SCREEN3 were lower than the NAAQS recommendations, the simulation results can be used as a base for reducing CO emission rates, because the long-term exposure to emissions of a cement plant imposes potentially significant health and environmental impacts.

Authors' contributions

Study concept, design, and critical revision of the manuscript for important intellectual content: G G, YOK, RR, MM, EAM; drafting of the manuscript and advisor YOK, GG, FK, MS, FM, SS, and performing experiments: MVS.

Competing interests

The authors declare that they have no competing interests.

Acknowledgments

The authors wish to thank the personnel of Doroud Cement Plant for their assistance in conducting this research (grant No. 1143).

References

1. Khaniabadi YO, Hopke PK, Goudarzi G, Daryanoosh SM, Jourvand M, Basiri H. Cardiopulmonary mortality and COPD attributed to ambient ozone. Environ Res 2017; 152: 336-41. doi: 10.1016/j.envres.2016.10.008.
2. Khaniabadi YO, Daryanoosh SM, Hopke PK, Ferrante M, De Marco A, Sicard P, et al. Acute myocardial infarction and COPD attributed to ambient SO_2 in Iran. Environ Res 2017; 156: 683-687. doi: 10.1016/j.envres.2017.04.028.
3. Omidi Khaniabadi Y, Daryanoosh SM, Amrane A, Polosa R, Hopke PK, Goudarzi G, et al. Impact of Middle Eastern Dust storms on human health. Atmos Pollut Res 2017; 8(4): 606-13. doi: 10.1016/j.apr.2016.11.005.
4. Khaniabadi YO, Fanelli R, De Marco A, Daryanoosh SM, Kloog I, Hopke PK, et al. Hospital admissions in Iran for cardiovascular and respiratory diseases attributed to the Middle Eastern Dust storms. Environ Sci Pollut Res Int 2017; 24(20): 16860-8. doi: 10.1007/s11356-017-9298-5.
5. Goudarzi G, Daryanoosh SM, Godini H, Hopke PK, Sicard P, De Marco A, et al. Health risk assessment of exposure to the Middle-Eastern Dust storms in the Iranian megacity of Kermanshah. Public Health 2017; 148: 109-16. doi: 10.1016/j.puhe.2017.03.009.
6. Sepahvand A, Godini H, Omidi Y, Tarrahi MJ, Rashidi R, Basiri H. Investigation of fungal bioaerosols and particulate matter in the teaching-medical hospitals of Khorramabad City, Iran during 2015. Iran J Health Environ 2016; 9(1): 115-26. [In Persian].
7. Mohammadi MJ, Goudarzi G, Geravandi S, Yari AR, Ghalani B, Shirali S, et al. Dispersion modeling of nitrogen dioxide in ambient air of Ahvaz city. Health Scope 2016; 5(2): e32540. doi: 10.17795/jhealthscope-32540.7.
8. Nourmoradi H, Omidi Khaniabadi Y, Goudarzi G, Daryanoosh SM, Khoshgoftar M, Omidi F, et al. Air quality and health risks associated with exposure to particulate matter: a cross-sectional study in Khorramabad, Iran. Health Scope 2016; 5(1): e31766. doi: 10.17795/jhealthscope-31766.
9. Daryanoosh SM, Goudarzi G, Khaniabadi YO, Armin H, Bassiri H, Khaniabadi FO. Effect of exposure to PM10 on cardiovascular diseases hospitalizations in Ahvaz, Khorramabad and Ilam, Iran during 2014. Iranian Journal of Health, Safety & Environment 2016; 3(1): 428-33.
10. Dobaradaran S, Geravandi S, Goudarzi G, Idani E, Salmanzadeh S, Soltani F, et al. Determination of cardiovascular and respiratory diseases caused by PM10 exposure in Bushehr, 2013. J Mazandaran Univ Med Sci 2016; 26(139): 42-52. [In Persian].
11. Omidi Y, Goudarzi G, Heidari AM, Daryanoosh SM. Health impact assessment of short-term exposure to NO2 in Kermanshah, Iran using AirQ model. Environ Health Eng Manag J 2016; 3(2): 91-7.
12. Khaefi M, Geravandi S, Hassani G, Yari AR, Soltani F, Dobaradaran S, et al. Association of particulate matter impact on prevalence of chronic obstructive pulmonary disease in Ahvaz, southwest Iran during 2009–2013. Aerosol Air Qual Res 2017; 17(1): 230-7. doi: 10.4209/aaqr.2015.11.0628.
13. Al Smadi M, Al-Zboon K, Shatnawi K. Assessment of air pollutants emissions from a cement plant: a case study in Jordan. Jordan of Civil Engineering 2009; 3(3): 265-82.
14. Zeleke Z, Moen B, Bratveit M. Cement dust exposure and acute lung function: a cross shift study. BMC Pulm Med

2010; 10: 19. doi: 10.1186/1471-2466-10-19.
15. Sari N, Tarumum S, Saryono. Pollutant dispersion modelling (Dust, CO, NOx, and SOx) from palm oil mill stack. Indonesian Journal of Environmental Science and Technology 2014; 1(1): 28-34.
16. Neisi A, Goudarzi G, Babaei A, Vosoughi M, Hashemzadeh H, Naimabadi A, et al. Study of heavy metal levels in indoor dust and their health risk assessment in children of Ahvaz city Iran. Toxin Rev 2016; 35(1-2): 16-23. doi: 10.1080/15569543.2016.1181656.
17. Yari AR, Goudarzi G, Geravandi S, Dobaradaran S, Yousefi F, Idani E, et al. Study of ground-level ozone and its health risk assessment in residents in Ahvaz City, Iran during 2013. Toxin Rev 2016; 35(3-4): 201-6. doi: 10.1080/15569543.2016.1225769.
18. Goudarzi G, Geravandi S, Mohammadi MJ, Salmanzadeh S, Vosoughi M, Sahebalzaman M. The relationship between air pollution exposure and chronic obstructive pulmonary disease in Ahvaz, Iran. Chronic Diseases Journal 2015; 3(1): 14-20.
19. Seangkiatiyuth K, Surapipith V, Tantrakarnapa K, Lothongkum AW. Application of the AERMOD modeling system for environmental impact assessment of NO2 emissions from a cement complex. J Environ Sci (China) 2011; 23(6): 931-40.
20. Guttikunda SK, Begum BA, Wadud Z. Particulate pollution from brick kiln clusters in the Greater Dhaka region, Bangladesh. Air Qual Atmos Health 2013; 6(2): 357-65. doi: 10.1007/s11869-012-0187-2.
21. Dimovska B, Šajn R, Stafilov T, Bačeva K, Tănăselia C. Determination of atmospheric pollution around the thermoelectric power plant using a moss biomonitoring. Air Qual Atmos Health 2014; 7(4): 541-57. doi: 10.1007/s11869-014-0257-8.
22. Khaniabadi YO, Goudarzi G, Daryanoosh S, Borgini A, Tittarelli A, De Marco A. Exposure to PM10, NO2, and O3 and impacts on human health. Environ Sci Pollut Res Int 2017; 24(3): 2781-9. doi: 10.1007/s11356-016-8038-6.
23. Mohebbi A, Baroutian S. A Detailed Investigation of particulate dispersion from Kerman Cement Plant. Iranian Journal of Chemical Engineering 2006; 3(3): 65-74.
24. Hess GD. Simulation of Photochemical Smog in the Melbourne Air shed: worst case studies. Atmos Environ (1994) 1989; 23(3): 661-9. doi: 10.1016/0004-6981(89)90014-0.
25. Mohebbi A, Baroutian S. Numerical Modeling of Particulate Matter Dispersion from Kerman Cement Plant, Iran. Environ Monit Assess 2007; 130(1-3): 73-82.
26. Nourmoradi H, Khaniabadi YO, Goudarzi G, Jourvand M, Nikmehr K. Investigation on the dust dispersion (PM10 and PM2.5) by Doroud Cement Plant and study of its individual exposure rates. Journal of Ilam University of Medical Sciences 2016; 24 (1): 64-75. [In Persian].
27. Zhong S, Zhou L, Wang Z. Software for environmental impact assessment of air pollution dispersion based on ArcGIS. Procedia Environ Sci 2011; 10(Part C): 2792-7. doi: 10.1016/j.proenv.2011.09.433.
28. U.S. Environment Protection Agency. SCREEN3 Model User's Guide. USA: EPA; 1995.
29. Abril GA, Wannaz ED, Mateos AC, Pignata ML. Biomonitoring of airborne particulate matter emitted from a cement plant and comparison with dispersion modelling results. Atmos Environ. 2014; 82: 154-63.
30. Abdulkareem A, Odigure J, Abenege S. Predictive model for pollutant dispersion from gas flaring: a case study of oil producing area of Nigeria. Energy Sources, Part A 2009; 31(12): 1004-15. doi: 10.1080/15567030801909318.
31. Visscher AD. Air Dispersion Modeling: Foundations and Applications. Philadelphia: John Wiley & Sons; 2013.
32. Abu-Allaban M, Abu-Qudais H. Impact assessment of ambient air quality by cement industry: a case study in Jordan. Aerosol Air Qual Res 2011; 11(7): 802-10. doi: 10.4209/aaqr.2011.07.0090 .
33. Kahforoshan D, Fatehifar E, Babalou AA, Ebrahimin AR, Elkamel A, Soltanmohammadzadeh JS. Modeling and evaluation of air pollution from a gaseous flare in an oil and gas processing area. WSEAS Conferences Santander; 2008 Sep 23-25; Santander, Cantabria; 2008.
34. Otaru AJ, Odigure JO, Okafor JO, Abdulkareem AS. Model prediction of particulate dispersion from a cement mill stack: case study of a cement plant in Nigeria. J Environ Sci Toxicol Food Technol 2013; 3(2): 97-110.
35. Schuhmacher M, Domingo JL, Garreta J. Pollutants emitted by a cement plant: health risks for the population living in the neighborhood. Environ Res 2004; 95(2): 198-206. doi: 10.1016/j.envres.2003.08.011.
36. Momeni S, Sekhavatjo M. Modeling of air pollution (case study: Lavan Island). 16th the National Conference on Environmental Health; 2013 Oct 1-3; Tabriz University of Medical Sciences, Tabriz; 2013.

Effects of noise pollution on Samen district residents in Mashhad city

Asiyeh Moteallemi[1], Bijan Bina[2*], Soheila Mortezaie[3]

[1]Department of Environmental Health Engineering, School of Nursing, Torbat Jam Faculty of Medical Sciences, Torbat Jam, Iran
[2]Department of Environmental Health Engineering, School of Health, Isfahan University of Medical Sciences, Isfahan, Iran
[3]Department of Occupational Health Engineering, School of Health, Isfahan University of Medical Sciences, Isfahan, Iran

Abstract
Background: Noise pollution is one of the most important environmental pollutions that affects human health in different dimensions. The current study aimed to survey the effects of noise pollution on residents of the Samen district in Mashhad.
Methods: To understand the psychological effects that noise pollution caused by vehicles has on people, 400 questionnaires designed to gather demographic data and information on attitudes about noise pollution, its effects on people's activities, and noise source annoyance were randomly distributed among the people living in the Samen district of Mashhad city. SPSS software was used for statistical analysis.
Results: According to the results of this study, the most important effects noise pollution had on the studied society were nervousness (29.1%), conversation problems (19.8%), amnesia (18.3%), and loss of concentration (12.8%). Furthermore, 54.8% of the respondents considered the environmental noises annoying, and 32.5% reported it very annoying. In this study, traffic noise was reported as the most important source of noise pollution.
Conclusion: Generally, the results showed that noise pollution is a serious issue in the Samen district, and the necessary actions should be taken to control noise and prevent the effects of noise pollution.
Keywords: Noise pollution, Psychological effects, Samen area, Mashhad city

***Correspondence to:**
Bijan Bina
Email: bbina123@yahoo.com

Introduction

Among different sources of environmental pollution, noise is very important because of its potential effects on human physiology and psychology (1). Noise pollution in terms of psychology is defined as an unpleasant, undesirable, or unwished sound which has various frequencies and acoustic pressures with no regular pattern (2). The World Health Organization (WHO) has identified noise pollution as a risk factor for poor health and one of the most important types of environmental pollution in large cities (3). The main sources of noise pollution are roads, railway traffic, and air traffic. Therefore, the most effective way to control noise pollution is to reduce it at its source (4).

Psychological or non-acoustical features, gender, age, health status, subjective noise sensitivity, lifestyle, activities, attitude toward noise pollution, acoustical factors of sound such as type of noise, noise level, duration of exposure, frequency and time of exposure (day, week, month, year) are all factors affecting the level of noise annoyance (5). The physiological and psychological effects of noise pollution appear on humans gradually and, in the long run, affect the human nervous system (6). Many researchers have reported that exposure to noise pollution increases the risks related to personal health, like irritability, muscle cramps, stress and anxiety, exhaustion, depression, headache and migraine, loss of body balance, pain, hypertension, cardiovascular problems, gastrointestinal disturbances, sleep disorders, and mental stress (7-12). Annoyance and sleep disorders are the most widely reported effects of noise pollution (13,14).

Many studies have assessed the effects of noise pollution in urban areas (15,16). According to these studies, there is a positive relationship between annoyance and increasing exposure to noise from different sources (17-19). For example, a study conducted in the city of Yazd investigated the consequences of noise pollution in different groups. The results revealed that police officers were most highly affected by high noise pollution levels (20). Omidvari and Nouri evaluated the effects of noise pollution on traffic policemen in Tehran city. The results showed that 67% and 60% of official policemen have suffered from insomnia and buzzing sounds in their ears, respectively (21).

Trombetta Zannin and Bunn studied noise annoyance through railway traffic in a large Latin American city. Their results revealed that railway traffic caused irritability, headaches, poor concentration, and insomnia; 88% of residents in the studied city claimed that nocturnal noise pollution is the most distressing type (22). In a survey by Lam et al, traffic noise was identified as the most annoying source of noise pollution by 60% of people living in highly noisy areas. It was also found that 40% of the people were exposed to unbearable noise and suffered confusion and distress (23). Goswami et al assessed and analyzed road traffic noise pollution in the city of Rourkela, India. Their results showed that traffic noise was the most important source of pollution. Subjects' responses on the questionnaire indicated that 50% of the respondents suffered from hypertension, headache, and sleep disorders (24).

Samen is one of the most important districts in Iran, because it houses the shrine of Imam Reza (Figure 1). Annually, many pilgrims from inside and outside the country visit the Imam Reza shrine, leading to heavy traffic in this area. Given that increased traffic noise affects human health in different dimensions, the current study evaluated the effects of noise pollution on residents of the Samen district in Mashhad city.

Methods

To understand the psychological effects that noise pollution caused by vehicles has on the citizens of Samen, a researcher-made questionnaire was used. After determining the validity and reliability of the questionnaire (Cronbach α: 0.83), a total of 400 questionnaires were randomly distributed to residents of this area. The response rate was approximately 89%, although answers were received from 400 respondents. Twenty-five questionnaires were excluded from the study because of erroneous or incomplete answers. The questionnaire included the following groupings: demographic data (gender, age, occupation, and education), definition of noise pollution from the perspectives of the respondents and the laws and regulations, effects on people's activities, knowledge of the consequences of noise pollution, and identification of the sources of noise pollution. The questionnaire comprised standard closed-ended questions (answered with yes, no, or I do not know), questions with given possible answers, and filter questions. The main questions of the questionnaire included:

1. Do you know what noise pollution is? (If answered no, describe to the respondent what it means)
2. What are the major sources of noise pollution in your area? (Light vehicles, heavy vehicles, motorcycles, religious places, bus stations, drilling)
3. What is your attitude about the degree of annoyance generated by noise sources during the day in your area? (very annoyed, annoyed, a little annoyed, not annoyed)
4. What are the most important effects of noise pollution on your health? (Nervousness, sleep disorders/ amnesia, conversation problems, headache, loss of concentration, stress, reduced ability to work)
5. How can we reduce noise pollution in this area? Or what are your suggestions to control noise pollution in Samen? (Educate people, reduce population, greenery, manage traffic, move industries)

The questionnaires were completed in 10-20 minutes. Statistical calculations were done using SPSS version 20 software and, to determine the relationship between respondent's annoyance and gender, the Mann-Whitney test was used.

Results

The results of questionnaires including degree of annoyance generated by noise sources during the daytime and nighttime, the effects of noise pollution, effects on people's activities, the performed noise studies in the Samen area, and solutions to reduce noise pollution are presented in Figures 2 to 7. According to Figures 2 and 3, the respondents in this study expressed the highest level of annoyance from traffic noises in the nighttime period. Also, the highest percentage of respondents considered traffic noise one of the worst abnormal environmental noises. Figure 4 shows the adverse reactions to

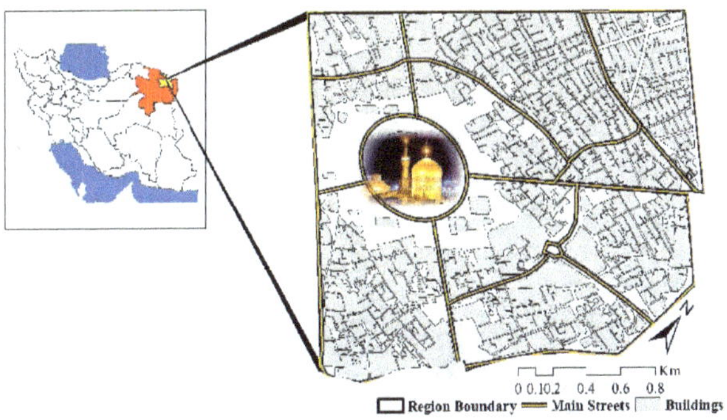

Figure 1. Location of the study area.

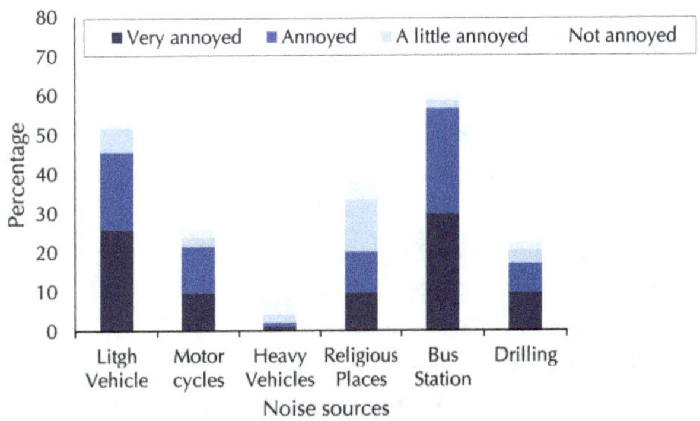

Figure 2. Degree of annoyance generated by noise sources during the day as reported by respondents.

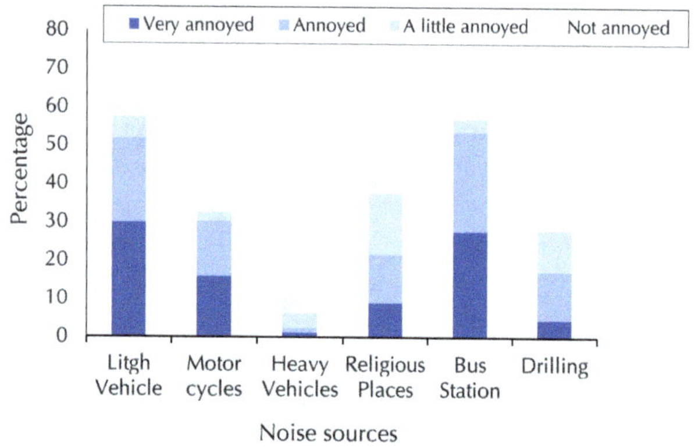

Figure 3. Degree of annoyance generated by noise sources during the night as reported by respondents.

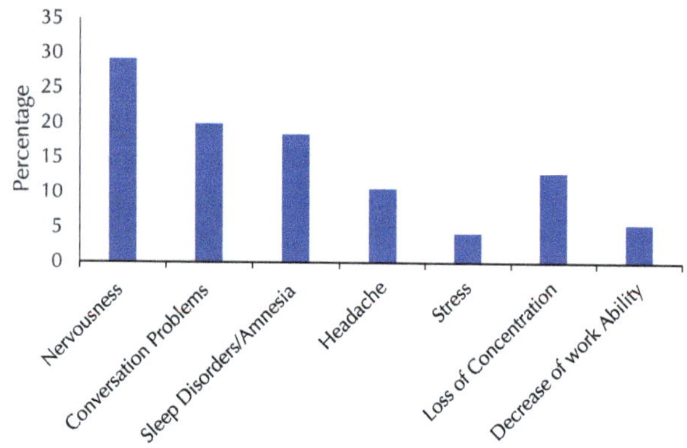

Figure 4. People's attitudes about the effects of noise pollution.

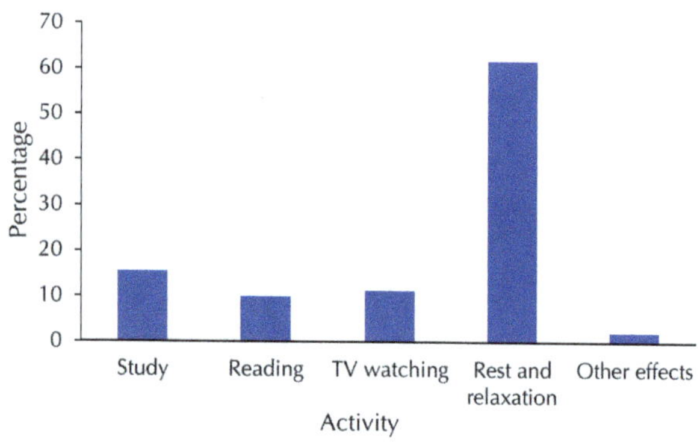

Figure 5. Activities most affected by noise pollution as reported by respondents.

environmental noises reported by respondents that affect their lives and daily activities: 29.1% reported nervousness, 19.8% conversation problems, 18.3% sleep disorders/ amnesia, 12.8% loss of concentration, 10.5% headache, 5.4% reduced work ability, and 4.1% stress.

As shown in Figure 5, the activities most affected by noise pollution were rest and relaxation (61.7%), studying (15.3%), TV watching (11.1%), and reading (9.8%), successively. Figure 6 shows that 38.4% of respondents had no information about any noise study performed in their residential area, and 52.7% of them chose to answer

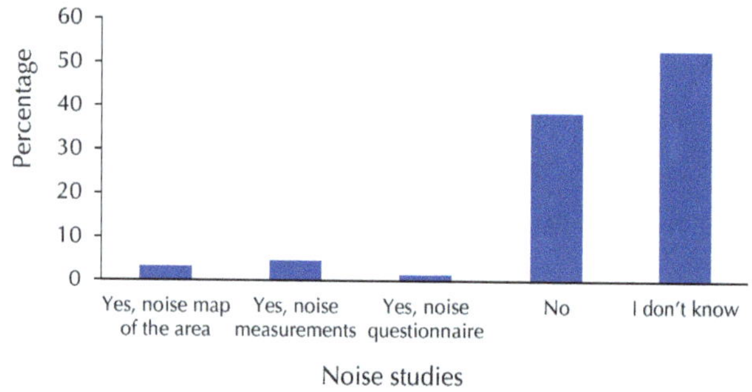

Figure 6. Knowledge of performed noise studies as reported by respondents.

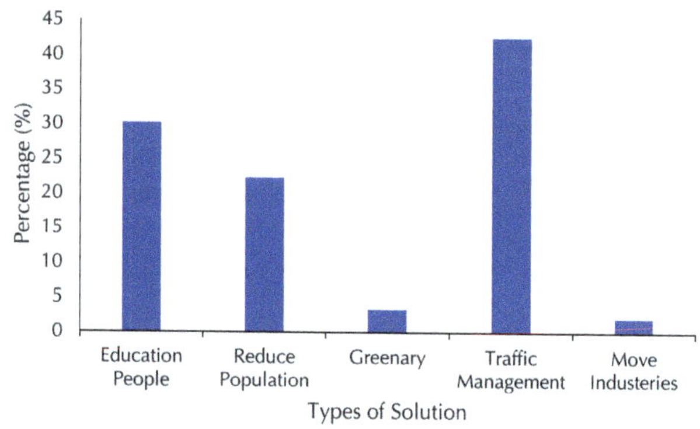

Figure 7. People's Views on Reducing Noise Pollution.

"I don't know." Of all respondents, 49.7% ranked educating people as the best way to control noise pollution, and traffic management and reducing population density ranked second (Figure 6).

Discussion

The first part of the questionnaire included questions about gender (65% male and 35% female) and age (15-30 years: 38%, 30-50 years: 55.5%, more than 50 years: 6.5%). The second part of the questionnaire revealed that 38% of respondents knew little about noise pollution and 43% had little knowledge of the relevant laws and regulations. Figures 2 and 3 show the degree of annoyance generated by different noise sources during the daytime and nighttime periods. According to the figures, respondents expressed the highest level of annoyance from traffic noises in the nighttime period. The highest percentage of respondents considered traffic noise one of the worst abnormal environmental noises. In addition to feeling annoyed by traffic noises, other sources of annoyance such as the bus station and religious places were reported as secondary sources of annoyance. Jakovljevic et al studied the relationship between noise annoyance and public transport in the city center of Belgrade, Serbia. They found that the presence of public transportation in both daytime and nighttime is a significant factor for high noise annoyance in an urban area (4). Similar findings were obtained by Mirzaie et al, Dzhambov et al and Klein et al (25-27).

Results of the current study showed that 54.8% of the respondents considered environmental noises annoying and 32.5% reported them as very annoying. To determine the relationship between respondent's annoyance and gender, the Mann–Whitney test was used. The test was significant with a 95% confidence interval. Men felt annoyance (73.86%) more than women (64.8%), which could be due to the men's job positions. Also, the test was significant with a 99% confidence interval for respondent's level of annoyance and age. Furthermore, it was found that the annoyance level increased as age increased.

As presented in Figure 4, the most important effect that noise pollution exerted on society was nervousness (29.1%), followed by conversation problems (19.8%), sleep disorder/amnesia (18.3%), and loss of concentration (12.8%). Tabraiz et al studied the physio-psychological effects of noise pollution on traffic wardens. Their results revealed that the most important psychological effects on wardens were depression 58%, stress 65%, public conflict 71%, irritation, annoyance 54%, behavioral affects 59%, and speech interference 56% (28). In another study, Yari et al evaluated the question of noise pollution and its effects in Ahvaz city. The results showed that the greatest effects of noise pollution were nervousness (40.15%) and sleep quality (17.88%) (29). Similar findings were reported by Perron et al (30).

As shown in Figure 5, 61.7% of the surveyed respondents reported that annoying noise affected their rest and relaxation period. In a study conducted in Amman, Jordan, it was reported that 81% of people working along main streets were exposed to suffering from traffic noises, and their daily activities were slowed down because of these noises (31). Moreover, according to the results of Jadaan et al (32), traffic noise has a negative effect on workers' and on patient outcomes. Their quiet hours (rest and relaxation) were affected by traffic noise (32,33).

The questionnaire in the current study contained a question about recent studies conducted in the Samen area to assess and reduce noise pollution. The results showed that 52.7% of respondents were not aware of any studies conducted in the studied district (Figure 6). According to Figure 7, the respondents reported that the best ways to control noise pollution are managing traffic (42.5%), educating people (30.1%), and reducing the population density (22.2%), successively. These results are in concordance with those of Popescu et al (16).

Conclusion

Given that high noise levels reduce quality of life and cause discontent among people, using local media to inform people about the effects of noise pollution and traffic management in urban areas will play a key role in reducing and controlling noise pollution.

Acknowledgements

The authors are grateful to the Isfahan University of Medical Sciences for the financial support of this project (No. 393633).

Competing interests

The authors declare that they have no competing interests.

Authors' contributions

All authors contributed equally and were involved in the study design, data collection, and article approval.

References

1. Fiedler PE, Zannin PH. Evaluation of noise pollution in urban traffic hubs—Noise maps and measurements. Environ Impact Assess Rev 2015; 51: 1-9. doi: 10.1016/j.eiar.2014.09.014.
2. Paunovic K, Jakovljevic B, Belojevic G. Predictors of noise annoyance in noisy and quiet urban streets. Sci Total Environ 2009; 407(12): 3707-11. doi: 10.1016/j.scitotenv.2009.02.033.
3. Fritschi L, Brown L, Kim R, Schwela D, Kephalopolous S. Burden of disease from environmental noise: Quantification of healthy years life lost in Europe. Geneva: WHO; 2011.
4. Jakovljevic B, Paunovic K, Belojevic G. Road-traffic noise and factors influencing noise annoyance in an urban population. Environ Int 2009; 35(3): 552-6. doi: 10.1016/j.envint.2008.10.001.
5. Shahid M, Bashir H. Psychological and physiological effects of noise pollution on the residents of major cities of Punjab (Pakistan). Peak Journal of Physical and Environmental Science Research 2013; 1(4): 41-50.
6. Dzhambov AM, Dimitrova DD. Exposure-response relationship between traffic noise and the risk of stroke: a systematic review with meta-analysis. Arh Hig Rada Toksikol 2016; 67(2): 136-51. doi: 10.1515/aiht-2016-67-2751.
7. Liu C, Fuertes E, Tiesler CM, Birk M, Babisch W, Bauer CP, et al. The associations between traffic-related air pollution and noise with blood pressure in children: results from the GINIplus and LISAplus studies. Int J Hyg Environ Health 2014; 217(4-5): 499-505. doi: 10.1016/j.ijheh.2013.09.008.
8. Hammer MS, Swinburn TK, Neitzel RL. Environmental noise pollution in the United States: developing an effective public health response. Environ Health Perspect 2014; 122(2): 115-9. doi: 10.1289/ehp.1307272.
9. Pathak V, Tripathi BD, Mishra VK. Evaluation of traffic noise pollution and attitudes of exposed individuals in working place. Atmos Environ 2008; 42(16): 3892-8. doi: 10.1016/j.atmosenv.2007.12.070.
10. Dzhambov AM, Dimitrova DD. Association between noise pollution and prevalent ischemic heart disease. Folia Med (Plovdiv) 2016; 58(4): 273-81. doi: 10.1515/folmed-2016-0041.
11. Dzhambov AM, Dimitrova DD. Children's blood pressure and its association with road traffic noise exposure - A systematic review with meta-analysis. Environ Res 2017; 152: 244-55. doi: 10.1016/j.envres.2016.10.024.

12. Roswall N, Raaschou-Nielsen O, Jensen SS, Tjonneland A, Sorensen M. Long-term exposure to residential railway and road traffic noise and risk for diabetes in a Danish cohort. Environ Res 2018; 160: 292-7. doi: 10.1016/j.envres.2017.10.008.
13. Sygna K, Aasvang GM, Aamodt G, Oftedal B, Krog NH. Road traffic noise, sleep and mental health. Environ Res 2014; 131: 17-24. doi: 10.1016/j.envres.2014.02.010.
14. Dzhambov AM, Dimitrova DD, Mihaylova-Alakidi VK. Burden of sleep disturbance due to traffic noise in Bulgaria. Folia Med (Plovdiv) 2015; 57(3-4): 264-9. doi: 10.1515/folmed-2015-0049.
15. Mohammadi G. An investigation of community response to urban traffic noise. In: Chou SY, Trappey A, Pokojski J, Smith S, eds. Global Perspective for Competitive Enterprise, Economy and Ecology: London: Springer; 2009. p. 673-680.
16. Popescu DI, Moholea IF. Monitoring the reaction and response of people to urban noise. Archives of Acoustics 2010; 35(2): 237-44. doi: 10.2478/v10168-010-0022-4.
17. Brink M, Wunderli JM. A field study of the exposure-annoyance relationship of military shooting noise. J Acoust Soc Am 2010; 127(4): 2301-11. doi: 10.1121/1.3337234.
18. Miedema HM, Oudshoorn CG. Annoyance from transportation noise: relationships with exposure metrics DNL and DENL and their confidence intervals. Environ Health Perspect 2001; 109(4): 409-16.
19. Miedema HM, Vos H. Exposure-response relationships for transportation noise. J Acoust Soc Am 1998; 104(6): 3432-45. doi: 10.1121/1.423927.
20. Oveysi E, Esmaeili Sari A, Ghasempouri M, Azad Falah P. Investigation on the effects of fleet noise pollution on general and psychlogical health of citizens in Yazd city. Journal of Environmental Studies 2007; 33(43): 50-1. [In Persian].
21. Omidvari M, Nouri J. Effects of noise pollution on traffic policemen. Int J Environ Res 2009; 3(4): 645-52. doi: 10.22059/ijer.2010.80.
22. Trombetta Zannin PH, Bunn F. Noise annoyance through railway traffic - a case study. J Environ Health Sci Eng 2014; 12(1): 14. doi: 10.1186/2052-336x-12-14.
23. Lam KC, Chan PK, Chan TC, Au WH, Hui WC. Annoyance response to mixed transportation noise in Hong Kong. Appl Acoust 2009; 70(1): 1-10. doi: 10.1016/j.apacoust.2008.02.005.
24. Goswami S, Swain BK, Panda SK. Assessment, analysis and appraisal of road traffic noise pollution in Rourkela city, India. J Environ Biol 2013; 34(5): 891-5.
25. Mirzaei R, Ansari-Mogaddam A, Mohammadi M, Rakhshani F, Salmanpor M. Noise pollution in Zahedan and residents' knowledge about noise pollution. J health Scope 2012; 1(1): 3-6.
26. Dzhambov A, Tilov B, Markevych I, Dimitrova D. Residential road traffic noise and general mental health in youth: The role of noise annoyance, neighborhood restorative quality, physical activity, and social cohesion as potential mediators. Environ Int 2017; 109: 1-9. doi: 10.1016/j.envint.2017.09.009.
27. Klein A, Marquis-Favre C, Champelovier P. Assessment of annoyance due to urban road traffic noise combined with tramway noise. J Acoust Soc Am 2017; 141(1): 231. doi: 10.1121/1.4973518.
28. Tabraiz S, Ahmad S, Shehzadi I, Asif MB. Study of physio-psychological effects on traffic wardens due to traffic noise pollution; exposure-effect relation. J Environ Health Sci Eng 2015; 13: 30. doi: 10.1186/s40201-015-0187-x.
29. Yari AR, Geravandi S, Goudarzi G, Idani E, Vosoughie M, Mohamadrezai Esfarjani N, et al. Assessment of noise pollution and its effect on residents health in Ahvaz, Iran in 2011. Archives of Hygiene Sciences 2016; 5(1): 56-60.
30. Perron S, Plante C, Ragettli MS, Kaiser DJ, Goudreau S, Smargiassi A. Sleep disturbance from road traffic, railways, airplanes and from total environmental noise levels in Montreal. Int J Environ Res Public Health 2016; 13(8):809. doi: 10.3390/ijerph13080809.
31. Banihani Q, Jadaan KS. Assessment of road traffic noise pollution at selected sites in Amman, Jordan: Magnitude, control and impact on the community. Jordan Journal of Civil Engineering 2012; 6(2): 267-78.
32. Jadaan KS, Msallam M, Abu-Shanab DA. The impact of road traffic noise on hospital workers. Indian Journal of Science and Technology 2016; 9(1): 1-8. **doi**: 10.17485/ijst/2016/v9i1/79259.
33. Alimohammadi I, Zokaei M, Sandrock S. The effect of road traffic noise on reaction time. Health Promot Perspect 2015; 5(3): 207-14. doi: 10.15171/hpp.2015.025.

27

Significance of physicochemical factors in the transmission of *Escherichia coli* and chloride

Sahar Akhavan[1], **Soheila Ebrahimi**[1*], **Maryam Navabian**[2], **Mahmoud Shabanpour**[3], **Ali Mojtahedi**[4], **Alireza Movahedi Naeini**[1]

[1]Department of Soil Sciences, Soil and Water Engineering School, Gorgan University of Agricultural Sciences and Natural Resources, Gorgan, Iran.
[2]Department of Water Engineering, School of Agriculture, University of Guilan, Rasht, Iran
[3]Department of Soil Science, School of Agriculture, University of Guilan, Rasht, Iran
[4]Department of Microbiology, School of Medicine, Guilan University of Medical Sciences, Rasht, Iran

Abstract
Background: Organic manures are the source of many pathogenic bacteria which could be dangerous for human health. Bacterial transmission and retention in soil is important for processes ranging from contaminant degradation during in situ bioremediation to transport of pathogenic bacteria into groundwater.
Methods: The aim of this study was to evaluate the transport of *Escherichia coli* and chloride (Cl) in the soil saturation conditions, considering the importance of preferential flow using synthetic macrospores (different diameters of macrospores including 0, 1 and 2 cm) and HYDRUS-2D model. Also, the effect of different salinity levels of water (including electrical conductivity of 1, 2 and 4 dSm^{-1}) on the transmission of *E. coli* was investigated. The preferential flow system was prepared and designed using two sand sizes including fine sand and coarse sands in the columns.
Results: The results showed that the retention of *E. coli* increased with the ionic strength of the solution, while the effect of *E. coli* in the fine sand was greater than that of the coarse sand. This bacterial transfer behavior was well described by numerical simulations. The importance of preferential flow in bacterial transfer showed that it increases at higher ionic strength, even if overall transmission is reduced. Although the bacterial transmission is facilitated in salinity, the results of this study showed that with increase of ionic strength of the soil solution, the amount of bacterial purification was increased that could be effective in controlling groundwater contamination with saline water management.
Conclusion: According to the results, with increase of ionic strength of the soil solution, the amount of bacterial purification was increased that could be effective in controlling groundwater contamination with saline water management, so that the least transition has taken place and the conditions for the use of unconventional water sources were also created, without the environmental problem of the risk of groundwater pollution.
Keywords: *Escherichia coli*, Soil, Water pollution

***Correspondence to:**
Soheila Ebrahi
Email: sohebrahimi@gmail.com

Introduction

Fertilizers are the source of some pathogenic bacteria that are harmful to human health and environment. Reaching this bio-pollutant to water resources is mainly due to human activities such as household, municipal and hospital wastes, waste disposal sites, wastewater wells, animal waste and animal fertilizers (1). Soil filtration removes or degrades bacterial pathogen in water as it passes through on its way to groundwater (2). But, macropores of soil increase the transmission of bacteria. Several studies have shown that bacteria could transport easily within the preferential flow direction (3-10). The transfer of bacteria in the soil is controlled by several mechanisms including advection, dispersion, attachment, detachment, inactivation (die-off), and straining (11,12). The inactivation of the bacteria is affected by various factors such as temperature, light, pH, toxic substances, oxygen, protozoa and antagonist (13).

Today, the use of alternative sources, especially unconventional water sources such as drainage waters from farms, saline water and surface and underground waters, has been seriously increased due to the growing restrictions of freshwater resources and consequent reduction soil fertility and quality. Although the application of saline water shows a significant difference compared with non-saline water conditions, but there are some options for the continuity and stability of agricultural activities, in order to provide a suitable bed for their sustainable consumption (14). Salinity is one of the important stressors for microorganisms. It decreases respiration, carbon dioxide levels, enzymatic activity and microbial biomass (15). Several studies have investigated the effects of saline water on the degradation or improvement of physical, chemical and biological properties of soils, with different and sometimes contradictory results. Ionic strength, electrolyte ion balance and soluble pH conditions are the three main factors affecting the reaction of the bacteria to the sand surface and their effect on bacterial retention has been investigated by many scholars, although the results of some studies were completely contradictory. For example, in theory, with increase of ionic strength, the maintenance of bacteria on the negative charge of subsurface deposits increases, because due to the compression of the double layer of compression electrostatic balance, equilibrium is established between superficial load of bacteria and sediment. However, different results were reported by Kim et al (16). They did not find any effect on ionic strength except at high pH on the retention of microorganisms. The electrolyte with bivalent cation can play the role of a bridge, and reacting with the surface load of the cell, keeps more bacteria in the porous medium, but the effect of negative loads of the multivalent ions is contradictory to the transmission or retention of the bacterium or virus under subsurface conditions. The factors influencing the reaction of the bacteria with the surface of the sand, are surface load change and hydrophobic properties (10). Also, surface absorption affects cell surface load, hydrophobicity, size and lipopolysaccharide surface structure (LPS) of the outer membrane of the cell wall of *E. coli*. It is due to this fact that liposaccharide of *E. coli* is the main factor in its absorption onto the mineral surfaces, absorption of metal ions and microbial stimuli, and sediment reactions and dissolution. Liposaccharide contains a phosphoric oligosaccharide hydrophobic fat and polysaccharide, which due to its low hydrophobic contact angle, leads to weak adhesion of *E. coli* (17). Also, various studies have shown that the main reason for the transfer of bacteria to undisturbed soils is preferential flows due to the continuity of coarse pores and cracks in the soil. During the transfer of bacteria, the presence of macropores and bio-pores allows fertilizer wastewater and microorganisms to quickly pass the soil matrix and reach deeper soils and possibly to subsurface drainage systems (18).

Measuring the parameters of soil and water is costly and time consuming. The prediction and simulation of these parameters using modeling, reduces the cost of water management (19). The HYDRUS-2D software has been developed to simulate the two-dimensional movement of water, heat and solvents in a porous medium and different humidity conditions. In this model, Richard's equations and flux-diffusion are used to explain the movement of water and solutes (20). Safadost et al examined the role of restoration of soil structure with physical weathering by testing columns for the transmission of *E. coli* and bromide. Observational data were analyzed using Mobile-Immobile (MIM) model by HYDRUS-2D software. The model estimates well the concentrations of wastewater. The results showed that the absorption coefficients of bacteria increased with clay content. The first peak in the breakthrough curve was observed for the weathered columns of the soil, which was attributed to the increase of the connection of pores with weathering and the presence of preferential flow. The balanced and symmetrical shape of the breakthrough curves of the soil columns showed that leaching mainly occurred through the matrix flow (21). Wang et al accurately described the precise transmission of *E. coli* in the column with the status and length of different synthetic macropores at two levels of ionic strength (1 and 20 mM NaCl) using the dual-permeability flow model in HYDRUS software, by optimizing the absorption parameters of the bacterium (10). The results showed that with decrease of macropores length, the apparent saturation hydraulic conductivity in the macroporous range was reduced. Also, the length of synthetic macropores greatly influenced the preferential transmission of *E. coli*, especially in high ionic strength conditions. In low ionic strength, a wider transport in the preferred pathway and an earlier time to reach *E. coli* than bromide was observed as a result of the size limitation (18). In another study, Unc et al, using modeling with HYDRUS, reported that the estimation of the migration rate of bacteria in the soil profile was consistent with the major hypothesis of bacterial transmission from macropores. The transfer rate of the bacteria was faster than that of water transfer in the soil pores. Suspended bacteria pass faster through the larger diameter of the pores and water in the pores (9). In this research, the transmission and retention of *E. coli* as an indicator of groundwater contamination in soil saturation conditions with regard to the importance of preferential flow were investigated using synthetic macroproes and simulated using HYDRUS-2D model. Also, the effect of different levels of salinity on the transmission of *E. coli* was investigated. The main aim of this research was to evaluate the transmission status of contaminant index (*E. coli*) in the presence of preferential flow with different diameters and different levels of water salinity in the experimental columns. In addition, the microbiological contaminant retention was evaluated at various soil depths.

Methods

Bacteria

Escherichia coli is the most common coliform of the cow manure that is considered as a bio-indicator of underground water pollution in the research. Features such as easy counting, hydrophilic and strong negative load of *E. coli* make it an indicator of underground fecal contamination assessment, especially in developing countries, with respect to the limited laboratory resources. *E. coli* is a gram-negative bacterium, rod shaped, 1.1-1.5 μm × 2-6 μm, single or pair and is a member of Enterobacteriaceae family (17).

Transport experiment

Preferential flow experiments were carried out in PVC containers with specific lengths and inner diameters (20 and 10 cm, respectively). After measuring some of the primary soil properties (Table 1), the preferential flow system was prepared and designed using two sand types including fine sand and coarse sands in the columns. To prepare the soil columns, first, about one third of the height of the column was filled with distilled water (autoclaved) and a plastic tube with a diameter of 30 cm with a desired diameter (1 and 2 cm) was placed in the center of the column. The fine sand was gradually added to the column matrix (outside of the plastic tube). Then, the extra water in the plastic tube was drained from the bottom. Afterwards, the tube was carefully drawn out of the column without disturbance around the sand structure, leaving a hole with a diameter of 2 cm in the center of the column. At this stage, the hole was filled up to a depth of 20 cm with coarse sand using a funnel to create the macropore structure of the desired preferential flow.

Before the bacterial transfer test, two pore volumes (PV) of NaCl solution (saline treatment) were selected and added to the sterilized columns using sterilized physiology serum and allowed the sand to reach a balance state with the solution (phase 0). Bacterial transfer experiments were carried out in two phases with boundary conditions and flow velocity, similar to phase 0. First, a pulse of bacterial suspension was added to the column at a constant velocity (phase 1). Then, an NaCl solution in the column was added with a flow rate and ionic strength similar to those in phase 1 until the concentration of the microbial wastewater returned to the initial amount (phase 2). Bacterial suspension was sprayed uniformly at the top of the sterile soil column along the flame using a sterile syringe. The bacterial suspension was prepared by McFarland Turbidity Standard by mixing 1.175% barium chloride dihydrate (0.048 M), with 9.95 mL of 1% sulfuric acid (0.36 N). Soil columns were washed for one hour and wastewater samples were collected from the bottom of the column at times of 0, 1, 2, 3, 5, 7, 10, 12, 15, 20, 25, 35, 40, 45, 50, 60 min. The experiment was performed with three replications for each treatment. After experiment, bacterial and chlorine concentrations were analyzed. The drained bacterial suspensions were prepared with dilutions of 10^{-1}, 10^{-2} and 10^{-3}. After dilution of the samples, 0.1 ml of the diluted solution was cultured in eosin methylene blue agar (EMB) plates. The bacterial concentrations in the effluent were estimated by the number of *E. coli* colonies in EMB agar after 24 hours incubation at 37°C, then, the concentration of the bacteria in the drained water was calculated and expressed with the unit of colony in milliliters (CFU/mL) (22).

In order to measure the concentration of bacteria in the soil profile, after the bacterial transfer experiment, the soil column was divided into three layers. The samples were taken from three depths. Then, 1 g of each sample was added to a 15 mm centrifuge tube with a 9 mL solution of 0.2% sodium hexametaphosphate. For isolation of the bacteria in the liquid phase from the solid phase, each sample was mixed in a vortex mixer for 15 minutes. To determine the concentration of bacteria in the uppermost solution, live counting method was used (22). The bacterial counting in the soil profile was done by measuring the concentration of bacteria in the wastewater.

To measure the chloride concentration of each sample, the drained water was measured by titration with silver nitrate (23). In this study, breakthrough curves (BTC) of the bacteria were drawn as output concentration (C) based on CFU/mL and the relative bacterial concentrations versus time were recorded using Excel software.

Theory and Model

Chloride transport

The transmission of non-reactive elements, such as chloride, is generally expressed in terms of mass-flow equation. For stable flow conditions, this equation can be as follows.

$$\frac{\partial c}{\partial t} = -v\frac{\partial c}{\partial z} + D\frac{\partial^2 c}{\partial z^2} \quad (1)$$

Where, C is the salt concentration in the liquid phase (ML^3), D, the diffusion coefficient (L^2T^{-1}), v, the average pore velocity of water (LT^{-1}), t, time and z is depth (L). First, the sensitive parameters of chloride breakthrough curve were detected by sensitivity analysis and their values were

Table 1. The primary characteristics of the soil column test

Material	Pore volume (PV) (cm³)	Vapor flow velocity ($\overline{V}$) (cm h⁻¹)	Stable flow rate (q) (cmh⁻¹)	Volumetric soil moisture (θ) (cm³cm⁻³)	Soil texture
Macropore	737.9	14.3	4.70	0.47	Loamy sand (LS)
Matrix	926.3	18.2	7.04	0.59	Sandy loam (SL)

estimated by the inverse modeling of HYDRUS-2D. The model for some hydraulic parameters of Van Genuchten equation and soil diffusion coefficients was calibrated using measured data of chlorine concentration of the drained water from the column during the experiment.

Bacteria transport

The general equation governing the absorption and transfer of bacteria in the soil was expressed by the two-site kinetic attachment-detachment model (24). This model describes the attachment-detachment processes with a first-order kinetic process. The kinetic absorption yield consists of two steps. In the first step, the so-called mass transfer, the bacteria are transferred from the liquid phase to the particle surface. In the second step, the bacteria are absorbed on the soil particle surface by the physical and chemical interactions. In a two-dimensional mode, the kinetic attachment-detachment model expresses the transfer of colloidal particles, bacteria and viruses as follows:

$$\frac{\rho_b}{\theta}\frac{\partial S_1}{\partial t} = k_{att1}C - k_{det1}\frac{\rho b}{\theta} - \mu_s \rho_b S_1 \quad (2)$$

$$\frac{\rho_b}{\theta}\frac{\partial S_2}{\partial t} = k_{att2}C - k_{det2}\frac{\rho b}{\theta} - \mu_s \rho_b S_2 \quad (3)$$

$$\frac{\partial C}{\partial t} + \frac{\rho_b}{\theta}\frac{\partial S_1}{\partial t} + \frac{\rho_b}{\theta}\frac{\partial S_2}{\partial t} = D\frac{\partial^2 C}{\partial z^2} - v\frac{\partial C}{\partial z} - \mu_1 C - \mu_s \rho_b (S_1 + S_2) \quad (4)$$

where C is the concentration of bacteria in the liquid phase (NL^{-3}), S, the concentration (colloid, bacteria or viruses) in the solid phase, the indexes of numbers 1 and 2, indicate kinetic sites 1 and 2, respectively, D, diffusion coefficient (L^2T^{-1}), v, pore velocity of water (LT^{-1}), θ, total porosity (L^3L^{-3}), ρ_b, soil bulk density (ML^{-3}), S, the concentration of bacteria adsorbed by the soil (NL^{-3}), K_{att}, the absorption rate of bacteria (T^{-1}), k_{det}, the detachment rate of bacteria from soil particles (T^{-1}), t, time, μ_1, inactivation of the bacteria in the liquid phase and μ_s, inactivation of the bacteria in the solid phase. According to the sensitivity analysis, K_{att} and k_{det} parameters were used for calibration.

Results

Transfer of chloride

The measured BTCs of chloride and the model fits with the HYDRUS-2D are demonstrated in Figure 1. The ascending line of the chloride breakthrough curve has a steep slope, therefore, chloride is rapidly observed in the drained water.

The optimal calibration parameters by HYDRUS-2D model are presented in Table 2. The residual moisture content (0.67) and saturated moisture content (0.5) in the matrix were greater than macropores. The saturation hydraulic conductivity in macropores was higher than the matrix (0.241 cmh^{-1}). DIFW, DISPT, DISPL parameters in both matrix and macro phases had constant values.

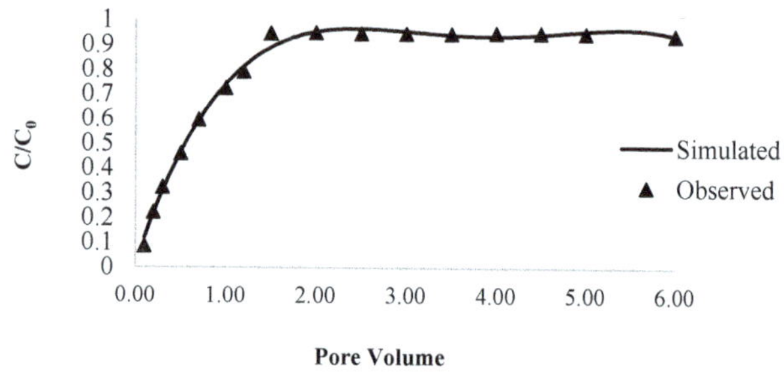

Figure 1. The measured chloride breakthrough curve (solid triangle) fitted with the HYDRUS-2D model (continuous line).

Transfer of bacteria

Estimated parameters of kinetic attachment-detachment model of bacteria by HYDRUS-2D are presented in Table 3. The results showed that soil column treatments with a pore diameter of 1 and 2 cm had a lower attachment coefficient than the saturated column without macropores diameter. This attachment rate was observed in both attachment sites. Therefore, by increasing the diameter of macropore, more conditions were provided for the transmission of the bacteria and its lower attachment.

As shown in Table 3, K_{att} value was 10 times more than k_{det}, indicating that the attachment of the bacteria in the saturated columns was almost irreversible. Two-site attachment parameters show that soil columns had two kinetic attachment sites (Table 3). The kinetic attachment site 1 was related to the salts with the same charge, such as sodium chloride, in which attachment process was very rapid and detachment was very slow. The attachment rate of the bacteria in the kinetic site 1 in the soil column was between 0.0015 and 0.0065 while the rate of detachment was zero in this site. However, in the attachment site 2, two processes of attachment and detachment were rapid. The attachment rate of bacteria in site 2 varied from 0.012 to 0.062 and the detachment rate ranged from 0.0042 to 0.0053.

The results showed that the effect of water salinity of 1 dsm^{-1} (the lowest salinity) on the concentration of the bacteria collected from the soil columns at the beginning of leaching, was the same (Figure 2). However, by increasing the leaching rate, the concentration of *E. coli* in the drained water collected from the soil columns was

Table 2. Values of the parameters obtained from chloride transfer in reverse modeling in two matrix and macro phases

Parameter	θ_r	θ_s	K_s (cmh^{-1})	DIFW (cm^2/day)	DISPT (cm)	DISPL (cm)
Matrix	0.067	0.50	0.015	0.05	0.05	0.05
Macropore	0.057	0.48	0.241	0.05	0.05	0.05

Table 3. The calibrated attachment-detachment model parameters of the bacteria

Soil Columns	EC (dsm^{-1})	Macrospore Diameter (cm)	K_{att1}	K_{det1}	K_{att2}	K_{det2}
A	1	0	0.0065	0	0.0051	0.00042
B	1	1	0.0045	0	0.0052	0.00052
C	1	2	0.0055	0	0.0062	0.00053
D	2	0	0.0049	0	0.0052	0.00052
E	2	1	0.0035	0	0.0032	0.00055
F	2	2	0.0035	0	0.0031	0.00049
G	4	0	0.0025	0	0.0022	0.00051
H	4	1	0.0015	0	0.0022	0.00048
I	4	2	0.0021	0	0.0012	0.00042

decreased.

The results of the evaluation of the simulated breakthrough curve showed that although the fitted data in the simulated breakthrough curve did not overlap with the measured values and there was an over-estimation in the simulation results, but the model was able to simulate the observed data well (Figure 3). The results showed that the optimized attachment parameters of the model were less than the values determined in the laboratory. This suggests that the model, with no consideration for the flow in the coarse pores of the soil, greatly reduces the amount of attachment parameters to simulate the movement of the bacteria in the soil. The measured breakthrough curves of the bacteria show that the concentration of bacteria in the drained water quickly reached peak concentration, and the breakthrough curve has a large dispersion, which can be due to the presence of sites with different attachment and detachment energies in the soil (Figure 3).

Also, the comparison of the measured and estimated breakthrough curve of the bacteria with bacterial attachment-detachment models is shown in Figure 4. As shown in Figure 3, the model had a very good estimation of the breakthrough curve of the bacteria. The coefficient of determination between the measured and estimated values of the breakthrough curve of the bacteria is presented in Figure 4. The results show that the coefficient of determination between the measured values of the breakthrough curve of the bacteria curve and its estimated values was 0.95.

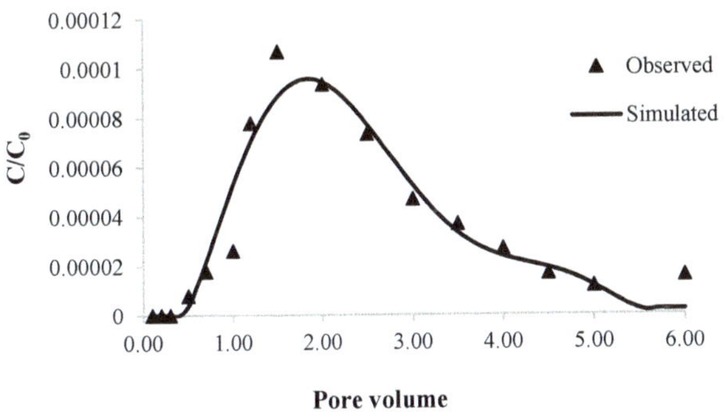

Figure 2. The measured breakthrough curve of the bacteria (solid triangle) and the calibrated breakthrough curve of the bacteria (continuous line) with HYDRUS-2D model.

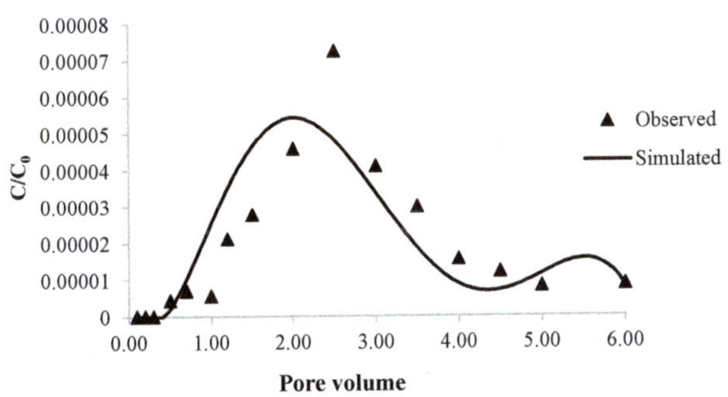

Figure 3. The measured breakthrough curve of the bacteria (solid triangle) and the simulated breakthrough curve of the bacteria (continuous line) with HYDRUS-2D model.

Discussion

Transfer of chloride

Figure 1 shows that the presence of large pores and the presence of preferential flow in the soil columns lead to early removal of chloride in the soil column. On the other hand, these curves have relatively long-tailed distribution due to the continuous flow of chloride. The elongation of breakthrough curve shows the important role of diffusion in the transfer of chloride to these soils. In saturated conditions, the chloride front quickly reaches the bottom of the soil column due to the mass and rapid flow through

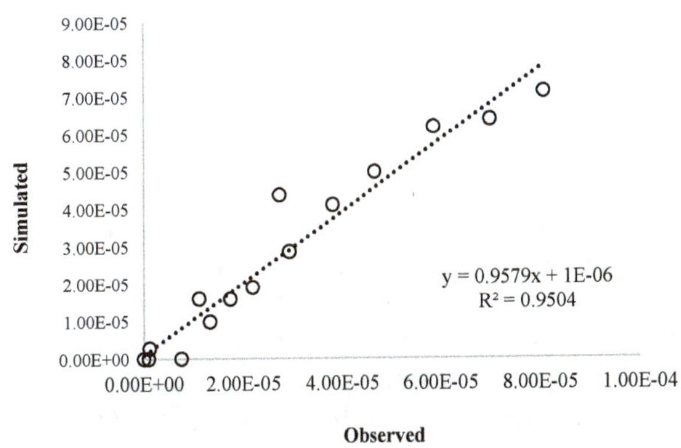

Figure 4. Comparison of the measured bacterial output with the simulated values using HYDRUS-2D model..

the macropores. In the early stages of the experiment, up to a pore volume of 0.8, the contamination through front piston and the preferential flow did not reached the bottom of the column and the chloride concentration in the effluent solution was negligible and close to zero. The steep slope of the curve approximately twice the pore volume can be due to the poor role of diffusion and distribution processes caused by the uniform distribution of pore size in the single-grained structure and the uniform distribution of chloride speed in saturated conditions. The superiority of the mass flow in the matrix and the preferential flow in the macropores caused the chloride to reach the bottom of the column at a very short time in 1/2 of the pore volume of the drained water, and in the pore volume equal to 1 of the drained water, the relative chloride concentration can be equal to 0.5, which represents the symmetry of the breakthrough curve. Therefore, in these conditions, delay was not observed in chloride transfer, due to the lack of interaction between the soil and chloride. Also, chloride is a passive tracer, it does not enter into exchange and precipitation reactions, and its absorption in the soil, especially in the studied soils with alkaline pH, is very low. The curve was S-shaped and completely symmetric and has a steep slope in $C/C0=0.5$, which is consistent with the results of Sebben et al (25). Their results showed that the breakthrough curve for homogeneous sandy soils and very light soils was S-shaped.

Transfer of bacteria

According to poiseuille [the poiseuille (symbol Pl) has been proposed as a derived SI unit of dynamic viscosity, named after the French physicist Jean Léonard Marie Poiseuille] rule, a large amount of the entire flow passes through the larger pores, resulting in the higher rate of bacterial transmission from the soil. Bacterial detachment is actually a risk for the return of pathogenic bacteria into the water and increases the risk of its contamination. Expressing the quantitative detachment of bacteria is necessary in determining the potential for transmission of bacteria. Field and laboratory observations showed that bacterial detachment caused the trailing of breakthrough curve to be longer (26). Jiang et al investigated several models and reported that two-attachment sites have higher performance (6).

Figure 2 shows that the salinity increased the ionic strength of the soil solution and compressed the diffused double layer (DDL). This action causes the bacteria to come closer to the surface of the soil particles and overcome the Van der Waals forces to absorb the bacteria on the surface of soil particles, therefore, with increasing solution concentration, transferring and leaching of the bacteria in the soil decreases. It seems that in lower salinity, a wider transition takes place in the preferential flow path and the arrival time is earlier. These results are consistent with the results of Liu et al (27).

As shown in Figure 3, bacterial transfer experiments have been carried out under steady state condition, the presence of fluctuations and various peak points and drops in the breakthrough curve of the bacteria and the distribution of data indicate a chemical and physical heterogeneity (28), because the soil columns were formed from different levels of salinity that have different attachment and detachment abilities. Also, it can indicate the preferential flow paths for bacterial transmission. The peak point of the breakthrough curve and also the area under the curve in the non-diameter treatment were higher and greater than that of the treatment with diameter of 1 cm, which indicates the occurrence of preferential flow and more consumed bacteria, and as a result, the high amount of its output from the macropores, which caused the relative concentration of the bacteria reaches about 0.00001. The peak point of the breakthrough curve in the treatment with a macropores diameter is far below the control, and these curves are relatively symmetrical in shape, indicating a lack of preferential flow in them (29). The presence of macropores results in the rapid appearance of the bacteria and the advance of the breakthrough curve shape, while the diffusion from fine pores (from the inside of the aggregate) into coarse pores leads to delays in the release of the solutes and shrinkage of the breakthrough curve shape (30). Given that the importance of the preferential flow in the transmission of bacteria, it was found that in higher ion strength, the effect of preferential flow increases even if overall bacterial transmission is reduced (10). Morales et al generally fitted two die-off and attachment/detachment indices as a particular variable in the trailing stage, to better test the model (31). Apart from the fitting method, the attachment rate that fitted with the model was higher in sandy and loamy sandy soils than clay soils. These results are consistent with the report of Unc et al (9). They showed the preferential flows in the movement and purification of bacteria in the soil. The soil's ability to purify the bacteria in the macropores decreased (32). Wang et al showed that the numerical simulations of *E. coli* in each of the different soluble chemistry conditions were very consistent with the experimental data, except for the ability to predict some differences in the transmission between different macropore settings (18). The two-site kinetics model of HYDRUS-1D was used to predict the transfer and attachment of bacteria in the soil column. The results showed that the two-site kinetics attachment-detachment model in comparison with the one-site model had better fitting with the data obtained from the bacterial transfer (21).

Conclusion

With regards to that the presence of oscillations and peak points and very high drop in the breakthrough curve of the bacteria in the studied soils, it was indicated that there are different attachment sites with different attachment and detachment energies. The rate of bacterial detachment in the soil columns was very low, which could indicate the role of salinity (sodium chloride) in the irreversible bacterial attachment. Therefore, the presence of salinity can be a significant factor in the inactivation and attachment of bacteria. It seems that the attachment of *E. coli* into the soil decreased with increasing salinity levels, which was due to increased competition for attachment sites. On the other hand, the preferential flows in the bacterial transmission can reduce the effect of tissue and soil attachment sites on the bacterial transmission process. The obtained results showed the effectiveness of preferential flows in different aspects of the study. It seems that in the inverse method, the attachment and detachment coefficients of the bacteria on the surface of the soil colloids were introduced into the model during the simulation process and the simulation was performed based on the attachment and detachment capacity of the bacteria. From the practical point of view, it can be concluded that when the soil is irrigated with saline water, the bacteria are exposed to preferential flows from the seams and gaps due to the contraction and expansion and are easily transmitted. But as time passes, the bacteria are disappeared through the transfer path due to high salinity and accumulate on the surface of the soil. Although the bacterial transmission is facilitated in salinity, the results of this study showed that increased ionic strength of the soil solution increased the rate of bacterial purification that could be effective in controlling groundwater contamination with saline water management, so that the least transition was taken place and the conditions for the use of unconventional water sources were also created, without the environmental problem threatening the risk of groundwater pollution.

Acknowledgments
This study was extracted from a Ph.D.'s thesis conducted at Guilan University of Medical Sciences, Rasht, Iran. The authors would like to gratitude Gorgan University of Agricultural Sciences and Natural Resources for its financial support and all others who involved improvement of this study.

Competing interests
The author declares that he has no competing interests.

Authors' contributions
The author contributed and was involved in the suggestion of the problem, design of experiments, data collection, analysis, and interpretation, and article approval.

References

1. Jackwood RW. Predicting fate and transport of fecal bacteria through soils using an advection-dispersion model. The University of Toledo; 2013.
2. Kadam AM, Oza GH, Nemade PD, Shankar HS. Pathogen removal from municipal wastewater in constructed soil filter. Ecol Eng 2008; 33(1): 37-44. doi: 10.1016/j.ecoleng.2007.12.001.
3. Cey EE, Rudolph DL, Passmore J. Influence of macroporosity on preferential solute and colloid transport in unsaturated field soils. J Contam Hydrol 2009; 107(1-2): 45-57. doi: 10.1016/j.jconhyd.2009.03.004.
4. Darnault CJG, Steenhuis TS, Garnier P, Kim YJ, Jenkins MB, Ghiorse WC, et al. Preferential flow and transport of *Cryptosporidium parvum* oocysts through the Vadose Zone: experiments and modeling. Vadose Zone J 2004; 3(1): 262-70. doi: 10.2136/vzj2004.2620.
5. Guber AK, Shelton DR, Pachepsky YA. Transport and Retention of Manure-Borne Coliforms in Soil. Vadose Zone J 2005; 4(3): 828-37. doi: 10.2136/vzj2004.0097.
6. Jiang S, Pang L, Buchan GD, Simunek J, Noonan MJ, Close ME. Modeling water flow and bacterial transport in undisturbed lysimeters under irrigations of dairy shed effluent and water using HYDRUS-1D. Water Res 2010; 44(4): 1050-61. doi: 10.1016/j.watres.2009.08.039.
7. Pang L, McLeod M, Aislabie J, Simunek J, Close M, Hector R. Modeling transport of microbes in ten undisturbed soils under effluent irrigation. Vadose Zone J 2008; 7(1): 97-111. doi: 10.2136/vzj2007.0108.
8. Pivetz BE, Steenhuis TS, Kelsey JW, Alexander M. A procedure to calculate biodegradation during preferential flow through heterogeneous soil columns. Soil Sci Soc Am J 1996; 60(2): 381-8. doi: 10.2136/sssaj1996.036159950060 00020008x.
9. Unc A, Goss MJ. Movement of faecal bacteria through the Vadose Zone. Water Air Soil Pollut 2003; 149(1-4): 327-37. doi: 10.1023/a:1025693109248.
10. Wang Y, Bradford SA, Simunek J. Transport and fate of microorganisms in soils with preferential flow under different solution chemistry conditions. Water Resour Res 2013; 49(5): 2424-36. doi: 10.1002/wrcr.20174.
11. Gargiulo G, Bradford SA, Simunek J, Ustohal P, Vereecken H, Klumpp E. Bacteria transport and deposition under unsaturated flow conditions: The role of water content and bacteria surface hydrophobicity. Vadose Zone J 2008; 7(2): 406-19. doi: 10.2136/vzj2007.0068.
12. Tufenkji N. Modeling microbial transport in porous media: Traditional approaches and recent developments. Adv Water Resour 2007; 30(6-7): 1455-69. doi: 10.1016/j.advwatres.2006.05.014.
13. Foppen JW, van Herwerden M, Schijven J. Measuring and modelling straining of Escherichia coli in saturated porous media. J Contam Hydrol 2007; 93(1-4): 236-54. doi: 10.1016/j.jconhyd.2007.03.001.
14. Feng G, Zhang Z, Wan C, Lu P, Bakour A. Effects of saline water irrigation on soil salinity and yield of summer maize (Zea mays L.) in subsurface drainage system. Agric Water Manag 2017; 193: 205-13. doi: 10.1016/j.agwat.2017.07.026.
15. Mamilov A, Dilly OM, Mamilov S, Inubushi K. Microbial eco-physiology of degrading aral sea wetlands: Consequences for C-cycling. J Soil Sci Plant Nutr 2004; 50(6): 839-42. doi: 10.1080/00380768.2004.10408544.
16. Kim KR, Owens G, Naidu R. Heavy metal distribution,

bioaccessibility, and phytoavailability in long-term contaminated soils from Lake Macquarie, Australia. Soil Research 2009; 47(2): 166-76. doi: 10.1071/SR08054.
17. Foppen JW, Schijven JF. Evaluation of data from the literature on the transport and survival of Escherichia coli and thermotolerant coliforms in aquifers under saturated conditions. Water Res 2006; 40(3): 401-26. doi: 10.1016/j.watres.2005.11.018.
18. Wang Y, Bradford SA, Simunek J. Physicochemical factors influencing the preferential transport of escherichia coli in soils. Vadose Zone J 2014; 13(1):1-10. doi: 10.2136/vzj2013.07.0120.
19. Mohammadi AA, Ghaderpoori M, Yousefi M, Rahmatipoor M, Javan S. Prediction and modeling of fluoride concentrations in groundwater resources using an artificial neural network: a case study in Khaf. Environ Health Eng Manag J 2016; 3(4): 217-24. doi: 10.15171/ehem.2016.23.
20. Simunek J, van Genuchten MT, Sejna M. The HYDRUS-2D Software Package for Simulating the Two-dimensional Movement of Water, Heat, and Multiple Solutes in Variably-saturated Media: Version 2.0. Colorado School of Mines; 1999. doi: 10.17221/1200-swr.
21. Safadost A, Mahbubi AA, Mossadeghi MR, Khodkaramian G, Heydari A. Transport of Escherichia coli in soil columns under different temperature and flow conditions. Water and Soil Science 2011; 15(57):183-97. [In Persian].
22. Mahon CR, Lehman DC, Manuselis G. Textbook of Diagnostic Microbiology. Elsevier Health Sciences; 2014. doi: 10.1016/0732-8893(85)90044-6.
23. Vogel AI. A Text-Book Of Quantitative Inorganic Analysis-Theory And Practice. 2nd ed. London: Longmans; 2013.
24. Schijven JF, Simunek J. Kinetic modeling of virus transport at the field scale. J Contam Hydrol 2002; 55(1-2): 113-35. doi: 10.1016/S0169-7722(01)00188-7.
25. Sebben ML, Werner AD. A modelling investigation of solute transport in permeable porous media containing a discrete preferential flow feature. Adv Water Resour 2016; 94: 307-17. doi: 10.1016/j.advwatres.2016.05.022.
26. United States Department of Agriculture. Soil taxonomy: A basic system of soil classification for making and interpreting soil surveys. Soil Science 1977; 123(4): 270. doi: 10.1097/00010694-197704000-00011.
27. Liu X, Gao C, Ji D, Walker SL, Huang Q, Cai P. Survival of Escherichia coli O157:H7 in various soil particles: importance of the attached bacterial phenotype. Biol Fertil Soils 2017; 53(2): 209-19. doi: 10.1007/s00374-016-1172-y.
28. Pang L, Simunek J. Evaluation of bacteria-facilitated cadmium transport in gravel columns using the HYDRUS colloid-facilitated solute transport model. Water Resour Res 2006; 42(12). doi: 10.1029/2006WR004896.
29. Li B, Pales AR, Clifford HM, Kupis S, Hennessy S, Liang W-Z, et al. Preferential flow in the vadose zone and interface dynamics: Impact of microbial exudates. J Hydrol 2018; 558: 72-89. doi: 10.1016/j.jhydrol.2017.12.065.
30. Liu HF, Genard M, Guichard S, Bertin N. Model-assisted analysis of tomato fruit growth in relation to carbon and water fluxes. J Exp Bot 2007; 58(13): 3567-80. doi: 10.1093/jxb/erm202.
31. Morales I, Atoyan JA, Amador JA, Boving T. Transport of pathogen surrogates in soil treatment units: Numerical modeling. Water 2014; 6(4): 818-38. doi: 10.3390/w6040818.
32. Sahraei N, Mahboobi AA. Investigating the Effect of Soil and Organic Fertilizer Building on the Movement of Escherichia coli in Soil Columns. Twelfth National Conference on the Health of Iran; 2009 Nov 3-5; Shahid Beheshti University of Medical Sciences, Tehran; 2009. [In Persian].

Biomedical waste disposal systems of health facilities in Ethiopia

Sisay Derso[1*], Girum Taye[2], Theodros Getachew[2], Atkure Defar[2], Habtamu Teklie[2], Kassahun Amenu[2], Terefe Gelibo[2], Abebe Bekele[2]

[1]Environmental Health Research Team, Ethiopian Public Health Institute, Addis Ababa, Ethiopia
[2]Health System Research Directorate, Ethiopian Public Health Institute, Addis Ababa, Ethiopia

Abstract
Background: Biomedical waste generated from health and health-related activities can be grouped as general waste and hazardous waste. This remains true if and only if there is proper on-site handling, such as the segregation and separation of waste based on the type and nature of the source.
Methods: A stratified random sampling design was used to provide representative results for Ethiopia, for various types of facility and management authorities, and for each of the 11 regions. Totally, 1327 health facilities were assessed using the World Health Organization (WHO) inventory tools.
Results: Nationally, medical waste in 32.6% of the studied health facilities was stored in covered containers, and in about 27% of them it was stored in another protected environment. About 40% of health facilities stored their medical waste in unprotected areas. Twenty-eight (2.6%) and 420 (39.3%) health facilities used 2-chamber industrial incinerators and 1-chamber drum incinerators, respectively. About 58% of health facilities used unsafe waste treatment methods. The proportion of using safe medical waste disposal method was high in referral hospitals (87.9%). This shows the utilization of safe medical waste disposal methods is in decreasing order from higher to lower levels of organization in health facilities.
Conclusion: The present study showed a preliminary finding on the waste disposal systems of health facilities at the national level. Dumping biomedical waste outside the health facility is common, and access to common waste facilities is limited. Therefore, a holistic approach to safe medical waste management practices, including the collection process (handling, sorting, and segregation), storage, treatment and final disposal is crucial in all types of health facilities, regardless of the level of organization, ownership, or geographic distribution.
Keywords: Health Facility, Biomedical Waste, Disposal, Incinerator, Ethiopia

***Correspondence to:**
Sisay Derso
Email: sisdres23@yahoo.com

Introduction

Healthcare waste can be defined as the total waste stream that is generated from healthcare establishments, health-related research facilities, and laboratories. Hospitals, clinics, laboratories, medical research centers, pharmaceutical manufacturing plants, pharmacies, blood banks, veterinary health care centers, and home healthcare activities are some of the generators of healthcare waste irrespective of volumes, characteristics, and composition (1,2).

Biomedical waste generated from health-related activities can be broadly grouped as general waste and hazardous waste. This remains true if and only if there is proper on-site handling, such as segregation, separation, and storing with a unique color-coded storage system. There are different estimates regarding the share of hazardous and non-hazardous constituents of healthcare waste. This difference was observed in a study conducted in Ethiopia. The results of a cross-sectional study conducted in selected hospitals in Addis Ababa indicated that the median waste generation rate varied between 0.361 and 0.669 kg/patient/d and was comprised of 58.69% non-hazardous and 41.31% hazardous wastes (3). This difference was also observed in health centers in rural and urban settings. A study conducted in Addis Ababa revealed that the mean (±SD) healthcare waste generation rate was 9.61 ± 3.28 kg/d, of which (38%) 3.64 ± 1.45 kg/d was general or non-hazardous waste and (62%) 5.97 ± 2.31 kg/d was hazardous (4). On the other hand, rural health centers contributed about 0.93 ± 0.3 kg/d (52.0%) general waste and 0.86 ± 0.33 kg/d (48.0%) hazardous waste (5). In general, the amount of waste generated increased as the number of patients increased. In addition, the rate of waste generation depended on the facility type; public health facilities generated a higher proportion of total healthcare waste than private facilities (3).

Waste generated at healthcare facilities needs an adequate and appropriate management mechanism before disposal, including all activities involved in waste generation, segregation, transportation, storage, treatment, and final disposal (6). Out of the many medical waste treatment technologies, incineration is the most preferable and common treatment method for medical waste in Ethiopia and elsewhere. Incineration ranks third in the waste management hierarchy, accompanied by source reduction, reuse, recycling, and final disposal/landfilling. Incineration is an engineered process that involves thermal decomposition through thermal oxidation at elevated temperatures (usually 900°C and greater) to destroy the organic fraction of the waste (7). However, the inadequate or inefficient incineration of medical waste can result in high concentrations of toxic pollutants being released into the atmosphere and in bottom and fly ash, which comprises toxic organic and inorganic compounds, threatening public health as well as the environment. The Environmental Protection Agency of the United States of America found in 1994 that emissions from incinerators in healthcare facilities were responsible for high levels of chemicals such as dioxin and furan in the atmosphere (8).

Next to incineration, landfills for medical waste are ranked second as a final waste management technology in the Ethiopian healthcare system. However, the use of landfills as refuse dumps is gradually expanding the problems of health hazards in the environment and among the general population. Selling biomedical waste to scavengers is another disposal method, but scavengers are always the victims of disease due to having contact with such wastes (9).

All individuals exposed to healthcare waste are at risk of being injured or infected. This includes the medical staff, inpatients and outpatients, support staff, waste handlers, waste scavengers, and the general public, particularly children who are exposed to materials from the disposed-of medical waste. However, in 2005 World Health Organization (WHO) study indicated that the rate of such injuries depends on the medical discipline. For instance, the prevalence of needlestick injury among healthcare providers in a university hospital in Germany was 46.9% (n=91/194) among medical staff in surgery and 18.7% (n=53/283) among HCWs in pediatrics. Of all occupational groups, physicians had the highest risk of experiencing needlestick injuries (55.1%, n = 129/234) (10). In general, the medical and ancillary staff as well as sanitary experts can be injured if the waste has not been safely packed. In this respect, sharps are considered one of the most dangerous categories of waste. Many injuries occur because syringe needles or other sharps have not been collected in safety boxes or because the boxes have been overfilled. At dumpsites, scavengers may also come in contact with infectious waste during their recycling activities if the waste has not been properly disposed of or treated (11).

Biomedical waste handling is a hazardous activity that requires a high standard of training and skill. It calls for specific training that depends on the nature of the work in the service delivery unit, the hazards and possibility of worker exposure, and the responsibilities of individual workers. A study conducted in Addis Ababa showed that only 19.8% of medical waste handlers were trained to handle medical waste and none was immunized against hepatitis B virus (HBV) (12). Due to the lack of adequate training and low awareness of biomedical waste handling and management, the HBV was detected in 8% of healthcare waste handlers and 0.8% of non-medical waste handlers in selected hospitals in Addis Ababa and 6.0% of healthcare waste handlers and 1.0% non-medical waste handlers in Gondar town health institutions (12,13).

The number of health facilities in Ethiopia has been greatly emphasized since the implementation of the health sector development program in 1990; in this program, the expansion of health service facilities was one of the program's pillars. Due to this and other related factors, the type and quantity of disposable medical equipment and logistics are increasing and may ultimately result in a higher rate of medical waste generation in the country. In Ethiopia, as in many other developing countries, little is known about safe waste disposal and the treatment of medical waste. Furthermore, there is no comprehensive, nationally representative data on the types of health facilities (hospitals, health centers, health posts, clinics), type of administration (governmental, non-governmental, and private), region, or urbanity in Ethiopia. Therefore, the main objective of the current study was to understand the existing waste disposal system in Ethiopian health facilities and to determine key influencing factors for safe waste management practices. The study also aimed to deliver information on the release through inefficient incineration of toxic pollutants, which may increase the risk of cancer and other teratogenic effects.

Methods

Data collection

The data for this study was taken from the 2014 Ethiopia Service Provision Assessment Plus (ESPA+) Survey. The sample for the survey was a stratified random sample designed to provide representative results for Ethiopia, for different facility types (hospitals, health centers, health posts, clinics), different management authorities (governmental, non-governmental, private), places of residence (rural/urban), and for each of the 11 regions of the country. The data was collected by a trained health professional recruited by the Ethiopian Public Health Institute. All field staff obtained detailed training on the survey, including theory, the administration of questionnaires and the observational checklist, computer programming, and practical and field pilot tests. Totally, 1327 health facilities were assessed. All hospitals, selected health centers, private clinics, and health posts were assessed using a structured questionnaire and an observational checklist.

Survey Instrument

The WHO healthcare waste management inventory tools were used to assess and capture data on waste management at different departments of each health facility. A facility inventory questionnaire was used to obtain information on how the facilities dispose of and manage healthcare wastes in each of the priority services. The facility inventory questionnaire collected information on the functional status of disposal systems, type of disposal system (maintenance and management), and service delivery environment. The data collectors interviewed the most knowledgeable persons at each facility and/or service. If another provider needed to give some specific information, that provider was invited (or visited, if appropriate) and questioned.

Data collection approaches

Following the preparation of the final questionnaires in English, the questionnaires were translated into three major local languages, Amharigna, Oromiffa, and Tigrigna. Both the English and the translated inventory questionnaires were loaded onto tablet computers which were used during interviews to ask questions and record responses (Computer Assisted Personal Interviewing–CAPI) in each respondent's preferred language.

Sampling

The sample size for this survey was determined by a combination of census and random samples. The Ethiopia health service system structure, organized into a 3-tier system: Level 1 (primary hospital, health center, and their satellite health posts) constituted the Primary Health Care Unit (PHCU); Level 2 was composed of general hospitals; and Level 3 was organized by teaching or specialized hospitals) was followed during sampling. The private-for-profit and NGO health sectors in Ethiopia have seen rapid expansion in recent years, and due to their importance, they were considered in sampling.

In general, the sample of this survey included all hospitals and a sample of health centers and private facilities. Health posts were selected independently. Due to their number and service, all hospitals were included in the survey, allowing for the inclusion of newly identified hospitals. A representative sample of health centers and clinics was selected for the survey. A total sample size of 1327 health facilities was selected, including 321 health posts and 10 newly identified hospitals.

Data analysis

The chi-square test was used to analyze bivariate data, and the logistic regression method was used for univariate and multivariate analysis. The medical waste treatment methods used in each health facility were considered as an outcome variable by categorizing them into safe medical waste disposal methods and unsafe medical waste disposal methods.

The independent variables for this analysis were facility type, managing authority, region, urban/rural, and the availability of waste disposal guidelines. Bivariate analysis revealed that, at a 5% level of significance, all independent variables (potential factors) had an association with medical waste disposal methods (safe/unsafe). Therefore, all independent variables were considered in both univariate and multivariate logistic regression models to identify the potential predictors of using safe medical waste disposal methods. The unit of analysis for this study was all health facilities covered in the SPA project. Both bivariate and multivariate statistical analyses were carried out to identify the potential determinants of using safe medical waste disposal methods in health facilities using SPSS version 20 software.

Hypothesis

To test the hypothesis, the following categorization gave the outcome variable:

- If the health facilities used Incinerator (2-chamber industrial), Incinerator (1-chamber drum/brick), open burning (pit or protected), dump no burning (covered pit or pit latrine), dump no burning (protected ground or pit), removal offsite (stored in covered container), or removal offsite (stored in other protected environment) and burned in other facility, they were recorded as using safe medical waste disposal methods.
- If the health facilities used open burning (flat ground no protection), dump no burning (flat ground, no protection), dump no burning (open pit no protection), removal off-site (stored unprotected) or barrel (Bermel), they were recorded as using unsafe medical waste disposal methods.

The independent variables considered were facility type, managing authority, region, urban/rural, and waste disposal guideline availability.

Results

Descriptive analysis

After medical waste is generated during the provision of healthcare services at health facilities, it needs to be handled and stored in a safe place to prevent nosocomial infections and to protect the public. Nationally, 32.6% of the health facilities stored medical waste in a covered container, and about 27% of health facilities stored it in another protected environment. The remaining 40% of health facilities stored their medical waste in unprotected areas, like an open field or barrel, and did not store waste completely, as shown in Table 1.

Table 2 presents the existing waste treatment methods in the studied health facilities. Twenty-eight (2.6%) and 420 (39.3%) health facilities used 2-chamber industrial incinerators and 1-chamber drum incinerators, respectively. The remaining 58% of health facilities (the majority) used unsafe waste treatment methods, including open burning and dumping in unsanitary ways.

Bivariate analysis

Table 3 presents the status of using safe medical waste disposal method in selected health facilities by background characteristics. At a 1% level of significance, the results indicate the status of using safe medical waste disposal methods is significantly associated with facility type, managing authority, region, urban/rural, and availability of guidelines for waste management in the service area. The use of safe medical waste disposal methods was high in referral hospitals (87.9%) followed by general hospitals (86.6%), health centers (79.5%), higher clinics (78.6%), primary hospitals (76.8%), medium clinics (64.3%), health posts (52.6%), and lower clinics (51%). This shows that the utilization of safe medical waste disposal methods has a generally decreasing trend with the decreasing level of health facilities from the higher to the lower tier of the Ethiopian health service structure.

Among the 1327 studied health facilities, 28 (87.5%) health facilities managed under the NGO authority

Table 1. Percentage of facilities by medical waste storage methods used

Methods used for medical waste storage	No. (%)
Storing in covered container	31 (32.6)
Storing in another protected environment	26 (27.4)
Unprotected storage	13 (13.7)
Barrel	8 (8.4)
Stored in other facility	3 (3.2)
Other	14 (14.7)
Total	95 (100)

Table 2. Percentage of facilities by medical waste treatment methods used

Methods used for medical waste treatment	No. (%)
Burn-in incinerator, 2 chambers industrial	28 (2.6)
Burn-in incinerator, 1 chamber drum	420 (39.3)
Open burning, flat ground-no protection	208 (19.4)
Open burning, pit or protected ground	346 (32.3)
Dump no burning, flat ground, no protection	20 (1.9)
Dump no burning, covered pit or pit latrine	13 (1.2)
Dump no burning, open pit, no protection	19 (1.8)
Dump no burning, protected ground or pit	16(1.5)
Total	1070 (100)

and 527 (68.6%) of the health facilities managed under government or public authority used safe medical waste disposal methods.

The use of safe medical waste disposal methods was high among facilities in Addis Ababa (106; 82.8%) followed by Tigray (95; 72%), S.N.N.P (130; 71%), Dire Dawa (58; 69%), Afar (53; 67.9%), Amhara (121; 65.8%), Harari (37; 60.7%), Somalia (51; 60.7%), Gambella (48; 60%), Oromiya (140; 59.3%), and Benshangul (44; 57.1%).

The proportion of health facilities using safe medical waste disposal methods was higher in urban areas (n = 465; 74.5%) compared with health facilities in rural areas (n = 418; 61.1%). In addition, the proportion of health facilities using safe medical waste disposal methods was high among those who had guidelines for waste management in the service area (n = 243; 82.7%) compared with those who did not (n = 640; 73.5%).

Multivariate analysis

Table 4 presents the adjusted and unadjusted odds ratios with 95% confidence intervals which were obtained from multivariate and univariate logistic regression models by considering the variables with the status of using safe medical waste disposal methods as an outcome variable. The results of univariate logistic regression at a 5% level of significance showed that facility type, managing authority, region, urban/rural, and guidelines availability were all statistically significant in determining whether the medical waste disposal methods used were safe or not. Therefore, all of the above background characteristics should be considered as explanatory variables in the multivariate logistic regression model.

The odds ratios shown in Table 4 were used to compare the probability of an event for two groups. In this study, it helps to test the following hypotheses.

Ho: There is no association between medical waste disposal methods in health facilities and background characteristics (*P* value > 0.05).

H1: There is an association between medical waste disposal methods in health facilities and background characteristics (*P* value < 0.05).

From Table 4, it can be seen that some *P* values for medical waste disposal methods by region had a less than 5% level of significance and its corresponding 95% CI for the odds ratio (OR) does not include one, implies somehow, there is an association between the two variables with the following interpretation.

The odds of using a safe medical waste disposal method in the assessed health facilities were 3.345 times greater among health facilities in the Dire Dawa region than facilities in the Tigray region.

At a 5% level of significance, almost all *P* values in measuring the association between medical waste disposal methods in the assessed health facilities and background characteristics were less than 0.05, and its corresponding 95% CI for OR does not include one, it indicates that there

Table 3. Status of using safe medical waste disposal methods in health facilities by background characteristics

Background Characteristics	Medical waste disposal methods		Chi-square	*P* value
	Safe, No. (%)	Unsafe, No. (%)		
Facility type (%)			**115.626**	**<0.01**
Referral hospital (2.5)	29 (87.9)	4 (12.1)		
General hospital (10.1)	116 (86.6)	18 (13.4)		
Primary hospital (4.2)	43 (76.8)	13 (23.2)		
Health centre (22.4)	237 (79.5)	61 (20.5)		
Health post (24.2)	169 (52.6)	152 (47.4)		
Higher clinic (5.3)	55 (78.6)	15 (21.4)		
Medium clinic (12.7)	108 (64.3)	60 (35.7)		
Lower clinic (18.6)	126 (51)	121 (49)		
Managing authority			**12.269**	**0.007**
Government or public (57.9)	527 (68.6)	241 (31.4)		
Other governmental (0.9)	7 (58.3)	5 (41.7)		
Private for profit (38.8)	321 (62.3)	194 (37.7)		
NGO (2.4)	28 (87.5)	4 (12.5)		
Region			**31.334**	**0.001**
Tigray (9,4)	95 (72)	37 (28)		
Afar (5.9)	53 (67.9)	25 (32.1)		
Amhara (13.9)	121 (65.8)	63 (34.2)		
Oromiya (17.8)	140 (59.3)	96 (40.7)		
Somalia (6.3)	51 (60.7)	33 (39.3)		
Benshangul (5.8)	44 (57.1)	33 (42.9)		
S.N.N.P (13.8)	130 (71)	53 (29)		
Gambella (6.0)	48 (60)	32 (40)		
Harari (4.6)	37 (60.7)	24 (39.3)		
Addis Ababa (9.4)	106 (82.8)	22 (17.2)		
Dire Dawa (6.3)	58 (69)	26 (31)		
Urban/Rural			**64.684**	**<0.01**
Urban (47.7)	465 (74.5)	159 (25.5)		
Rural (52.3)	418 (61.1)	266 (38.9)		
Guideline availability			**10.084**	**0.001**
Yes (25.2)	243 (82.7)	51 (17.3)		
No (74.8)	640 (73.5)	231 (26.5)		

is an association between the two variables.

Moreover, the results can be interpreted as showing that among the assessed health facilities, general hospitals are 7.537 times more likely to use safe medical waste disposal methods than referral hospitals. In addition, primary hospitals, health centers, health posts, and medium clinics are 5.914, 4.335, 4.639, and 8.227 times more likely, respectively, to use safe medical waste disposal methods compared to a referral hospital.

At a 5% level of significance, there was no association between medical waste disposal methods in health facilities and facility type, managing authority, availability of guidelines for waste management in the service area, or urban/rural background characteristics.

Discussion

Biomedical waste generated from health and health-related activities can be broadly grouped as general waste and hazardous waste. This remains true if and only if there is proper on-site handling, segregation, and separation of waste with regard to the type and nature of the source. The present study revealed that about 33% of health facilities use covered containers, and 27% of them store their medical waste in protected environments. Conversely, about 40% of the studied health facilities stored their waste in an unprotected environment (Table 1). Waste produced in healthcare facilities in developing countries has raised serious concerns because of inappropriate treatment and final disposal practices, which can impose negative impacts on public health and the environment (14). Having this concept in mind, the present healthcare waste storage practices in Ethiopian health facilities could threaten the public as well as the environment. In addition, the unimproved waste storage practices of health facilities could lead to insufficient waste incineration and complicated final disposal of medical waste.

In general, poor medical waste handling and storage practices potentially create risks to health workers, clients, the environment, and human health. One study conducted in Ethiopia indicated that due to the lack of adequate waste handling and biomedical waste storage practices, the HBV was detected in waste handlers (8% of healthcare waste handlers and 0.8% in non-medical waste handlers) in selected hospitals in Addis Ababa and 6.0%

Table 4. Adjusted odds ratios with 95% confidence intervals for using safe medical waste disposal methods in health facilities

Background Characteristics	Adjusted OR	95% CI for adjusted OR	*P* value
Facility type			
Referral Hospital	1		
General Hospital	7.537	(1.297,43.807)	0.024
Primary Hospital	5.914	(1.782,19.626)	0.004
Health Centre	4.335	(1.097,17.134)	0.036
Health post	4.639	(1.299,16.567)	0.018
Higher clinic	1.617	(0.453,5.771)	0.459
Medium clinic	8.227	(1.888,35.846)	0.005
Lower clinic	1.767	(0.977,3.194)	0.060
Managing authority			
Government or public	1		
Other governmental	0.236	(0.048,1.151)	0.074
Private for profit	0.294	(0.044,1.954)	0.205
NGO	0.596	(0.167,2.131)	0.426
Region			
Tigray	1		
Afar	1.398	(0.683,2.861)	0.360
Amhara	1.932	(0.822,4.541)	0.131
Oromiya	0.938	(0.492,1.787)	0.845
Somalia	0.671	(0.361,1.247)	0.207
Benshangul	1.024	(0.46,2.278)	0.954
S.N.N.P	0.964	(0.456,2.039)	0.923
Gambella	1.233	(0.642,2.368)	0.530
Harari	1.198	(0.558,2.572)	0.643
Addis Ababa	0.698	(0.318,1.530)	0.369
Diredawa	3.345	(1.142,9.798)	0.028
Urban/Rural			
Urban	1		
Rural	1.23	(0.82,1.843)	0.317
Guideline availability			
Yes	1		
No	1.078	(0.704,1.651)	0.704

of healthcare waste handlers and 1.% non-medical waste handlers in Gondar town health institutions (12,13). Such findings are in agreement with the WHO estimation that injections with contaminated syringes caused 21 million HBV infections (32% of all new infections), 2 million hepatitis C virus (HCV) infections (40% of all new infections), and 260000 HIV infections (5% of all new infections) globally (15).

Furthermore, the improper medical waste handling and storage practices of the majority of Ethiopian health facilities could result in needlestick and sharp object injuries. All individuals exposed to healthcare waste are at risk of being injured or infected. This includes medical staffs, inpatients and outpatients, support staff, waste handlers, scavengers, and the public, particularly children or scavengers who are exposed to materials from disposed-of medical waste. However, the study showed that the rate of such injuries depends on the medical discipline; for instance, the prevalence of needlestick injury among healthcare providers in a university hospital in Germany was 46.9% (n=91/194) among medical staff in surgery and 18.7% (n=53/283) among healthcare workers in pediatrics. Of all occupational groups, physicians have the highest risk of experiencing needlestick injuries (55.1%; n = 129/234) (10).

Incineration is the most preferable and common treatment method for medical waste in Ethiopia and elsewhere. Incineration ranks third in the waste management hierarchy, accompanied by source reduction, reuse, recycling, and final disposal/landfilling. About 94% of health facilities in the present study used burning as their preferred treatment method for medical waste; 3% used 2-chamber incinerators, 39% used 1-chamber incinerators, and the remaining health facilities, a substantial number, used open burning as their medical waste treatment (Table 2). Inadequate or inefficient incineration of medical waste can result in the release of high concentrations of toxic pollutants into the atmosphere and to bottom and fly ash, which comprises toxic organic and inorganic compounds. These toxic releases comprise organic emissions such as polychlorinated dibenzo-dioxins/furnace (PCDD/Fs) and polycyclic aromatic hydrocarbons (PAHs), inorganic emissions, and ashes containing toxic metals. These products are carcinogenic and affect the development, reproduction, and immune systems of humans (7). Historically, health concerns raised by incineration focused on communities living near the incinerator. Recently, the WHO identified three potentially exposed populations: the local population through inhalation, workers at the facility, and the larger regional population through the food chain and bioaccumulate pollutants (16). Furthermore, incinerators dangerously pollute technologies that will virtually undermine the objectives of the treaty on persistent organic pollutants (POPs). The Stockholm Convention on POPs, which was ratified by Ethiopia (2003) and entered into action (2004), identifies waste incinerators as the principal source of dioxins and furans, which are among the initial 12 substances being targeted for continuing minimization and ultimate elimination by the global community (17). Considering this, many countries have taken action to treat and dispose of health facility waste using environmentally safer, non-combustion technologies. Ethiopia, as a global entity, could follow this approach as well.

In this study, the result of bivariate analysis shown in Table 3 indicates that at a 1% level of significance, the status of using safe medical waste disposal method was significantly associated with facility type, managing authority, region, urban/rural, and availability of guidelines for waste management in the service area. This finding is in agreement with a study conducted in India which revealed that biomedical waste management practices were better among hospital staff in comparison with private medical practitioners and marginally higher among those in urban areas in comparison with those in rural areas (18).

The management of healthcare waste is an integral part of a national healthcare system. The waste management system consists of all activities related to the handling, treatment, disposal, or recycling of waste materials. The purpose of a waste management system is to make sure that waste materials are removed from the source or location where they are generated and treated, disposed of, or recycled in a safe and proper manner (19). However, in this study, the multivariate logistic regression analysis revealed that general hospitals were 7.537 times more likely to use safe medical waste disposal methods than referral hospitals. Furthermore, primary hospitals, health centers, health posts, and medium clinics were 5.914, 4.335, 4.639, and 8.227 times more likely, respectively, to use safe medical waste disposal methods than referral hospitals (Table 4). As a result, a holistic approach to healthcare waste management including a clear delineation of responsibilities, occupational health and safety programs, waste minimization and segregation, the development and adoption of safe and environmentally sound technologies, and capacity building should be considered in all types of health facilities in both rural and urban settings.

Education and awareness of waste and waste management are increasingly important from a global perspective of resource management. The role of sustainable waste management is to reduce the amount of waste that is discharged into the environment by reducing the amount of waste generated. In Ethiopia, medical waste is mostly dumped in the open field or burned in open fires, which may contribute to air pollution and the pollution of other environmental compartments, including groundwater sources and soil due to leachate and recharging. To improve such situations, strategies must be designed for all types of health facilities with special emphasis on those using less safe waste management methods, regardless of facility type, location, or managing authority. Waste pollutes the environment and threatens human health; therefore, tackling such problems requires rigorous and continual public health education. Educating personnel will also improve the efficiency of waste management systems and minimize the possible health and environmental risks (19).

This study also showed that the availability of healthcare waste management guidelines contributes to safe waste handling and management (Figure 1). The current results indicated that more health facilities with waste management guidelines are practicing safe waste management than health facilities without guidelines. The results further illustrated that 231 health facilities that did not have guidelines during the survey managed their medical waste in an unsafe manner in a higher proportion than those with guidelines (51 health facilities only). Another study conducted in Ethiopia, which is in agreement with the current findings, indicated that the management of healthcare waste requires well-organized documents, including policy documents, regulations, and technical guidelines, but the existing healthcare

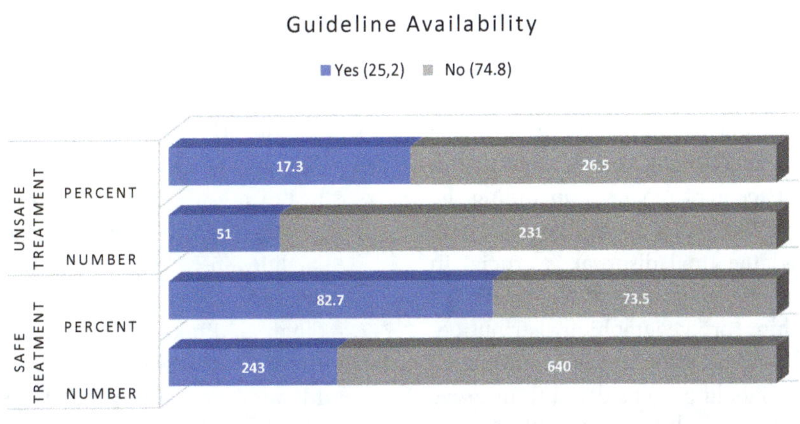

Figure 1. Availability of guidelines in health facility and its contribution to waste management.

waste management practices do not obey the principles of waste management in general. In addition, mandate overlapping and limited cooperation between various stakeholders and responsible sectors were identified as major barriers to safe medical waste management (20). Some aspects of healthcare waste management can be improved by providing training for medical staff, waste handlers, support staff, and the public on proper waste management and source reduction. Another step toward improvement is the preparation of wholesome legislation and policy documents on healthcare waste management with a clear description of the mandates to different interested parties. However, significant financial and infrastructure challenges remain. These include the costs for special containers, human resources, administrative and regulatory capacities, as well as disposal systems and technologies.

Conclusion

The present study showed a preliminary finding on the waste disposal systems of health facilities at a national level. The results revealed that 60% of health facilities stored waste in a protected environment, and the remaining 40% stored it in an insanitary way. About 94% of the studied facilities used burning medical waste as a major treatment method, among which only about 42% used a standard incinerator; the remaining facilities practiced open burning.

Utilization of safe medical waste disposal methods is significantly associated with facility type, managing authority, region, urban/rural, and availability of guidelines for waste management in the service area. This study showed that the utilization of safe medical waste disposal methods had a decreasing trend with the decreasing levels of organization of the health facilities. At a 5% level of significance, the bivariate analysis showed that all background characteristics considered in this study (facility type, managing authority, region, urban/rural, and guideline availability) were associated with the respective medical waste disposal methods in the selected health facilities. Based on the multivariate analysis, however, it seems that, at a 5% level of significance, general hospitals are more likely to use safe medical waste disposal methods than referral hospitals.

Dumping biomedical waste outside the health facility is a common practice, and access to common waste facilities is still limited. Therefore, a holistic approach to safe medical waste management practices, including the collection process (handling, sorting, and segregation), storage, treatment, and the final disposal is crucial in all types of health facility, regardless of their level of organization, ownership, or geographic distribution. Furthermore, surveillance, monitoring, and continuous awareness-raising tasks should be considered to improve waste management systems in all health facilities across the country.

Acknowledgments

The authors would like to acknowledge the Ethiopian Public Health Institute for its financial and logistic support of this research paper.

Competing interests

The authors have declared that they have no conflicts of interest.

Authors' contributions

SD performed the overall manuscript writing. GT helped with data analysis and application of software. TG participated in data collection and the overall coordination of the survey. AD, HT, KA, and TG participated in data collection. AB guided and managed the data collection and manuscript preparation.

References

1. Khajuria A, Kumar A. Assessment of Healthcare Waste Generated by Government Hospital in Agra City, India. Our Nature 2007; 5(1): 25-30. doi: 10.3126/on.v5i1.794.
2. Pruss A, Giroult E, Rushbrook P. Safe Management of Wastes from Health-care Activities. Geneva: World Health Organization; 1999.
3. Debere MK, Gelaye KA, Alamdo AG, Trifa ZM. Assessment of the health care waste generation rates and its management system in hospitals of Addis Ababa, Ethiopia, 2011. BMC Public Health 2013; 13: 28. doi: 10.1186/1471-2458-13-28.
4. Tadesse ML, Kumie A. Healthcare waste generation and management practice in government health centers of Addis Ababa, Ethiopia. BMC Public Health 2014; 14: 1221. doi: 10.1186/1471-2458-14-1221.
5. Azage M, Kumie A. Healthcare waste generation and its management system: the case of health centers in West Gojjam Zone, Amhara Region, Ethiopia. Ethiop J Health Dev 2010; 24(2):119-26. doi: 10.4314/ejhd.v24i2.62960.
6. Odette RH, Masika J, Venance T, Soatiana JE, Christiane NA, Lamine CM, Bin L. Assessment of healthcare waste generation and its management systems: a prevalence survey of the healthcare facilities in Madagascar. J Environ Sci Toxicol Food Technol 2014; 8: 20-9.
7. Singh S, Prakash V. Toxic environmental releases from medical waste incineration: a review. Environ Monit Assess 2007; 132(1-3): 67-81. doi: 10.1007/s10661-006-9503-3.
8. Malkan S, Nelson J. Global trends in responsible

healthcare waste management-A perspective from health Care without harm. Waste Manag 2005; 25(6): 570-2.

9. Hussein H, Musah BA, Guo E. Disposal of health facility waste in landfill sites and its effects on the people of Gbalahi community in the Tamale metropolis. Int Res J Public Environ Health 2014; 1(1): 1-9.

10. Wicker S, Jung J, Allwinn R, Gottschalk R, Rabenau HF. Prevalence and prevention of needlestick injuries among health care workers in a German university hospital. Int Arch Occup Environ Health 2008; 81(3): 347-54. doi: 10.1007/s00420-007-0219-7.

11. Manual G. Preparation of national healthcare waste management plans in sub-Saharan countries. Geneva: World Health Organization; 2005.

12. Shiferaw Y, Abebe T, Mihret A. Hepatitis B virus infection among medical waste handlers in Addis Ababa, Ethiopia. BMC Res Notes 2011; 4(1): 479. doi: 10.1186/1756-0500-4-479.

13. Anagaw B, Shiferaw Y, Anagaw B, Belyhun Y, Erku W, Biadgelegn F, et al. Seroprevalence of hepatitis B and C viruses among medical waste handlers at Gondar town Health institutions, Northwest Ethiopia. BMC Res Notes 2012; 5: 55. doi: 10.1186/1756-0500-5-55.

14. Diaz LF, Savage GM, Eggerth LL. Alternatives for the treatment and disposal of healthcare wastes in developing countries. Waste Manag 2005; 25(6): 626-37. doi: 10.1016/j.wasman.2005.01.005.

15. World Health Organazation. WHO core principles for achieving safe and sustainable management of health-care waste. Geneva, Switzerland: WHO; 2007.

16. Batterman S, Water S. Findings on an Assessment of Small-scale Incinerators for Health-care Waste. Geneva: WHO; 2004.

17. Convention S. Stockholm convention on persistent organic pollutants. UNEP; 2001.

18. Rao PH. Report: Hospital waste management--awareness and practices: a study of three states in India. Waste Manag Res 2008; 26(3): 297-303. doi: 10.1177/0734242x08088693.

19. Demirbas A. Waste management, waste resource facilities and waste conversion processes. Energy Convers Manag 2011; 52(2): 1280-7. doi: 10.1016/j.enconman.2010.09.025.

20. Haylamicheal ID, Desalegne SA. A review of legal framework applicable for the management of healthcare waste and current management practices in Ethiopia. Waste Manag Res 2012; 30(6): 607-18. doi: 10.1177/0734242x11419891.

Risk assessment of noise pollution by analyzing the level of sound loudness resulting from central traffic in Shiraz

Hadi Negahdari[1], Sirus Javadpour[2*], Faramarz Moattar[1], Hashem Negahdari[3]

[1]Department of Environmental Engineering, Faculty of Natural Resources and Environment, Science and Research Branch, Islamic Azad University, Tehran, Iran
[2]Material Science and Engineering Department, School of Engineering, Shiraz University, Shiraz, Iran
[3]Department of Civil Engineering, School of Engineering, Islamic Azad University, Shiraz Branch, Shiraz, Iran

Abstract
Background: Today, the effects of environmental pollution on human life and human needs, which reduces the level of community health caused by traffic noise in large cities, are clearly visible by creating irritation and pathogenic conditions. The aim of this study was to assess the risk of noise pollution resulted from central traffic in Shiraz by analyzing its indicators and related components.
Methods: By specifying the high traffic jam in Shiraz, the sound and its frequency in 156 points of the city were analyzed using a sound analyzer (Tes-1358C model). The sound pressure levels (L_A and L_p) and the one and one-third octave band were continuously measured in A and C networks. Then, data were extracted and analyzed using Excel 2016 and Minitab 18.1. Eventually, phon and sone indexes were calculated for the heavy traffic jam in some of the central streets of Shiraz and the results were statistically calculated and their charts were prepared with comfort disturbance ranges.
Results: The highest harmful frequency of traffic in Shiraz was 50 Hz and 83.3 dB. The sound pressure level ranged from 70 to 92.7 dB in network A and 87.8 dB in network C. The maximum sound level was 87 phon and the maximum sone was 26 at 14 stations.
Conclusion: According to the results, the sound pressure levels exceeded the environmental standards of Iran and the values of phon and sone were higher than the standard of comfort at night and day.
Keywords: Noise pollution, Environmental pollution, Loudness perception, Health risk assessment, Shiraz.

***Correspondence to:**
Sirus Javadpour
Email: Javadpor@shirazu.ac.ir

Introduction

Today, with the rapid advances in technology and increasing human needs, the kind of popular look to sound has changed. Some people enjoy loud sound in their jobs (such as musicians), on the other hand, some find it annoying. One of the most damaging and neglected factors in the environment, life, and work is noise pollution (1). One of the major problems of large cities in Iran is noise pollution. Recent studies have shown that in Tehran and other large metropolitan areas of Iran, the level of noise pollution has reached an intolerable level so that the residents of these cities should gradually think about providing hearing protectors to protect their ears from loud sound, while attending the city, or accept that they gradually lose their hearing ability (1). Noise pollution is not a new issue for large cities, and public health authorities warned that the level of noise pollution and its consequences are raising above the tolerance level in large cities.

Noise-induced hearing loss (NIHL) is known as an occupational disease in the world (2). The living conditions of humans are such that they interact with noise daily based on their activity and place of live (3). According to the Environmental Protection Agency (EPA), the balance of sound level meter should not exceed 35 dB at night and 45 dB in day (3). Studies have shown that the average sound pressure level in different parts of a hospital is 56.3 dB (4). Using noise maps, noise pollution level (NPL), and traffic noise index (TNI) can help intelligent traffic control planning, because these maps can represent the movement of people in different times and parts of a city (5).

From a practical point of view, scientists have progressively realized that noise pollution in large cities of Iran was higher than the Iran's Environmental Protection Organization (IEPO) standard such as Kashan, Zahedan, and Qom (6-8). According to a study by Mosaferi et al, the main cause of noise pollution in Tabriz is motor vehicles, thus, control procedures are necessary in this area (9). In a similar study conducted in Tehran, the analysis of sound pressure level showed that the equivalent sound level (Leq) in all regions during night, the day average sound level only in the Simetry Jey area, and the night average sound level in all regions except Dorahi Ghopan, were more than the acceptable one (10). According to Safari Variani et al study, exposure to high levels of noise can affect the businesses and people who are exposed to high noise levels for a long time in the area, including traffic police. High noise levels also increase mental fatigue, and reduce tolerance thresholds and focus in the ear of traffic police, business activists, and drivers (11,12). Sound is a sociopolitical phenomenon that plays an important role in the quality and socio-economic structure of societies. So, the risk assessment of traffic plans is necessary (13). According to a study conducted in Zanjan, clock changes completely follow the traffic habits of people and traffic loads in the commercial areas of the cities (14). In various health studies, the effects of noise pollution on heart rate (15), blood pressure and cardiovascular disease, especially in high-noisy industries (16), neuroticism, sensitivity, and creating extroversion to low frequencies (17) in hot climates was investigated and it was known as an effective elements on health factors and cognitive performance. Noise pollution has special physiological effects on sensitive groups such as pregnant women (18). In another study on the effects of sound on the health of outdoor workers such as taxi drivers (19), it was revealed that it created mistakes in the reaction time and sensitive occupations (20), high levels of sound pressure in large and medium cities (21), and occupational hearing loss at low frequencies (22).

The noise level in low and high traffic areas in Shiraz city was higher than the standard levels that increases the sleep disorders and decreases the quality of people's life (23). Although air pollution and traffic jams and droughts over the past few years have left no place for concern about noise pollution, but if this situation continues, in the near future, noise pollution will also be on the brink of a crisis, as climate and drought are now among the top ecological and critical issues. Noise pollution is one of the neglected aspects of environmental pollution. According to the reports of the World Health Organization (WHO) and other related organizations such as the International Labour Organization (ILO), National Institute for Occupational Safety and Health (NIOSH), and American Conference of Governmental Industrial Hygienists (ACGIH), noise pollution is the third most harmful and dangerous type of pollution in large cities after air and water pollution (24-26). Therefore, this study was performed due to the importance of this issue.

In developed countries, for controlling the noise, a minimum level of relaxation in the front view of the building called "quiet side", is provided by compiling the requirements for building insulation and decreasing the level of sound pressure to 5 to 10 dB and no sound increase more than 55 dB (17), so that the difference between a loud and slow sound be at least 10 dB as a base. However, there is growing evidence that the indoor sound environment for residents of homes adjacent to high-traffic areas, especially for those living in apartments, is discomfort (27).

Some disorders especially sleep disorders as the first stage of the negative effects of the environmental noise penetration to the residential homes are of great importance. But other sleep indicators (e.g., heartbeat changes, sleep stages, etc.) have shown complex relationships with the value and level of sound pressure (28). There is some evidence that some traffic events commonly do not occur at night (29). It is worth noting that noise events at the end of sleep have a greater effect on the overall quality of sleep and as a result, traffic in the morning has the most important effect (29). Today, according to the modern urban perspective, people's perceptions of the concept of sound have been changed and the indoor noise at home has changed with the modernization of life. Therefore, sound planning in a modern city involves new evaluations and comments to accommodate these differences. The quality of sound in public space is identified and evaluated as an integral part of the urban environment within the scope and specific uses imposed by the urban space. Physical characteristics of the environmental sound required to assess this quality far exceeds the overall noise level and includes spectrum and structure (30-32). Today, the efforts to develop appropriate physical indicators are continuing, but it seems that physical indicators are never enough, it means that a listener who is dependent on sound is very important (33).

Given the fact that the urban public spaces are often located in the center of city, overall quality of sound including traffic noise, mobile phone, people's talks, etc., must be evaluated. An important reason for conducting this study is that the availability of high-quality urban spaces, for example, a green and quiet space in the city that helps to the health of urban citizens, has not been evaluated by the authorities in modern perspectives in the cities of Iran. Today, in particular, some architects have suggested the potential for mental reconstruction by creating natural relaxation areas. Therefore, by considering the environmental goals, the risk assessment of traffic noise has become more vital in urban management and planning.

Various studies have discussed the problem of pathogenicity and discomfort and annoyance due to noise pollution, and what contemporary society is facing seriously is that if the authorities do not react to reduce and control noise pollution, the use of hearing protection equipment (e.g., earplug or earmuff) will become inevitable for people especially those who have industrial occupation in the near future. Therefore, in order to find the fundamental solutions for control and reduction of noise pollution in terms of engineering and management, it is necessary to identify the indicators and criteria for assessing the risk of noise pollution in the majority of large cities and metropolitan areas. So far, many studies have been conducted on health issues and harmful effects of noise pollution on health and work efficiency, but few studies have been conducted on sound loudness. The aims of this study were to measure the frequency and loudness of the traffic noise and evaluate the traffic-induced noise pollution.

This study is the first one evaluated loudness of the urban traffic noise in Shiraz. Acoustic analyses are used in many areas. The common goal of many acoustic analyses is to study the sound characteristics emitted from a source, to find how it is propagated in the environment, and in some cases, to adapt the acoustic conditions to what is required by local standards or laws (34). One of the ways for performing acoustic analysis is to examine related criteria such as sound loudness. In this regard, it is necessary to use analytical indicators such as sound loudness (sone) and phon according to the global criteria In this study, for the first time, these valuable criteria were used to assess the risk of noise pollution in the central and high traffic areas of Shiraz at different hours of the day and night.

Materials and Methods

This study was performed on a number of the most crowded and heavy traffic streets and highways in the downstream and center of Shiraz along with 6 streets connected to the main road that have heavy traffic during the day. Measurements were completed on 2016 July to 2017 December at 156 measuring stations. Totally, 156 urban centers were selected acoustically for business-residential situations along roads, sidewalks, and shopping areas and at least two points along each of the main and secondary streets and the city center. The majority of the population is inhabited in regions 6, 7, and 8, and the central part of Shiraz including areas 1, 2, 4, and 5, which is the more heavily populated, has the highest level of noise pollution.

As shown in Figure 1, the population size of the passengers and pedestrians at public transportation stations of Shiraz was higher at morning peak hours in the areas 1, 3, and 6. This makes it necessary to protect residents and workers from noise pollution caused by urban traffic (see Figure 1B).

Sound loudness level (Sone)

Sound loudness is a mental issue that reflects the power of perception of sound by the ear. In other words, it is the intensity of sound. The intensity of sound should be focused by the sensitivity of the ear to the specific sound frequencies. This kind of sensitivity is the information that exists in the narrow curves for the human ear (3,34). A general rule for sound loudness is that the power should be increased by about ten times to make the sound twice longer. To more realistically measure sound loudness, hearing sensitivity curves are used to measure sound loudness on a phon scale. Then, the 10th rule of thumb can be used to produce the sone scale of sound loudness. In particular, in measuring the sound level, weighting network filters such as weighting networks A, B, and C are used for measuring instruments like ear structure (3,34).

Sound loudness level (phon)

Sound loudness unit is sone and sound loudness level is expressed by phon. In this study, the following equation was used to calculate the cumulative content (35):

$$SL(Phone) = 33.2 \log S + 40 \quad (1)$$

Where SL is the sound loudness level and S is the absolute loudness or sone.

It was also found that sone is a function of the same curve that is obtained from the following equation:

$$St = I_m(1-k) + k\sum_{i=1}^{n} I_i \quad (2)$$

(A)

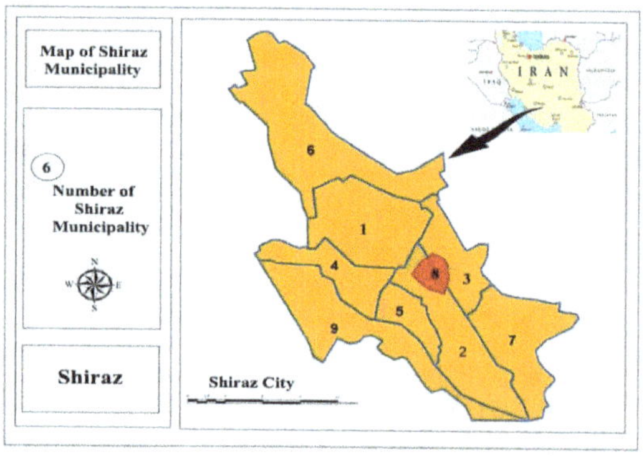

(B)

Municipal areas	Residential with permanent residence	Residential with temporary residence	Police Services	Industrial - Workshop	Transportation and warehousing	Infrastructure	Cultural-artistic	Educational	Health - Therapy	Sports	Official	Non-urban applications	Access network
1	35.02	0.22	3.35	0.0	0.3	0.15	0.72	6.75	1.09	0.47	1.79	10.1	29.7
2	39.03	0.09	1.67	1.04	4.20	0.87	0.29	3.23	0.75	1.61	2.33	15.39	25.55
3	38.91	0.23	1.21	2.52	1.09	0.21	0.92	3.06	0.29	0.62	1.74	13.70	28.87
4	22.67	0.03	1.18	3.26	2.96	1.24	0.15	0.53	0.1	0.16	0.14	42.56	17.69
5	20.99	0.00	0.34	0.07	0.06	0.11	0.01	0.62	0.13	0.27	0.24	55.70	16.96
6	42.89	0.14	3.98	0.0	0.89	0.04	0.1	1.73	0.05	0.08	3.07	12.07	28.87
7	30.56	0.00	0.62	5.03	0.91	0.07	0.0	1.80	0.03	0.49	0.74	29.03	25.62
8	49.96	0.67	9.57	0.42	0.95	0.09	1.37	2.75	0.32	0.06	1.90	10.49	16.01

Figure 1. A) The population size of the passengers and pedestrians at public transportation stations of Shiraz during morning peak hours (adapted from studies by Shiraz Municipality in 2006). B) Percentage of urban land use in Shiraz city (reported by the city council in 2003).

Where the total sum loudness (St), the maximum loudness (I_m) and I_i of each high value of the sound loudness (including the maximum peak) were obtained from the same magnitude curves and sound band weighting factor (K) is equal to 0.3 for octave and 0.15 for one-third octave bands. Based on the results of previous studies and also using the following formula, the number of sampling stations was determined (36):

$$n = \frac{Z_{\alpha/2}^{2} \times S^{2}}{d^{2}} \quad (3)$$

Where a constant value ($Z_{\alpha/2}$) indicates the confidence level, α, the error rate, in this case (0.3 for octave and 0.15 for S2, the prototype variance, and d, the measurement accuracy. The statistical calculations based on equation (3) showed that the 120 measurements may lead to 96 to 99% accuracy and precision, which are more precise and also due to the possibility that a number of measurements may not be usable during the measurement. The number of measurements was 30% higher. The number of test stations was 156. The duration of calibration, according to ISO 9613 standard, determined for each measurement was about 90 seconds (37). Appropriate charts were produced using statistical analysis by Excel 2016 software.

In the next step, in order to measure the sound in the vicinity of highways and around the building, according to the Australian Standard Method, as well as the provisions of ISO 9613, first, the appropriate location was determined, then, according to ISO 9613, noise was measured (see Figure 2A and 2B) (38). The sound measurement positions were determined according to the EPA guidelines for accuracy and precision, not disturbing by airflow. Two sound level meters (TES-1358c, Taiwan) and (BSWA 308/309 , class A and B, China) with the ability to measure LP, Leq, LN, SD, SEL, Max, Min, and Peak were used in this research. Calibration was carried out using a TES-1358C sound level calibrator, at each stage of the measurement. After sound measurement and frequency analysis, the TES-1358 was turned off and the results were accurately extracted from the memory of the machine and the manual data collection sheets and entered into the software (39).

The above-mentioned method has been confirmed by other researchers in terms of speed of measuring sound level and reducing waste of time but at high temperatures and altitudes, two important contradictions of microphone resistance against low temperatures and the impossibility of measuring sound level at high altitudes for accurate examination were observed. These contradictions were the main challenges to the present study.

Collected data were analyzed using Cox appropriate-hazards model multivariate method. The Cox model is considered as a semi-parametric model for fitting the risk function. The relationship between the variables and survival time. The risk function for X variable is:

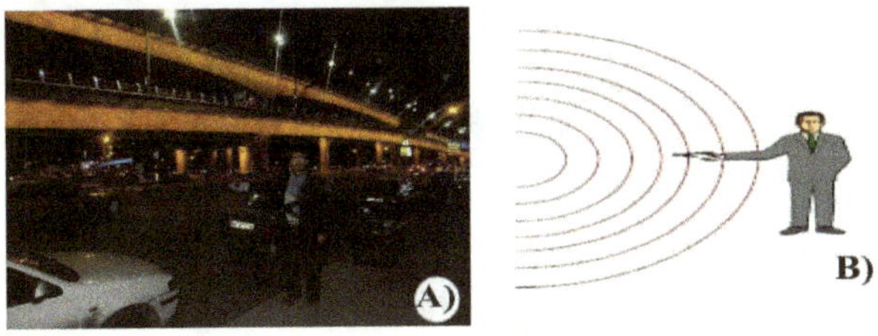

Figure 2. (A) Moalli Abad Bridge, measurement at 10 PM. (B) How to manually measure sound according to the Australian standard (38).

$$\lambda(t;x) = \lambda_0(t)\exp(x\beta) \quad (4)$$

Data were statistically analyzed using Minitab 18.1 and statistical significant level was considered at $P<0.05$. In order to predict the risk of hearing loss in citizens of the study areas, it was necessary to consider variables such as occupation, business experience, noise exposure, and smoking. Industrial results of risk assessment in previous studies showed that the higher the contact with disturbing and annoying sound, the greater the risk of cardiovascular disease and hearing loss will be. Cox regression model is one of the most widely used models for modeling the factors affecting the risk of various events by considering censored observations (40). In order to reduce the risk of hearing loss in a wide range of age with exposure to traffic noise, cultural and collaborative efforts to maintain and enhance hearing conservation programs are required.

Results

The results of environmental measurements in more than 156 points in the weighting network A and C are shown in Figure 3 and 4. According to these figures, all stations under study were at risk and no safety limit was recorded. The highest average sound pressure level belonged to the downtown and center stations and was equal to 83.3 dB. It was also revealed that among 120 employees in the administrative center and 170 shopkeepers in this study, half of them had a history of hearing loss with a mean hearing threshold of 29.5±3.5 dB. It should be noted that at the time of the measurement of the sound pressure level, no periodical or medical examination was performed and data were extracted only from the HSE departments and medical records. Work experience in the cases with normal hearing status was 5±1.2 years and in those with hearing loss was 15±2.7 years. As shown in Table 1, the risk of hearing loss in administrative workers was lower than that of commercial workers and taxi drivers. Here, the comparisons are purely with the environmental standards, not with occupational health standards.

Figure 3 shows the comparison of 7 different stations together. As shown in this table, the most frequency changes have been at frequencies below 150 Hz. Figure 4 shows the change in sound pressure level (L_p, C) in slow mode in the study stations. The results suggest that

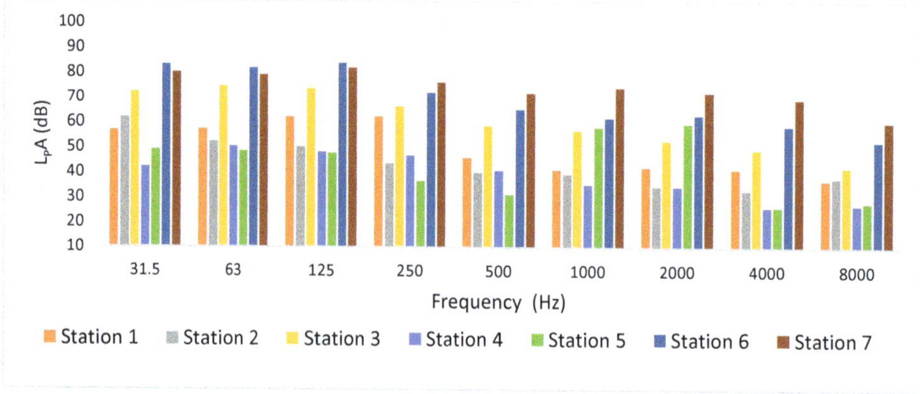

Figure 3. Sound pressure level (L_p A) changes in the octave band weighting network in fast mode at 156 stations measured in Shiraz during 2015-2016.

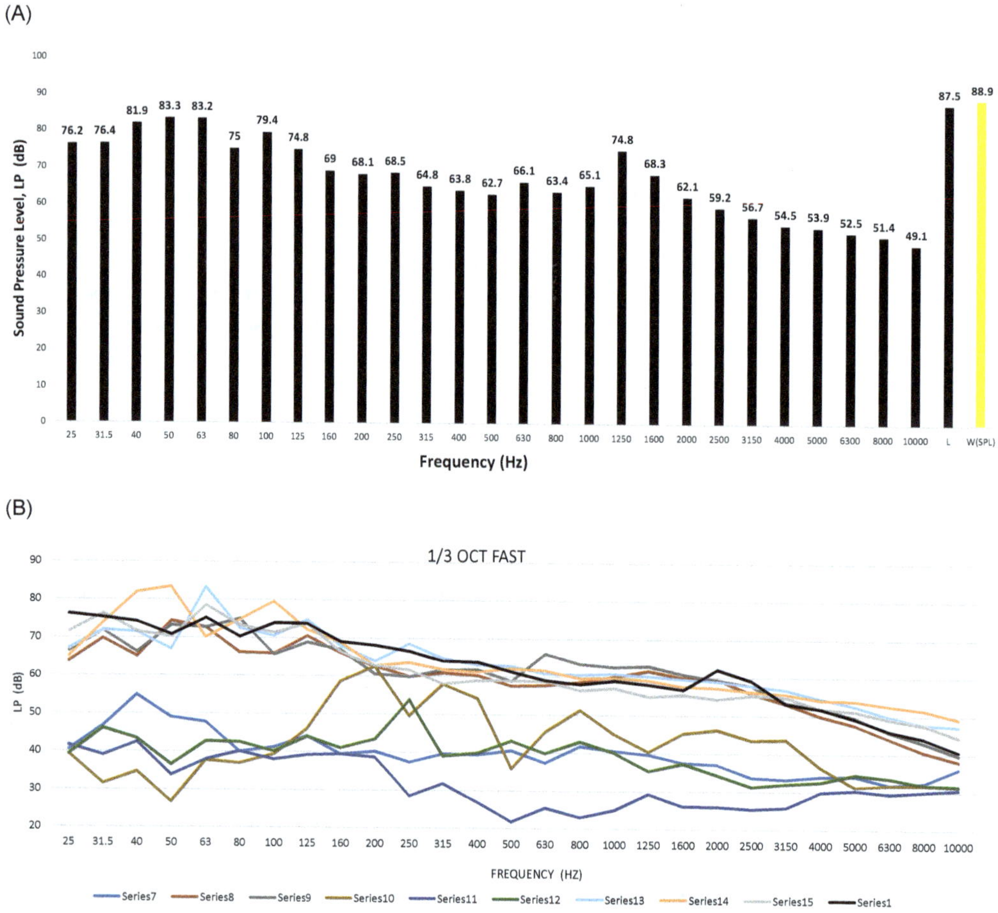

Figure 4. A) The maximum sound pressure level (L_p, C) variations in one-third octave band weighting network in fast mode at 156 stations. B) Sound pressure level changes in one-third octave band weighting network in fast mode at 156 stations measured in Shiraz during 2015-2016.

changes in the sound pressure level varied from 27 to 88.4 dB. According to Table 2, all results obtained from the study stations were higher than the Iran's environmental standard.

As shown in Figure 4, the highest level of sound pressure in a weighting system of one-third octave band was 83.33 dB. This result showed that noise pollution was higher than the Iran's environmental standard. According to frequency analysis and conventional methods, intrusive frequency of traffic in Shiraz was less than 250 Hz.

The sound pressure level (LP) varied from 80 to 97.9 dB in these areas. The maximum and minimum level of LP were 88.9 and 53 dB, respectively. Figures 3 and 4 show that the LP had a maximum level of 84.4 dB, indicating

Table 1. The variables affecting Noise-induced Hearing Loss (NIHL) using the Cox model in Shiraz citizens during 2015-2016

	Job Description	Regression Coefficient (β)	*P* value	Relative Risk
Job Type	Taxi drivers	1.10	0.042	3.36
	Shop-keepers	1.077	0	2.5
	Administrative-commercial	0.092	-	1.11
	Commercial	0.093	0.672	1.15
Smoking Cigarettes	Smoker	0.558	-	1.8
	Non-smoker	-	-	1.2

Table 2. Free sound standards in Iran

Zone Type	Night: 10 PM to 7 AM Leq (30), dB (A)	Day: 7 AM to 10 PM Leq (30), dB (A)
Residential	45	55
Residential - Commercial	50	60
Commercial	55	65
Residential - Industrial	60	70
Industrial	65	75

Table 3. The noise rating equalizer in the octave band based on the ISO proposal

Range	Description
<15 dB	Very low level Zone
15-45 dB	Comfort Zone
>85 dB	Danger Zone

that the traffic noise violated the state noise standard for residential, commercial, and other areas (Tables 1-3). Figure 4 shows that the houses around the highways tolerated a high level of sound pressure (88.4 dB).

Noise pollution in large cities is a growing problem with the fact that the urban environment is becoming more crowded and noisy. In this study, the sound levels in the center of Shiraz were measured at 156 points along with 6 related streets. Simultaneously with noise measurements, the frequency analysis showed an annoying frequency of 50 to 250 Hz. It was also revealed that the undesirable noise, the traffic noise and the crowd, were due to the noise of the streets and the construction. This result is consistent with the results of other studies. The findings showed an increase in traffic noise as reported by others.

As shown in Figure 5, the cumulative sone in Shiraz with a maximum value was equal to 26 at several heavy traffic stations, while the calculations showed that the loudness level at two stations (11 and 12) was 87 phon. Transmission of data to the noise rating (NR) diagram showed that all stations except station 5 were in danger zones (Table 3). At station 5, the results were higher than the comfort zone and less than the danger zone. In total, no area with low-frequency sound pressure levels was observed. Analysis of sone and phon charts at a heavy traffic station using Excel 2016 software showed a gentle downward slope to high frequencies, this means that as we go towards lower frequencies, we see an increase in the amount of sone and sound loudness. This result is consistent with the results of low-frequency sound pressure levels (Figure 6).

For proper environmental risk analysis, the sound pressure level is compared with bulk curves and the environmental effects are determined. In this regard, the frequency ranged from 16 to 500 Hz was divided into two sections of 16 to 100 Hz and 125 to 500 Hz. The frequency analysis along with the calculated sone and phon values are plotted in Figures 7 and 8. These figures show that the Sone amount at frequencies below 20 Hz has constant level at heavy traffic stations, but with increasing frequencies to 31.5 and 40 Hz at five stations and in other cases at frequencies of 50 and 63 Hz, it had the largest amount.

Data analysis showed that the sound loudness at both frequencies (below and above 100 Hz) was high and lower values were observed in only four stations (Figure 7A and 7B). This fact clearly showed that sound loudness level was higher than the sound comfort, therefore, it was in danger range. Administrators, especially those who are involved in commercial and residential construction, can use the phon and sone charts for acoustic design of the buildings so that they can provide the quiet side for the users and consider the permissible environmental limit (Figures 7 and 8).

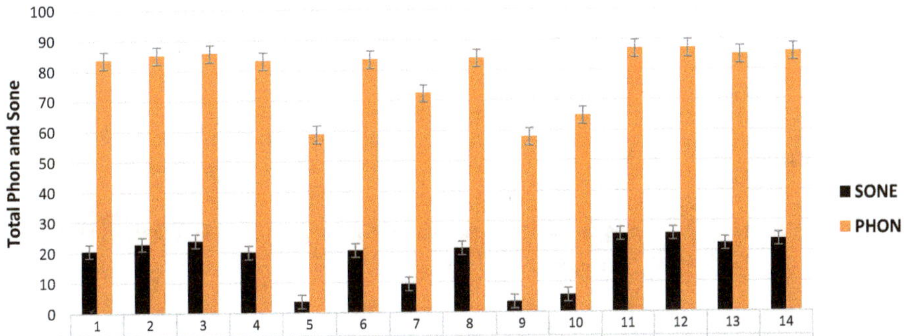

	1	2	3	4	5	6	7	8	9	10	11	12	13	14
SONE	20.5165	22.8028	23.737	19.9535	3.6707	20.4625	9.3535	21.1152	3.44585	5.5835	25.714	25.8425	22.3918	23.8318
PHON	83.56	85.08	85.66	83.16	58.74	83.52	72.23	83.9	57.8	64.79	86.8	86.89	84.822	85.72

Figure 5. Cumulative phon and sone values of 14 heavy traffic stations in Shiraz during 2015-2016.

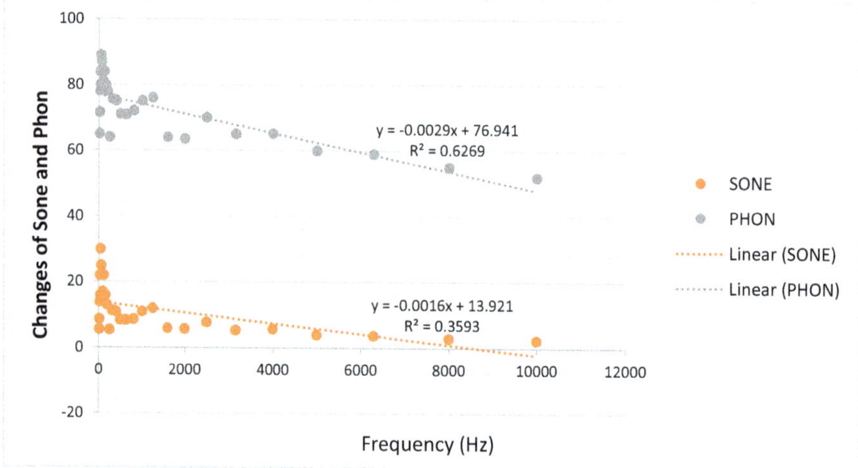

Figure 6. Linear changes of cumulative sone and phon of frequency at 14 heavy traffic stations in Shiraz during 2015-2016.

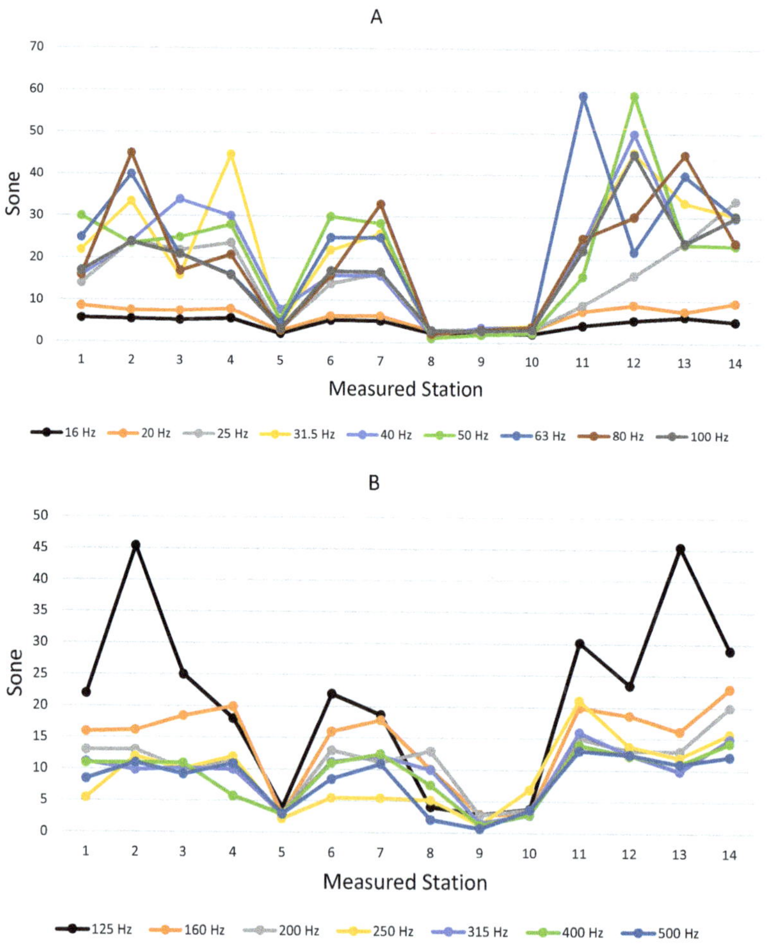

Figure 7. A) Sound loudness rate (sone) at frequencies below 100 Hz in Shiraz. B) Sound loudness rate (sone) at frequencies above 100 Hz in Shiraz during 2015-2016..

Discussion

Based on the analysis of the data obtained from the model, the amount of hearing loss in citizens exposed to sound depends on traffic habits, the presence of nearby sound generation resources, and other variables such as age, smoking behavior, gender, and the use of personal protective equipment (that is not customary in the citizens). Hearing loss in the vicinity of noise centers increased, therefore,

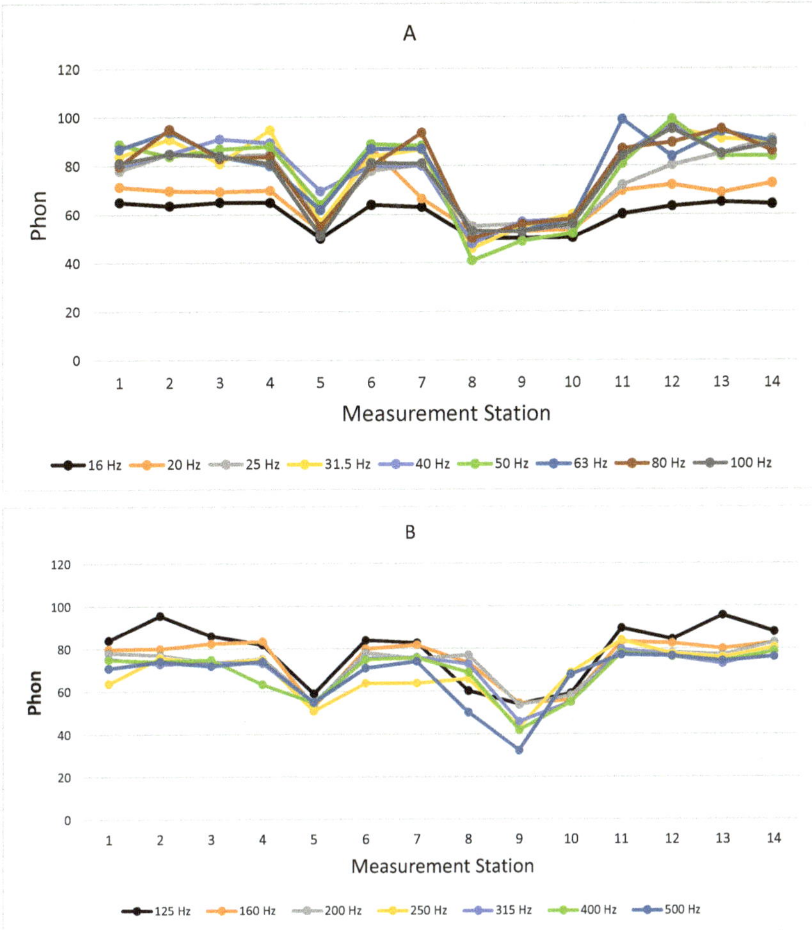

Figure 8. A) The rate of sound loudness level (phon) at frequencies below 100 Hz in 14 heavy traffic stations in Shiraz. B) The rate of sound loudness level (phon) at frequencies above 100 Hz in 14 heavy traffic stations in Shiraz during 2015-2016.

there is a need for a hearing conservation program as well as controlling and preventing noise transmission. Occupational variables and noise exposure had the most effect on the risk of hearing loss. High pressure levels of noise are one of the important variables in causing hearing loss.

As shown in Figure 4, the maximum frequency amount was below 1000 Hz (Max=50 Hz). Weighting network of the one-third octave band as a pre-requisite of planning of engineering designs, showed the highest changes in the sub-250 Hz range. According to Figure 1 and Table 1, if the citizens of Shiraz be considered in the central part of the city as commercial-residential, the environmental standard has not yet been observed and the results showed much higher values.

In shopkeepers, L_{eq} was equal to 83.7. According to the environmental standard in Iran, these values are higher than the standard. Because the use of personal protective equipment for hearing loss is not common in people, therefore, in order to predict the risk of hearing loss, only the daily exposure and smoking variables were considered. It seems that the results of this study while confirming the results of other researchers, showed a slight difference. The research also showed an increase in noise pollution in Shiraz. The researchers were able to determine harmful environmental frequency of Shiraz traffic. So sone and phon were determined. It seems that the reason for these changes can be due to the following:

- Changing in the technology of making internal combustion engines with low-frequency output.
- The impact of high buildings on highway sound reflection and increasing the sound pressure level.
- Examining the index parameters with frequency analysis.
- Crowded cities with new noise resources.

It should be noted that in the past, a few research has pointed to harmful frequency, but many studies have been performed on the type of sound pressure level. To our knowledge, the sound pressure level does not generally reflect the frequency value. In any case, despite the above, noise was still recognized as a disturbing environmental factor.

Conclusion

Therefore, due to the high level of sound pressure level and the amount of sone and phon in Shiraz, noise pollution in the city has imposed economic and social costs and high risk on the citizens. Since the highest rate of noise pollution happened at low frequencies in Shiraz, therefore, low-frequency noise control with thin-layer adsorbents is very hard in this area. In this frequency range, no new sound absorber or sound control method (except classical methods with high cost and inconvenience, which in many cases are not applicable to buildings) has been introduced or applied in Iran. According to the results, the environmental and health risks in the city are clearly evident. The knowledge about the effect of low-frequency noise can help readers analogy this kind of effect with the results. The obtained results are consistent with the results of other studies (41-43).

The use of risk-based health impact assessment models on health such as Cox can be effective in analyzing relevant environmental data and decisions. According to ACGIH's reports, the errors of decentralization in both industrial and educational (office) sectors are clearly due to the effect of noise on the focus. Cox regression model well describes the quantitative effect of exposure conditions of citizens, especially workers who are permanently exposed to noise, on the risk of hearing loss. Accordingly, the noise in the environment of citizens has become a neglected factor in the large cities. The use of risk-forecasting tools and methods for controlling the sound transmission can provide useful information for planners and managers to improve traffic schedules and promote community health.

Acknowledgements

The authors would like to gratitude all people who have cooperated with the research team.

Competing interests

The authors declare that they have no conflict of interests.

Authors' contributions

All authors contributed equally and were involved in the study design, data collection, and article approval.

References

1. Mansoori N. Environmental Pollution (Air, Water, Soil, Sound). Tehran: Etehad Publication; 2011. [In Persian].
2. John ME. Patties Industrial Hygiene and Toxicology. 3rd ed. USA: Wiley-inter Science Publication; 1978. p. 813-20.
3. Golmohammadi R. Sound and Vibration Engineering. Hamedan: Daneshjoo of Hamedan Publication; 1999. [In Persian].
4. Ohrstrom E, Skanberg A, Svensson H, Gidlof-Gunnarsson A. Effects of road traffic noise and the benefit of access to quietness. J Sound Vib 2006; 295(1-2): 40-59. doi: 10.1016/j.jsv.2005.11.034.
5. Fiedler PE, Zannin PH. Evaluation of noise pollution in urban traffic hubs—noise maps and measurements. Environ Impact Assess Rev 2015; 51: 1-9. doi: 10.1016/j.eiar.2014.09.014.
6. Paravar A, Monazzam MR, Mansouri N, Motalebi Kashani M. Evaluation of noise pollution and traffic noise index using geographical information system in the main streets of Kashan, Iran. Health System Research 2015; 11(4): 688-93. [In Persian].
7. Mirzaei R, Ansari-Moghaddam A, Mohammadi M, Rakhshani F, Salmanpor M. Noise pollution in Zahedan and residents' knowledge about noise pollution. Health Scope 2012; 1(1): 3-6. doi: 10.5812/jhs.4544.
8. Yari AR, Dezhdar B, Koohpaei A, Ebrahimi A, Mashkoori A, Mohammadi MJ, et al. Evaluation of traffic noise pollution and control solutions offering: a case study in Qom, Iran. Journal of Sabzevar University of Medical Sciences 2016; 23(4): 600-7. [In Persian].
9. Mosaferi M, Rasulzadeh Y, Nazari J, Taghipour H, Diyanat I. Study of noise pollution in downtown area of Tabriz during heavy traffic times. Medical Journal of Tabriz University of Medical Sciences 2012; 34(4):112-19. [In Persian].
10. Yousefzadeh A, Nassiri P, Rahimi Foroushani A. The relationship between air traffic noise and its induced annoyance in the southwest area in Tehran, Iran. Journal of Health and Safety at Work 2016; 6(3): 15-28. [In Persian].
11. Safari Variani A, Nikpay A, Ghalenoei M, Emamjomeh MM. Comparison of equivalent noise pollution and traffic noise index in different cities of Qazvin province (2010). Journal of Qazvin University of Medical Sciences 2013; 16(4): 69-74. [In Persian].
12. Ghanbari M, Nadafi K, Mosaferi M, Yunesian M, Aslani H. Noise pollution evaluation in residential and residential-commercial areas in Tabriz-Iran. Iranian Journal of Health and Environment 2011; 4(3): 375-84. [In Persian].
13. Nadrian H, Taghdisi MH, Shojaeizadeh D, Nedjat S. Impacts of Sanandaj urban traffic and transport on social determinants of health from the perspective of key informants: a qualitative study. Journal of Education and Community Health 2018; 5(1): 49-60. doi: 10.21859/jech.5.1.49. [In Persian].
14. Majidi F, Khosravi Y. Noise pollution evaluation of city center of Zanjan by Geographic Information System (GIS). Iranian Journal of Health and Environment 2016; 9(1): 91-102. [In Persian].
15. Dehghan H, Gharib S. The effect of noise exposure on heart rate in the hot and humid conditions in climatic chamber. Journal of Occupational Hygiene Engineering 2016; 3(3): 1-8. doi: 10.21859/johe-03034. [In Persian].
16. Yaghoobi K, Alimohammadi I, Aboulghasemi J, Shirin Shandiz M, Aboutaleb N, Ashtari Nezhad A. The effect of noise on blood pressure and heart rate in an automotive industry. Journal of Occupational Hygiene Engineering 2016; 4(1): 26-34. doi: 10.21859/johe-04014. [In Persian].
17. Babamiri M, Motamedzadeh M, Golmohammadi R, Derakhshan J, Farhadian M. Role of personality type in the effects of low frequency sound on cognitive performance of the students. Journal of Occupational Hygiene Engineering

2017; 4(2): 59-66. doi: 10.21859/ johe.4.2.59. [In Persian].

18. Soury S, Golmohamadi R. A review of the auditory and non-auditory effects of exposure to noise on women's health. Journal of Occupational Hygiene Engineering 2017; 4(2): 53-8. doi: 10.21859/johe.4.2.53. [In Persian].
19. Biabani A, Aliabadi M, Golmohamadi R. Study of performance of acoustic fixture for using in noise reduction rate tests of hearing protection devices. Journal of Occupational Hygiene Engineering 2016; 3(1): 60-6. doi: 10.21859/johe-03018. [In Persian].
20. Jafari S, Ansari H, Raee T, Mohammadian U, Hajizadeh R, Fazli B. Survey of noise-induced hearing loss among Fereidonkener taxi drivers in 2013. Journal of Health 2016; 7(1): 51-7. [In Persian].
21. Beheshti MH, Koohpaei A, Mousavian Z, Mehri A, Zia G, Tajpour A, et al. The effect of sound with different frequencies on selective attention and human response time. Iran Occupational Health Journal 2018; 15(3): 118-28. [In Persian].
22. Mohammadi AK, Alidadi H, Delkhosh MB, Fallah SH, Amouei A, Asgharnia HA, et al. Noise pollution measurement in crowded areas of Neyshabur during primary three months of 2015. Journal of Research in Environmental Health 2016; 2(4): 276-84. [In Persian].
23. Zamanian Z, Azad P, Porkar S, Pirami H, Abdollahi M, Kouhnavard B. Study of noise pollution caused by traffic and its effect on sleep disturbances and quality of life for the citizens city of Shiraz. Occupational Medicine Quarterly Journal 2017; 8(4): 58-66.
24. World Health Organization (WHO). Global Health Observatory (GHO) data. [cited 2018 Aug 2] Available from: https://www.who.int/gho/publications/en/.
25. United States Environmental Protection Agency (US EPA). Information on levels of environmental noise requisite to protect public health and welfare with an adequate margin of safety. Washington DC: Government Printing Office; 1974.
26. Nwali EI, Agunwamba JC. Analysis of the environmental and socio-economic impact of noise pollution in ELEME petrochemical company limited. Nigerian Journal of Technology 2005; 24(1): 67-78.
27. Klaeboe R. Are adverse impacts of neighbourhood noisy areas the flip side of quiet area benefits? Appl Acoust 2007; 68(5): 557-75. doi: 10.1016/j.apacoust.2005.05.007.
28. Griefahn B, Brode P, Marks A, Basner M. Autonomic arousals related to traffic noise during sleep. Sleep 2008; 31(4): 569-77.
29. Griefahn B, Marks A, Robens S. Experiments on the time frame of temporally limited traffic curfews to prevent noise induced sleep disturbances. Somnologie 2008; 12(2): 140-8. doi: 10.1007/s11818-008-0341-0.
30. Raimbault M, Lavandier C, Berengier M. Ambient sound assessment of urban environments: field studies in two French cities. Appl Acoust 2003; 64(12): 1241-56. doi: 10.1016/S0003-682X(03)00061-6.
31. Dubois D, Guastavino C, Raimbault M. A cognitive approach to urban soundscapes: using verbal data to access everyday life auditory categories. Acta Acust United Acust 2006; 92(6): 865-74.
32. Botteldooren D, De Coensel B, De Muer T. The temporal structure of urban soundscapes. J Sound Vib 2006; 292(1-2): 105-23. doi: 10.1016/j.jsv.2005.07.026.
33. Luz GA. Maslow's hierarchy of needs as a model for the process of the development of national noise regulations. 9th International Congress on Noise as a Public Health Problem (ICBEN); 2008 Jul 21-25; ICBEN, USA; 2008.
34. Loudness - HyperPhysics Concepts. "Rule of Thumb" for Loudness. [cited 2018 May 28] Available from: http://hyperphysics.phy-astr.gsu.edu/hbase/Sound/loud.html.
35. Kuttruff H. Acoustics, an Introduction. Translated by Abbassi AM. Tehran: Tehran University Publication; 2015. [In Persian].
36. Mohammadfam I. Research Design and Statistics for Safety and Health. Tehran: Fanavaran Publication; 2006. [Persian].
37. International Organization for Standardization (ISO). ISO 9613-2:1996. Acoustics -- Attenuation of sound during propagation outdoors -- Part 2: General method of calculation. Geneva, Switzerland: ISO; 1996.
38. Environmental Performance and Coordination Branch, Department of Environment and Heritage Protection. Noise Measurement Manual. [cited 2018 May 28] Available from: https://environment.des.qld.gov.au/licences-permits/pdf/noise-measurement-manual-em1107.pdf.
39. TES Electrical Electronic Corp. Sound analyzer real time 1\1 and Octave band analysis. [cited 2018 Aug 3] Available from: http://www.tes.com.tw/en/product_detail.asp?seq=380.
40. Klein JP, Moeschberger ML. Survival Analysis: Techniques for Censored and Truncated Data. Springer Publication; 2003.
41. Moteallemi A, Bina B, Mortezaie S. Effects of noise pollution on Samen district residents in Mashhad city. Environmental Health Engineering and Management Journal 2018; 5(1): 23-7. doi: 10.15171/ehem.2018.04.
42. Mohammadi G. An investigation of community response to urban traffic noise. Iranian Journal of Environmental Health Science and Engineering 2009; 6(2): 137-42
43. Environmental Protection Agency (EPA). Guidance Note for Strategic Noise Mapping For the Environmental Noise Regulations 2006. [cited 2018 Nov 29] Available from: https://www.epa.ie/pubs/advice/noisemapping/EPA%20Guidance%20Note%20for%20Strategic%20Noise%20Mapping%20(version%202).pdf.

30

Estimating greenhouse gas emissions using emission factors from the Sugarcane Development Company, Ahvaz, Iran

Amir Zahedi[1], **Sorour Ghodrati**[2], **Mehdi Ahmadimoghaddam**[3], **Nematollah Jaafarzadeh**[4*]

[1]Committee Research, Department of Environmental Health Engineering, School of Health, Ahvaz Jundishapur University of Medical Sciences, Ahvaz, Iran
[2]Department of Environmental Assessment and Land Use Planning, School of Environment and Energy, Islamic Azad University, Science and Research Branch, Tehran, Iran
[3]Environmental Technologies Research Center, Department of Environmental Health Engineering, School of Health, Ahvaz Jundishapur University of Medical Sciences, Ahvaz, Iran
[4]Environmental Technologies Research Center, Department of Environmental Health Engineering, School of Health, Ahvaz Jundishapur University of Medical Sciences, Ahvaz, Iran

Abstract
Background: Greenhouse gas (GHG) emissions are increasing worldwide. They have harmful effects on human health, animals, and plants and play a major role in global warming and acid rain.
Methods: This research investigated carbon dioxide (CO_2) and CH_4 emissions obtained from different parts of the Hakim Farabi, Dobal Khazaei, and Ramin factories which produce ethanol and yeast. Seasonal rates of CO_2 at the soil surface at the studied sites were estimated from measurements made on location and at intervals with manual chambers. This study aimed to assess the production rate of GHG emissions (CH_4, CO_2) in the sugar production units of Hakim Farabi, Dobal Khazaei, and Ramin factories.
Results: Mean concentrations of CO_2 and CH_4 emissions are respectively 279 500.207 and 3087.07 tons/year from the Hakim Farabi agro-industry, 106 985.24 and 1.14 tons/year at the Dobal Khazaei ethanol producing factory, and 124 766.17 and 1.93 tons/year at the Ramin leavening producing factory.
Conclusion: Sugar plant boilers and the burning of sugarcane contributed the most CO_2 and CH_4 emissions, respectively. Moreover, lime kilns and diesel generators showed the least carbon dioxide and methane emissions, respectively.
Keywords: Carbon Dioxide, Methane, Ethanol, Farms, Global Warming

***Correspondence to:**
Nematollah Jaafarzadeh
Email: Jaafarzadeh-n@ajums.ac.ir

Introduction

Greenhouse gases (GHGs) cause a significant amount of pollution in the atmosphere (1). They are harmful to human health, animals, and plants, and they play a major role in global warming and acid rain (2). During recent decades, public concern has arisen regarding the presence of air pollutants both outdoors and indoors, and their potential to damage human health has increased (3,4). Carbon dioxide (CO_2) and CH_4 are the main GHGs today; CO_2 emissions from fossil fuels are the main cause of global warming (5,6). Other studies showing the importance of CO_2 and CH_4 rates in global warming have been conducted in some industrial and agricultural countries (7-11). The great development of the sugarcane and ethanol production industries, including agricultural industries and other technologies, seen in recent decades has created a need for recalculating the emission of pollutants and energy balances. Methane and CO_2 are the main emissions of the agricultural/industrial levels (12). In the last 10 years, atmospheric concentrations of CO_2 have increased by almost 40%, from a preindustrial concentration of approximately 280 ppmv (parts per million volume) to almost 384 ppmv in 2007 (13). Large reductions in GHG emissions are expected to prohibit serious climate destabilization, however, GHG emissions from fixed and transport sources are growing more quickly than other energy-using sectors and are predicted to increase GHG emissions by 80% between 2007 and 2030 (14). CH_4 is produced during the production and transport of coal, natural gas, oil, and other natural resources such as fertilizer and landfills with open-path technology and other anaerobic waste treatment systems (15,16). Municipal landfills are great resources of CH_4 emissions; in municipal solid waste landfills, CH_4 is about

30 times more potent as a heat-trapping gas (17). About 3.6% to 7.9% of natural gas released to the atmosphere is CH_4 gas (18). The main GHGs included SOx, NOx, PM, CO_2, and HCs, all of which cause global warming and increase atmospheric temperatures. Today, the proportion of CO_2 and CH_4 directly emitted by each country has been much discussed, have focused on CO_2 emissions, as the most important GHG. Specifically, emphasis has been placed on CO_2 emissions as the exhaust of fossil fuel combustion, cement and the other industrial manufactories, which is termed CO_2 here, referring to fossil carbon. Increasingly, CO_2 and CO emissions from land-use change and forestry (LUCF) are garnering much attention. However, it is not just CO_2 that is causing global warming; a suite of human activities resulting in the emission of GHGs is termed climate-altering pollutants (CAPs). Among GHGs, CO_2 emissions cause about one-half of total global warming (7). The resulting contrary health outcomes cause governments to work collectively with resolution to reduce and remove GHG emissions. What has been less widely understood, though, is that policies to decrease GHG emissions (climate change mitigation policies) could pave the way for great effects on the health of people in a society (8,19). GHGs in industry are emitted from two main sections. These emissions including direct and indirect emissions that are produced at the facility and occur off-site, respectively (20). After 10 years of an annual average growth rate of 4%, the years 2012 and 2013 showed a decrease to about 1%, also global CO_2 emissions abated 0.5% in 2014 to the record level in 2013. In 2014, the Environmental Protection Agency (EPA) reported that industry emissions accounted for approximately 21% of the total GHG emissions in the world (21). Carbon is the most abundant element in the production of sugarcane that can be changed to CO_2 and CH_4 pollution as the result of burning. Some fossil fuels are used in industry and agriculture; some bagasse, for example, is used as fuel in other parts, and a portion of the bagasse is used inside the factory as fuel for the boilers used in sugar production. The current study evaluated the emission factors of GHG emissions of (CO_2) and (CH_4) in the production of Hakim Farabi agriculture and industry, which includes raw sugar and sugarcane, and Dobal Khazaei and Ramin factories that produce alcohol and yeast. Industries, factories, and farms emit large quantities of CO_2 and CH_4 during the various stages of production. The main sources of CO_2 and CH_4 emissions are fuel-consuming equipment, such as boilers, lime kilns, diesel generators, electrical equipment in factories, and sugarcane burning for the elimination of waste; thus, CO_2 is emitted during the process of producing alcohol.

Methods

Description of the study area

This study was performed in Ahvaz city located in southwest Iran, which includes an estimated area of 220 km^2 and an estimated density of 4815.73 people per square kilometer. The climate in Ahvaz is tropical with a limited downfall period and an extended dry period lasting generally 9 months per year (22). One of the biggest industries in this city is the Hakim Farabi agro-industry, which is in southeastern Ahvaz, located on the Kilometer 35 Road of Ahvaz-Abadan. With the geographical coordinates of zone 39R, 267920.09 m E and 3426751.75 m N, this area has 12 thousand hectares of arable land. In addition, this complex has several units, including a sugar production unit with the capacity to produce 100 000 tons of sugar per year, the alcohol production units of Dobal Khazaei, and an agricultural part including 10 000 ha of arundinaceous farms. Figure 1 shows the location of the studied stations.

Energy input and GHG emissions

For this research, CO_2 and CH_4 emissions were obtained from different parts of the Hakim Farabi, Dobal Khazaei, and Ramin factories that produce ethanol and yeast. Sampling time and the number of samples were one year and 144, respectively. Seasonal rates of CO_2 at the soil surface at the sites were estimated from measurements made on location and at intervals with manual chambers. The soil CO_2 rate was measured continuously with six automatic chambers. The rate of CH_4 in the above yield was measured continuously using a micrometeorological gradient method. In addition, the emission and conversion factors were used for the CO_2 and CH_4 stack and emitted gasses from different sections such as boilers; field burners were vented to ambient air. One method for estimating CO_2 and CH_4 emissions is the ratio of energy output and input to GHG emissions, which demonstrates the quantity of CO_2 and CH_4 by measuring the concentrations of these gases in the fuel.

Results

The results of this study showed that CO_2 and CH_4 emissions from the Hakim Farabi agro-industry are 279 500.207 and 3087.07 tons/year, respectively, from the Dobal Khazaei ethanol producing factory are 106 985.24 and 1.14 tons/year, respectively, and from the leavening producing factory is 124 766.17 and 1.93 tons/year, respectively. Sugarcane is cultivated in an area of

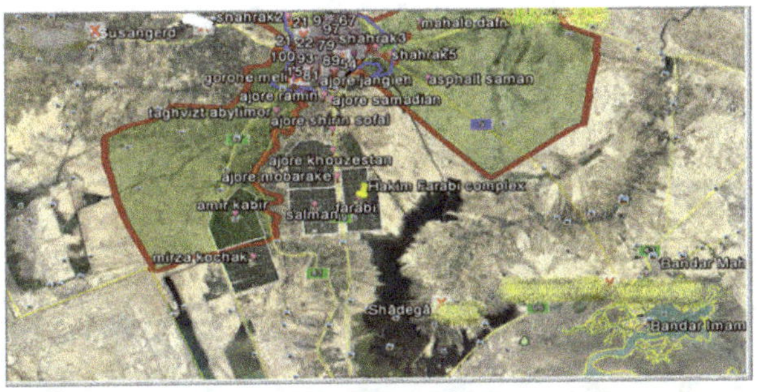

Figure 1. Locations of the studied stations.

Table 1. CO_2 and CH_4 emission factors in sugarcane factories

Emission resource	Gas	Emission factor	Unit	Reference
Sugarcane straw Burning in the field	CO_2	1.66	g/kg	CEPA (23)
	CH_4	2.7	g/kg	CEPA
Trash burning in the field	CO_2	1.3 – 1.4	kg/tones	EPA (24)
	CH_4	2.7	kg/tones	IPCC (24)
Boiler emission	CO_2	1891	g/m^3 fuel	CAPP (25)
	CH_4	0.03	g/m^3 fuel	CAPP
Limestone burning emission	CO_2	3.14	kg/m^3 fuel	Canada can met energy diversification research laboratory (26)
	CH_4	0.12	Ton CO_2/1000 m^3 fuel	CAPP
Diesel generator	CO_2	2.68	Kg CO_2/L fuel	SEIA (27)
	CH_4	0.13	g CH4/L fuel	Canada national inventory report

12000 hectares in the Farabi farm. The main sources of GHG emissions in this complex are open burning in the field, boilers, limestone burning, diesel generators, and electrical equipment. Emission rates for the different parts were calculated using the following formula. Table 1 indicates the emission factor for CO_2 and CH_4 gases in sugarcane factories as different guidelines. Emission factor and emission rate are common and simple indices used to show GHG emissions. Table 2 indicates the CO_2 and CH_4 emission rates at different units of the Dobal Khazaei factory.

Emission rate = emission factor * fuel type (22)

The emission factors in different parts of the factory based on type of fuel are as follows:

Emission factor = Emission rate / Fuel type

Figure 2 shows the carbon dioxide and methane emission rates during harvest; this emission factor obtained from bagasse burning that occurred as open-field burning at the Hakim Farabi farm.

Dobal Khazaei factory is one of the main factories in the region. It produces the largest amounts of ethanol and leaven in the country. In this factory, there are 3 sources of CO_2 emissions (boilers, the ethanol unit, and electrical equipment) and two sources of CH_4 emissions (boilers and electrical equipment). Figure 3 shows a comparison of CO_2 and CH4 emission rates from different emission sources at the Hakim Farabi factory. Figure 4 shows the CO2 and CH4 emission rates at the Dobal Khazaei factory.

Methane and carbon dioxide emissions

Methane and carbon dioxide are emitted from different parts of the Hakim Farabi and Dobal Khazaei complexes, including the burning of sugarcane fields before harvest,

Table 2. CO_2 and CH_4 emission rates from Dobal Khazaei factory

Emission resource	Gas	Emission (ton/year)
Boiler (ethanol production)	CO_2	10892.16
	CH_4	0.20
Leaven production process	CO_2	14000
Boilers (Leaven production process)	CO_2	7412.72
	CH_4	0.14

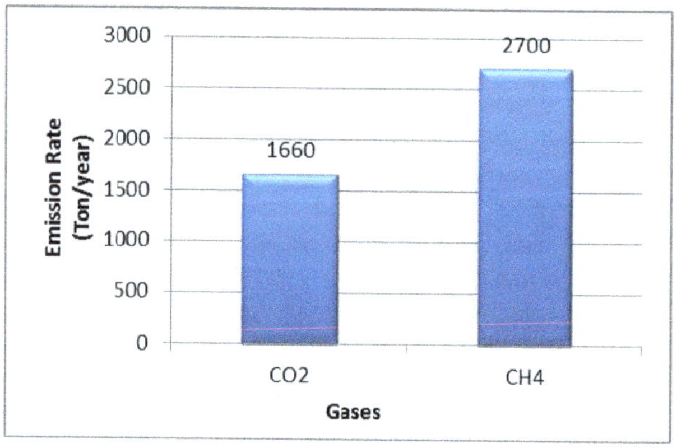

Figure 2. Open-field burning at Hakim Farabi farm.

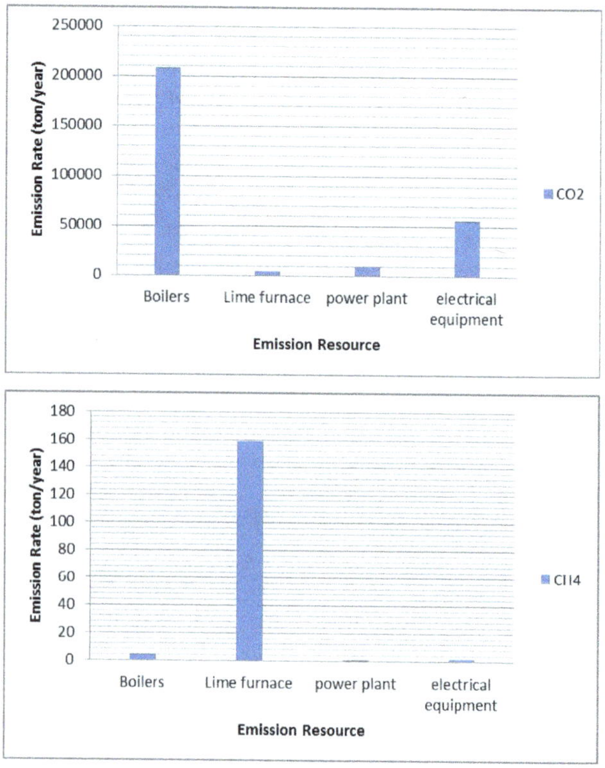

Figure 3. Comparison of CO_2 and CH_4 emissions from different sources at Hakim Farabi Sugar factory

using stillage as fertilizer, boilers, and burning ethanol in ethanol engines. Results of this study indicate the emission factor for CH_4 and CO_2 in Hakim Farabi farm. During the burning of sugarcane trash in the field, CH_4 is the main gas produced and emitted; CO_2 emissions are insignificant. Therefore, the bulk of CH_4 emissions are produced in field by trash burning, whereas CO_2 emissions resulting from open burning in the field are related to bagasse and cane waste. Figure 5 shows the comparison of CO_2 and CH_4 emissions from different sources. A recent study that analyzed emission factors for sugarcane and simulated burning in a wind tunnel indicated that GHG emissions were 0.32 kg/t (dry fuel) in the case of a spreading fire and 0.59 kg/t (dry fuel) for fire in a pile. In transient or disturbed boiler processes, CH_4 emissions are produced only from unburnt organics.

Discussion

In this study, GHG emissions from five main factory sources were investigated, including the sugarcane farm, boilers, limestone burning, diesel generators, and electrical equipment. The Farabi cane crop was transferred from the farm to the Farabi, Dobal Khazaei, and Ramin factories to become the final products such as ethanol and sugarcane. Therefore, sugarcane mills produce sugar, ethanol, Leaven, which are splatted and sent to respond to market needs. Straw and sugarcane that are cut and burned on the Hakim Farabi farm produce the greatest amounts of CO_2 and CH_4 emissions. In addition, bagasse, the residue of sugarcane sap dewatered from sugarcane, is combusted in sugar factories to produce steam and electricity. Nguyen and Gheewala showed in their study that the methane emission rate from sugarcane burning is 3.5 kg/ton. They also revealed that open burning on the farm caused a CH_4 emission rate of 2.2 kg/ton. Their results were obtained by the emission factor (28). The Hakim Farabi and Dobal Khazaei factories are major producers of sugar, leaven, and ethanol, and their activities produce a large quantity of CO_2 and CH_4 emissions. Ordinarily, GHG emissions are produced in winter, which is the harvest season. The GHGs emissions from these factories along with particulate matter (PM) are considered synergistic agents. The California Environmental Protection Agency revealed that the CO_2 and CH_4 emission rates from the open burning of sugarcane for the production of ethanol are 315.973 and 514.1 g/ton, respectively (29), but in the current study, CO2 and CH4 emission rates of 1660 and 2700 g/ton were determined (Figure 2). Boilers are another part of the factories that release high concentrations of CO_2 and CH_4 emissions into the atmosphere. Boilers, lime furnaces, diesel generators, and electrical equipment are internal units in the Hakim Farabi Complex And are used in the production of sugar and ethanol. The GHG emissions in these processes are caused by the internal burner. This unit of the factory uses natural gas and gasoline; therefore, the emission and energy rates related to gasoline are affected by the class of the crude oil, the petroleum refinery configuration, and

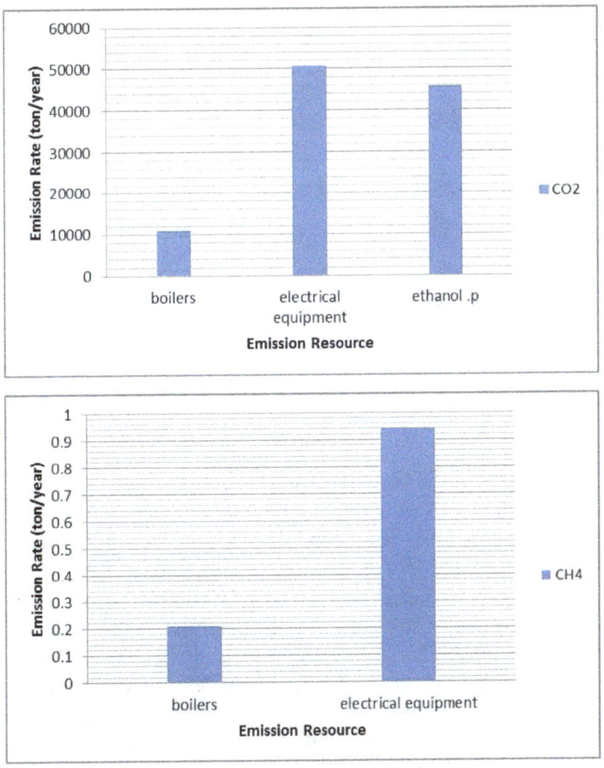

Figure 4. Comparison of CO_2 and CH_4 emissions from different sources at Dobal Khazaei factory

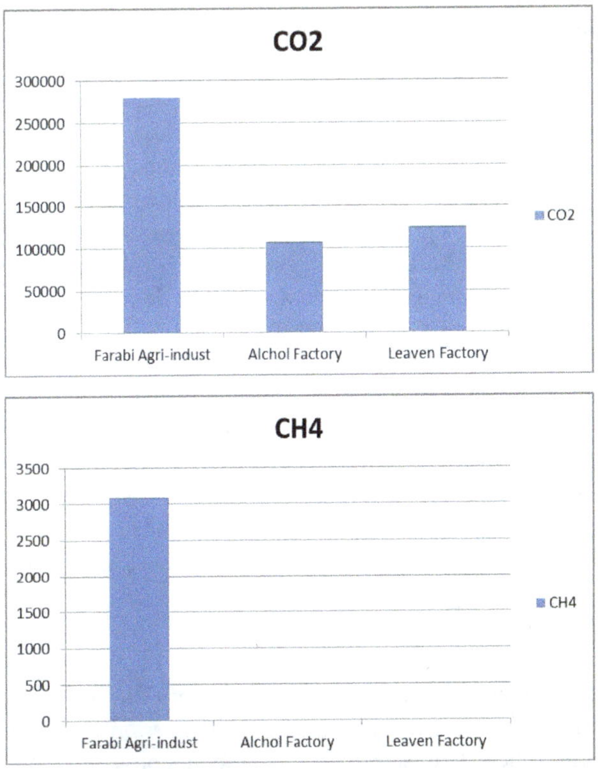

Figure 5. Comparison of CO_2 and CH_4 emissions from different sources in the whole complex

such factors as natural gas, petrol, and gasoline quality (11). The lime furnace uses natural gas, and therefore produces a high amount of CH_4. The power plant unit is one of the main parts of the Hakim Farabi complex. It uses six diesel generators to supply electricity to the entire Hakim Farabi complex. In this unit, the use of gasoline fuel could not be determined as local reliable documents were not available. Thus, international consolidated data about energy consumption and GHG emissions in the production of oil-derived fuels was used in this study. The electrical equipment is another main unit in the Hakim Farabi factory. This unit supplies electrical energy for the entire Hakim Farabi complex.

Total bagasse production is almost 1129 222 tons/year (2014) at 50% moisture. It is the sum of bagasse which percentage of bagasse will be lost in different ways, and this is used as fuel in some industries such as paper pulp and food industries. However, the main part of bagasse is used in sugar mills as an energy resource to produce sugar or ethanol. Also some of bagasse are used to produce sugar and ethanol. The bagasse to sugar ratio is 1:1, and the bagasse to ethanol ratio is 0.5:1.

Sugarcane farming correlates with a significant amount of GHG emissions such as CO_2 and CH_4, from both upstream processes such as fertilizer production and from the field itself. The nitrogen in bagasse (i.e. straw) on the farm is also the N in fertilizer and emits N_2O. Open field burning was done in farm, by physical harvesting of sugarcane, and transportation logistics. These two activities are the main GHG emission sources in the sugarcane ethanol life cycle. In the last decade, mechanical harvesting increased the speed of operations. This technology also increased fuel consumption by 20%; however, the use of bigger equipment and new technology is replacing these methods. Automatic harvesting will increase to 50% in the next 8 years (10). However, mechanical harvesting will increase GHG emissions in the atmosphere. Moreover, an increase in green cane reaping will produce a huge volume of trash. This could increase GHG emissions due to open burning in the field. Most boilers do not have wet scrubbers, and CH_4 emissions have not been reported. The most significant pollutants emitted by bagasse boilers are CO_2 and PM, which can travel long distances in the atmosphere and be transferred to Ahvaz city atmosphere. Due to the higher volume of gases emitted from this agro-industry complex, it is suggested that this factory should use scrubbers and filters to control gases and use biofilters to remove gases through the use of microorganisms.

Conclusion

The Hakim Farabi, Dobal Khazaei, and Ramin are the most important sugar and ethanol factories in Iran, and they release a great amount of GHG emissions into the atmosphere. In these factories, GHG emissions come from five main sources: the sugarcane farm boilers, limestone burning, diesel generators, and electrical equipment. In these factories, straw and bagasse are burned in the field, and open burning released significant concentrations of CO_2 and CH_4 into the atmosphere. Ordinarily, GHG emissions are produced in winter, which is the harvest season. The GHG emissions from these factories along with PMs are considered synergistic agents. The emission rates for the different parts of the factories were calculated. The results showed that in the Hakim Farabi factory, boiler emissions, electrical equipment, diesel generator, limestone burning emissions, sugarcane straw burning in the field, and trash burning in the field released the highest concentrations of CO_2, respectively. Furthermore, sugarcane straw burning and trash burning in the field produced the biggest percentage of methane emissions. In open burning, the CH_4 emissions are greater than the CO_2 emissions. In the Dobal Khazaei factory, electrical equipment, ethanol, and boilers released the highest concentrations of CO_2 into the atmosphere. Also, the electrical equipment produced the highest rate of CH_4 emissions into the atmosphere.

Acknowledgments

This research project was financially supported by the Environmental Technologies Research Center, Ahvaz Jundishapur University of Medical Sciences (grant No. ETRC 9012).

Competing interests

The authors declare that they have no competing interests.

Authors' contribution

All authors contributed equally and participated in the collection, analysis, and interpretation of the data. All authors critically reviewed, refined, and approved the manuscript.

References

1. Samaras C, Meisterling K. Life cycle assessment of greenhouse gas emissions from plug-in hybrid vehicles: implications for policy. Environ Sci Technol 2008; 42(9): 3170-6. doi: 10.1021/es702178s.
2. Weisser D. A guide to life-cycle greenhouse gas (GHG) emissions from electric supply technologies. Energy 2007; 32(9): 1543-59. doi: 10.1016/j.energy.2007.01.008.
3. Bastianoni S, Pulselli FM, Tiezzi E. The problem of assigning responsibility for greenhouse gas emissions. Ecol Econ 2004; 49(3): 253-7. doi: 10.1016/j.ecolecon.2004.01.018.
4. Jaafarzadeh N, Amiri H, Ahmadi M. Factorial experimental design application in modification of volcanic ash as a natural adsorbent with Fenton process for arsenic removal. Environ Technol 2012; 33(2): 159-65. doi:

10.1080/09593330.2011.554887.
5. Davis SJ, Caldeira K. Consumption-based accounting of CO2 emissions. Proc Natl Acad Sci U S A 2010; 107(12): 5687-92. doi: 10.1073/pnas.0906974107.
6. Stocker TF, Qin D, Plattner GK, Tignor M, Allen SK, Boschung J, et al. Climate change 2013: The physical science basis. Intergovernmental Panel on Climate Change, Working Group I Contribution to the IPCC Fifth Assessment Report (AR5). New York: Cambridge Univ Press; 2013.
7. Smith KR, Desai MA, Rogers JV, Houghton RA. Joint CO2 and CH4 accountability for global warming. Proceedings of the National Academy of Sciences 2013; 110(31): E2865-74. doi: 10.1073/pnas.1308004110.
8. Taylor M, Tam C, Gielen D. Energy efficiency and CO2 emissions from the global cement industry. Korea 2006; 50(2-2): 61-7.
9. de Carvalho Macedo I. Greenhouse gas emissions and energy balances in bio-ethanol production and utilization in Brazil (1996). Biomass and Bioenergy 1998; 14(1): 77-81. doi: 10.1016/S0961-9534(97)00038-X.
10. Denmead OT, Macdonald B, Bryant G, Naylor T, Wilson S, Griffith DWT, et al. Emissions of methane and nitrous oxide from Australian sugarcane soils. Agric For Meteorol 2010; 150(6): 748-56. doi: 10.1016/j.agrformet.2009.06.018.
11. Macedo IC, Seabra JE, Silva JE. Green house gases emissions in the production and use of ethanol from sugarcane in Brazil: The 2005/2006 averages and a prediction for 2020. Biomass Bioenergy 2008; 32(7): 582-95. doi: 10.1016/j.biombioe.2007.12.006.
12. Rafiei M, Gadgil AS, Ghole VS, Gore SD, Jaafarzadeh N, Mirkazemi R. Assessment of air pollution and its effects on the health status of the workers in beam rolling mills factory (Iran National Steel Industrial Group) from Ahvaz-Iran. Indian J Occup Environ Med 2009; 13(1): 20-2. doi: 10.4103/0019-5278.50719.
13. Doney SC, Fabry VJ, Feely RA, Kleypas JA. Ocean acidification: the other CO2 problem. Ann Rev Mar Sci 2009; 1: 169-92. doi: 10.1146/annurev.marine.010908.163834.
14. Woodcock J, Edwards P, Tonne C, Armstrong BG, Ashiru O, Banister D, et al. Public health benefits of strategies to reduce greenhouse-gas emissions: urban land transport. Lancet 2009; 374(9705): 1930-43. doi: 10.1016/s0140-6736(09)61714-1.
15. Burba G, Anderson T, Ediger K, von Fischer J, Gioli B, Ham J, et al , eds. Latest on Mobile Methane Measurements with Fast Open-Path Technology: Experiences, Opportunities & Perspectives. Vienna: EGU General Assembly; 2016.
16. Ge S, Liu L, Xue Q, Yuan Z. Effects of exogenous aerobic bacteria on methane production and biodegradation of municipal solid waste in bioreactors. Waste Manag 2016; 55: 93-8. doi: 10.1016/j.wasman.2015.11.024.
17. Jorgenson AK. Global Warming and the Neglected Greenhouse Gas: A Cross-National Study of the Social Causes of Methane Emissions Intensity, 1995. Social Forces 2006; 84(3): 1779-98. doi: 10.1353/sof.2006.0050.
18. Howarth RW, Santoro R, Ingraffea A. Methane and the greenhouse-gas footprint of natural gas from shale formations. Clim Change 2011; 106(4): 679-90. doi: 10.1007/s10584-011-0061-5.
19. Searchinger T, Heimlich R, Houghton RA, Dong F, Elobeid A, Fabiosa J, et al. Use of U.S. Croplands for Biofuels Increases Greenhouse Gases Through Emissions from Land-Use Change. Science 2008; 319(5867): 1238-40. doi: 10.1126/science.1151861.
20. Satterthwaite D. Cities' contribution to global warming: notes on the allocation of greenhouse gas emissions. Environ Urban 2008; 20(2): 539-49. doi: 10.1177/0956247808096127.
21. Newell RG, Raimi D. Implications of Shale Gas Development for Climate Change. Environ Sci Technol 2014; 48(15): 8360-8. doi: 10.1021/es4046154.
22. Shahsavani A, Naddafi K, Jafarzade Haghighifard N, Mesdaghinia A, Yunesian M, Nabizadeh R, et al. The evaluation of PM10, PM2.5, and PM1 concentrations during the Middle Eastern Dust (MED) events in Ahvaz, Iran, from April through September 2010. J Arid Environ 2012; 77: 72-83. doi: 10.1016/j.jaridenv.2011.09.007.
23. Crilly D, Zhelev T. Emissions targeting and planning: An application of CO2 emissions pinch analysis (CEPA) to the Irish electricity generation sector. Energy 2008; 33(10): 1498-507. doi: 10.1016/j.energy.2008.05.015.
24. Venkatram A. A critique of empirical emission factor models: a case study of the AP-42 model for estimating PM10 emissions from paved roads. Atmos Environ 2000; 34(1): 1-11. doi: 10.1016/S1352-2310(99)00330-1.
25. Chambers A, Strosher M, Wootton T, Moncrieff J, McCready P. DIAL measurements of fugitive emissions from natural gas plants and the comparison with emission factor estimates. 15th Annual Emission Inventory Conference, US Environmental Protection Agency New Orleans; 2006.
26. Ordorica-Garcia G, Croiset E, Douglas P, Elkamel A, Gupta M. Modeling the Energy Demands and Greenhouse Gas Emissions of the Canadian Oil Sands Industry. Energy Fuels 2007; 21(4): 2098-111. doi: 10.1021/ef0700984.
27. Murray SN, Walsh BP, Kelliher D, O'Sullivan DTJ. Multi-variable optimization of thermal energy efficiency retrofitting of buildings using static modelling and genetic algorithms – A case study. Build Environ 2014; 75: 98-107. doi: 10.1016/j.buildenv.2014.01.011.
28. Nguyen TLT, Gheewala SH. Life cycle assessment of fuel ethanol from cane molasses in Thailand. Int J Life Cycle Assess 2008; 13(4): 301. doi: 10.1007/s11367-008-0011-2.
29. Detailed C. GREET pathway for California reformulated gasoline blendstock for oxygenate blending (CARBOB) from average crude refined in California, Version 2.1. Sacramento, CA: California Air Resources Board; 2009.

31

Assessing some heavy metals pollutions in sediments of the northern Persian Gulf (Bushehr province)

Mehdi Bibak[1*], Masoud Sattari[1,2], Ali Agharokh[3], Saeid Tahmasebi[4], Javid Imanpour Namin[1]

[1]Department of Fisheries, School of Natural Resources, University of Guilan, Sowmehsara, Iran
[2]Department of Marine Sciences, Caspian Sea Basin Research Center, University of Guilan, Sowmehsara, Iran
[3]Research Center for Persian Gulf, School of Persian Gulf, University of Persian Gulf, Bushehr, Iran
[4]Department of Statistics, School of Basic Sciences, University of Persian Gulf, Bushehr, Iran

Abstract

Background: Land and water pollution by heavy metals is a universal issue. Although the pollution affects all countries, but its range and severity vary hugely. The pollution of the marine environment by heavy metals is a worldwide problem. Marine sediments can be sensitive indicators for monitoring contaminants in aquatic environments.

Methods: The concentration of 10 elements (As, Cd, Cr, Cu, Al, Fe, Ni, Pb, Sb, and Zn) was determined in the sediments of four shoreline stations including Imam Hassan port, Ameri port, Bushehr port, and Nayband Bay at the west Persian Gulf from March to December 2017. The elements were measured by inductively coupled plasma mass spectrometry (ICP-MS). Data were analyzed using SPSS version 16.

Results: The contamination of the sediments was assessed based on the geoaccumulation index (Igeo) and enrichment factor (EF). Spearman correlation matrix was calculated between all the trace metals and major elements as well as corresponding sampling regions. Statistically significant inter-elemental correlations (e.g., Cr-Fe, Cr-Al, Cr-Ni, Cr-Zn, and Cr-Cu) were found between some metals. High EF levels for Fe, Al, and Pb suggest that metals in the sediments of the northern Persian Gulf could have originated from anthropogenic sources.

Conclusion: The contamination pattern of sediments is affected by factors such as sedimentation patterns, physical and chemical properties of the sediments. For example, sediments with fine-grained and high surface area-to-volume ratio can act as good absorbents for many pollutants.

Keywords: Heavy metals, Geologic sediment, Persian Gulf, Bushehr

***Correspondence to:**
Mehdi Bibak
Email:
mehdi.bibak65@yahoo.com

Introduction

The pollution of marine environment by heavy metals is a worldwide problem. Although the pollution affects all countries, but its range and severity vary hugely. In this regard, marine sediments can be sensitive indicators for monitoring contaminants in aquatic environments (1,2). The sediments are used as a stock for heavy metals and thus, need special investigation in projecting aquatic pollution research. Accumulation of heavy metals happen in upsaid sediments in aquatic environments by biological mechanisms. Sediment is a habitat and major nutrient source for aquatic organisms. These processes become toxic to sediment-dwelling organisms, resulting in death, reduced growth, reproductive impairment, and prevent species diversity (3,4). Heavy metals pollute marine sediments and other aquatic ecosystems, which happen due to industrialization (5,6).

Great quantities of pollutants, directly or indirectly, are discharged into the marine environment every day. In this regard, heavy metals are considered as serious pollutants of the aquatic environments due to their accumulative behavior (7,8). Heavy metals are one of the constituents that affect the marine ecosystems. Potential toxicity of heavy metals in an aquatic ecosystem is determined by their chemical form. Some elements are necessary for human health in trace amounts (Co, Cu, Cr, and Ni), while others are carcinogenic or toxic, mainly affecting the central nervous system (Hg, Pb, and As), the kidneys or liver (Hg, Pb, Cd, and Cu), or skin, bones and teeth (Ni, Cd, Cu, and Cr) (9). Heavy metals that have been recognized in the polluted environment include As, Cu, Cd, Pb, Cr, Ni, Hg, and Zn. The toxicity of trace metals

arises from their interference with an organism's uptake of essential metal ions such as sodium and calcium. For example, cadmium and zinc block the uptake of calcium ions, which are important for bone and teeth growth.
The interaction of some heavy metals with enzymes and their tendency to bind to the protein and other biological tissues also cause trace metal poisoning in organisms (10,11).
The Persian Gulf is a relatively shallow semi-enclosed sea with poor flushing characteristics. Thus, pollution discharges into the sea are diluted more slowly than into open marine ecosystems (12). The Persian Gulf has been facing many environmental challenges like biodiversity loss, industrial pollution, and harmful effluents (13). Additionally, environmental incidents, ship traffic, transportation, oil pollutants, and oil spills can cause different pollutants including heavy metals (14,15). Iran has the longest water joint border in the Persian Gulf and it has a way through the Strait of Hormuz and Makran Sea (Oman) to the Indian Ocean from the east. It leads to Arvand River in Khuzestan province from the west, which is composed of two Tigris and Euphrates rivers in Iraq as well as Karun River attachment in Iran (16).
The aim of this study was to determine the concentration of 10 metals (As, Cu, Cd, Pb, Cr, Ni, Zn, Fe, Al, and Sb) in sediments of the Persian Gulf.

Materials and Methods

Bushehr is located at 28° 55′ 19.84″ N and 50° 50′ 4.76″ E in southwestern Iran and around the northern of the Persian Gulf. In this study, 12 sampling sites in four regions of Imam Hassan port, Bushehr port, Ameri port, and Nayband Bay (Figure 1) were selected during March to December 2017.
Samples were obtained from the upper layer (5 cm depth) of sediments. Ten square meters of each area was sampled. The sediments were collected from the intertidal areas once low tides. Sediments were transferred to polyethylene containers and transported to the laboratory at 4°C. The

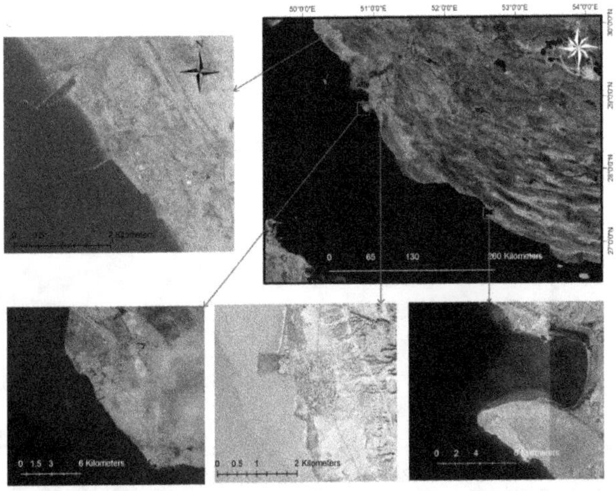

Figure 1. Sampling areas.

samples were dried at 105°C for at least 24 hours (17). The samples were sieved through a 63 micron stainless steel sieve and agitated vigorously to produce homogeneity (18). One gram of each sample was digested in a mixture of concentrated HNO3 (65%) and HClO4 (60%) in the ratio of 4:1, first, at a low temperature (40°C) for 1 hour and then, at a high temperature (140°C) for 4 hours (19). The digested samples were then diluted to a certain capacity (25 mL) with double distilled water (DDW). The sample was then filtered through Whatman No. 40 filter paper. The heavy metals concentrations were determined by inductively coupled plasma mass spectrometry (ICP-MS) (scheme code was MMS-01: Detection limited were in ppm) in Zarazma Co.
The geoaccumulation index (Igeo) is used to determine the level of contamination in sediments (20). For this purpose, the current concentrations is compared to pre-industrial levels using the following equation:

$$I_{geo} = \log_2 C_n / 1.5B_n$$

where *Cn* is the measured concentration of the element n in the pelitic sediment fraction (< 2 Am) and *Bn* is the geochemical background value in fossil argillaceous sediment (average shale). The quality of the sediments is divided into six classes by Igeo: unpolluted (Igeo < 0), unpolluted to moderately polluted (0 < Igeo < 1), moderately polluted (1 < Igeo < 2), moderately to strongly polluted (2 < Igeo < 3), strongly polluted (3 < Igeo < 4), strongly to extremely polluted (4 < Igeo < 5), and extremely polluted (5 < Igeo). Concentrations of the geochemical background are increased each time by the constant 1.5 in order to allow value fluctuations of a given substance in the environment as well as very small anthropogenic influences (21).
The enrichment factor (EF) is based on the standardization of a tested element against a reference one. According to contamination standards based on the EF, the following classes are obtained: EF<2 (deficiency to minimal enrichment), 2 ≤ EF < 5 (moderate enrichment), 5 ≤ EF < 20 (significant enrichment), 20 ≤ EF<40 (very high enrichment), and EF ≥ 40 (extremely high enrichment) (22). A reference element is the one characterized by low-frequency current variability. The most common reference elements are Sc, Mn, Ti, Al, and Fe (23). The EF is calculated using the following expression:

$$EF = [(Me)_s / (Fe)_s] / [(Me)_b / (Fe)_b]$$

where $(Me)_s$ and $(Me)_b$ are the concentrations of metal and normalizer, respectively. Also, $(Fe)_s$ and $(Fe)_b$ denote the sample and background sediments, respectively. Data were analyzed using SPSS version 16.

Results

Table 1 shows the concentrations of heavy metals in sediment samples collected from intertidal zone from four regions in the Bushehr province.
The obtained Igeo values for these four regions are shown

Table 1. Mean concentrations of each metal analyzed (mg/kg)

Metals	Region			
	Ameri Port	Bushehr Port	Imam Hassan Port	Nayband Bay
As	16.24±8.76	5.03±0.15	3.31±2.65	1.55±0.49
Cr	16.82±3.05	14.29±7.79	10.96±3.30	10.19±5.97
Cu	5.5±0.88	5.5±2.83	3.75±0.49	3.45±0.77
Pb	12.27±4.59	2.77±0.38	3.03±0.02	6.35±4.30
Zn	14.20±1.41	11.45±8.13	8.45±1.06	4.75±0.78
Al	3980±462.4	4189±5 3143.09	3828.5±688.01	695±173.2
Fe	8420±1824.3	5360±3309.26	4141±642.05	773.5±193.04
Ni	18.07±2	13.4±6.36	11.8±3.25	8.19±2.25
Sb	0.45±0.07	0.35±0.21	0.35±0.07	0.55±0.07
Cd	0.07±0.04	0.18±0.01	0.10±0.04	BDL*

*BDL: Below detection limit.

in Table 2.

Spearman correlation matrix was calculated between all the trace metals (and also major elements) and corresponding sampling regions (Table 3).

EF was used as an index to evaluate anthropogenic influences of heavy metals in sediments. When $0.5 \leq EF \leq 1.5$, the trace metals might have originated entirely from crustal materials or natural weathering processes, while when EF>1.5 suggested that a significant portion of trace metals is provided by other sources (24).

Discussion

In this study, sediment pollution was assessed using geoaccumulation index (Igeo) and EF. As can be seen in Table 1, metal levels in all areas of the sample sites in terms of frequency were Fe> Al> Cr> Ni> Zn> As> Pb> Cu> Sb> Cd. The relatively high concentrations of heavy metals during winter coincide principally with decreasing rate of organic matter decomposition, due to a low water temperature (25). The highest concentrations of Fe and Al were found in Ameri port while the lowest values of Cd were reported in Nayband Bay. Fe, Al, and Pb levels were found to be higher than the other metals in the four regions (Table 2). Approximately, 42% of the samples were included in Class 0. A small percentage of the samples was included in Class 2, 3, and 4 for Al, Fe, Cd, and Pb. There were significant inter-elemental correlations (e.g., Cr-Fe, Cr-Al, Cr-Ni, Cr-Zn, and Cr-Cu). Inverse correlations

Table 2. Index of geoaccumulation for sampling regions

Region	Class								
	Fe	Al	Cd	Pb	Ni	As	Zn	Cu	Sb
Imam Hassan	0	2	0	0	0	1	0	0	1
Bushehr	3	3	2	2	0	1	0	0	1
Ameri	4	3	0	3	0	1	0	0	1
Nayband	3	2	0	2	0	0	0	0	1

Table 3. The Spearman correlation matrix between element levels in the sediment of the Persian Gulf

	Cr	Al	Fe	Ni	As	Cu	Pb	Zn	Sb	Cd
Cr	1									
Al	.934	1								
Fe	1.000**	.927	1							
Ni	.997**	.901	.998**	1						
As	.857	.639	.865	.891	1					
Cu	.947	.999**	.940	.917	.667	1				
Pb	.131	-.233	.150	.213	.557	-.195	1			
Zn	.996**	.961*	.995**	.986**	.816	.971	.046	1		
Sb	-.724	-.923	-.711	-.664	-.310	-.907	.589	-.780	1	
Cd	.317	.570	.303	.253	.072	.546	-.715	.381	-.756	1

*Correlation is significant at the 0.05 (2-tailed); ** Correlation is significant at the 0.01 (2-tailed).

Table 4. Enrichment factor in sampling regions

Metals Region	As	Cr	Cu	Pb	Zn	Al	Fe	Ni	Sb	Cd
Imam Hassan	EF<2	EF<2	EF<2	EF<2	EF<2	EF<2	EF<2	EF<2	EF<2	EF<2
Bushehr port	EF<2	EF<2	EF<2	EF<2	EF<2	2<EF<5	2<EF<5	EF<2	EF<2	EF<2
Ameri port	EF<2	EF<2	EF<2	2<EF<5	EF<2	2<EF<5	2<EF<5	EF<2	EF<2	EF<2
Nayband Bay	EF<2	EF<2	EF<2	EF<2	EF<2	EF<2	EF<2	EF<2	EF<2	EF<2

were observed between Sb and Cd with almost all other elements, suggesting a positive strong significant correlation among Cr, Al, Fe, Ni, and Cu, which were clustered in the first class. Sb had a negative correlation with other elements in the first class. High EF level for Fe, Al, and Pb demonstrated that the levels of metals in sediments of the Persian Gulf could have originated from anthropogenic sources (Table 4). According to these results, the presence of these metals in the same groups might reflect a similar behavior or suggest common bio-originated sources.

The highest mean concentrations of Pb (12.27 mg/kg), Ni (18.07 mg/kg) and As (16.24 mg/kg) were reported in the Ameri port. This concentration was similar to the results of Ganugapenta et al (26) and Zhuang & Gao (27) but lower than that of El Tokhi et al (21). The pollution in the Ameri port was higher than other ports, due to the increase in the amount of agricultural wastewater, industrial wastewater, oil pollution and shipping in this port compared to the other ports.

Conclusion

Oil extraction and recent regional wars in the Persian Gulf have released millions of oil barrels, including detectable trace metals, to the sea. Seawater desalination plants in the Persian Gulf with a capacity of millions cubic meters freshwater per day are another sources of heavy metal pollution in the area. In addition to pollutants, the contamination pattern of sediments is affected by factors such as sedimentation patterns, physical and chemical properties of the sediments. For example, sediments with fine-grained and high surface area-to-volume ratio can act as good absorbents for many pollutants.

Acknowledgements

The authors wish to thank all who assisted in conducting this research.

Competing interests

The authors declared no competing interests.

Authors' contributions

All authors contributed in all aspects of this research like performing surveys and experiments, preparing the figures and tables, designing the experiments, analyzing the data graphical elaborations, writing the manuscript, and providing critical revision of the paper.

References

1. Pekey H, Karakas D, Ayberk S, Tolun L, Bakoglu M. Ecological risk assessment using trace elements from surface sediments of Izmit Bay (Northeastern Marmara Sea) Turkey. Mar Pollut Bull 2004; 48(9-10): 946-53. doi: 10.1016/j.marpolbul.2003.11.023.
2. Sinem Atgin R, El-Agha O, Zararsız A, Kocataş A, Parlak H, Tuncel G. Investigation of the sediment pollution in Izmir Bay: trace elements. Spectrochim Acta Part B At Spectrosc 2000; 55(7): 1151-64. doi: 10.1016/S0584-8547(00)00231-7.
3. Rubio B, Nombela MA, Vilas F. Geochemistry of major and trace elements in sediments of the Ria de Vigo (NW Spain) an assessment of metal pollution. Marine Pollution Bulletin 2000; 40(11): 968-80.
4. Reimann C, de Caritat P. Intrinsic flaws of element enrichment factors (EFs) in environmental geochemistry. Environ Sci Techno 2000; 134(24): 5084-91.
5. Yang H, Rose NL. Distribution of mercury in six lake sediment cores across the UK. Sci Total Environ 2003; 304(1-3): 391-404. doi: 10.1016/s0048-9697(02)00584-3.
6. Capillo G, Silvestro S, Sanfilippo M, Fiorino E, Giangrosso G, Ferrantelli V, et al. Assessment of electrolytes and metals profile of the Faro Lake (Capo Peloro Lagoon, Sicily, Italy) and its impact on *Mytilus galloprovincialis*. Chem Biodivers 2018; 15(5): e1800044. doi: 10.1002/cbdv.201800044.
7. Abdolahpur Monikh F, Maryamabadi A, Savari A, Ghanemi K. Heavy metals' concentration in sediment, shrimp and two fish species from the northwest Persian Gulf. Toxicol Ind Health 2015; 31(6): 554-65. doi: 10.1177/0748233713475498.
8. Forouhar Vajargah M, Mohamadi Yalsuyi A, Hedayati A, Faggio C. Histopathological lesions and toxicity in common carp (Cyprinus carpio L. 1758) induced by copper nanoparticles. Microsc Res Tech 2018; 81(7): 724-9. doi: 10.1002/jemt.23028.
9. Olubunmi FE, Olorunsola OE. Evaluation of the status of heavy metal pollution of sediment of Agbabu bitumen deposit area, Nigeria. Eur J Sci Res 2010; 41(3): 373-82.
10. Torre A, Trischitta F, Faggio C. Effect of CdCl2 on regulatory volume decrease (RVD) in *Mytilus galloprovincialis* digestive cells. Toxicol In Vitro 2013; 27(4): 1260-6. doi: 10.1016/j.tiv.2013.02.017.
11. Savorelli F, Manfra L, Croppo M, Tornambe A, Palazzi

D, Canepa S, et al. Fitness Evaluation of Ruditapes philippinarum Exposed to Ni. Biol Trace Elem Res 2017; 177(2): 384-93. doi: 10.1007/s12011-016-0885-y.
12. Burgos-Aceves MA, Cohen A, Smith Y, Faggio C. MicroRNAs and their role on fish oxidative stress during xenobiotic environmental exposures. Ecotoxicol Environ Saf 2018; 148: 995-1000. doi: 10.1016/j.ecoenv.2017.12.001.
13. Fernandez JM, Hayes PJ, Smith MR. Comprehensive Analytical Chemistry. Elsevier; 1992. p. 345-47.
14. Khoshnood Z, Mokhlesi A, khshnood R. Bioaccumulation of some heavy metals and histopathological alterations in liver of Euryglossa orientalis and Psettodes erumei along North Coast of the Persian Gulf. Afr J Biotechnol 2010; 9(41): 6966-72. doi: 10.5897/AJB10.944.
15. Sabzalizadeh S, Dehghan Madise S. Assessment of heavy metals pollution in the sediments of Lifeh-Busaf (northwest of Persian Gulf) using Geo-accumulation Index. Iranian Scientific Fisheries Journal 2010; 19(3): 51-60. [In Persian].
16. Pourang N, Nikouyan A, Dennis JH. Trace element concentrations in fish, surficial sediments and water from northern part of the Persian Gulf. Environ Monit Assess 2005; 109(1-3): 293-316. doi: 10.1007/s10661-005-6287-9.
17. Tatina M, Oryan S, Gharibkhani M. Surveying the amount of heavy metals (Ni, Pb,Cd & V) accumulation derived from oil pollution on the muscle tissue of Pelates quadrilineatus from the Persian Gulf. Mar Biol 2009; 1(1): 28-39. [In Persian].
18. Dehghan Chenari A, Lak R. Effects of heavy metals from petroleum pollutions on carbonate surface sediments of the Persian Gulf. Int J Environ Res 2014; 8(2): 297-304. doi: 10.22059/ijer.2014.720.
19. Ismail A, Badri MA, Ramlan MN. The background levels of heavy metal concentration in sediments of the west coast of Peninsular Malaysia. Sci Total Environ 1993; 134 (Suppl 1): 315-23. doi: 10.1016/S0048-9697(05)80032-4.
20. Muller G. Index of geoaccumulation in sediments of the Rhine River. GeoJournal 1969; 2: 108-18.
21. El Tokhi M, Amin BM, Alaabed SA. Environmental assessment of heavy metals contamination of bottom sediments of Oman Gulf, United Arab Emirates. J Pollut Eff Cont 2017; 5(4): 203. doi: 10.4172/2375-4397.1000203.
22. Tanner PA, Leong LS, Pan SM. Contamination of heavy metals in marine sediment cores from Victoria Harbour, Hong Kong. Marine Pollution Bulletin 2000; 40(9): 769-79.
23. Zhuang W, Gao XL.Acid-volatile sulfide and simultaneously extracted metals in surface sediments of the southwestern coastal Laizhou Bay, Bohai Sea: concentrations, spatial distributions and the indication of heavy metal pollution status. Mar Pollut Bull 2013; 76(1-2): 128-38.
24. Taylor SR, McLennan SM. The geochemical evolution of the continental crust. Rev Geophys 1995; 33(2): 241-65. doi: 10.1029/95RG00262.
25. Bazzi AO. Heavy metals in seawater, sediments and marine organisms in the Gulf of Chabahar, Oman Sea. J Oceanogr Mar Sci 2014; 5(3): 20-9. doi: 10.5897/JOMS2014.0110.
26. Ganugapenta S, Nadimikeri J, Chinnapolla SRRB, Ballari L, Madiga R, Nirmala K, et al. Assessment of heavy metal pollution from the sediment of Tupilipalem Coast, southeast coast of India. International Journal of Sediment Research 2018; 33(3): 294-302. doi: 10.1016/j.ijsrc.2018.02.004.
27. Zhuang W, Gao X. Integrated assessment of heavy metal pollution in the surface sediments of the Laizhou Bay and the coastal waters of the Zhangzi Island, China: comparison among typical marine sediment quality indices. PLoS One 2014; 9(4): e94145. doi: 10.1371/journal.pone.0094145.

32

Adsorption of copper, lead and cadmium from aqueous solutions by activated carbon prepared from saffron leaves

Shidvash Dowlatshahi[1], Ahmad Reza Haratinezhad Torbati[2], Mahshid Loloei[1*]

[1]Instructor, Environmental Health Engineering Research Center and Department of Environmental Health, School of Public Health, Kerman University of Medical Sciences, Kerman, Iran
[2]M.Sc Student of Environmental Health Engineering, Department of Environmental Health, School of Public Health, Kerman University of Medical Sciences, Kerman, Iran

Abstract
Background: Industrial development has caused the release of various pollutants including heavy metals into the environment. These toxic compounds are extremely dangerous to living beings and the environment due to their non-biodegradability, severe toxicity, carcinogenicity, the ability to be accumulated in nature and the ability to contaminate groundwater and surface water. The aim of the present research was to provide an appropriate and cost-effective adsorbent to remove heavy metals from aqueous solutions.
Methods: The activated carbon was produced from the dried. Batch experiments were performed on real and synthetic samples at room temperature. The effect of pH, adsorbent dose, initial concentration, and contact time were studied, and the adsorption isotherms of heavy metals were determined. The removal efficiency was evaluated on real wastewater.
Results: The maximum removal efficiency of heavy metals (copper, cadmium and lead) by activated carbon adsorbent prepared from saffron leaves was obtained in pH 7. The optimum amount of adsorbent was 0.6 g, and the optimum contact times were 45 min for copper and cadmium ions and 90 min for lead ion, respectively. In these optimum conditions the removal efficiencies were 76.36%, 91.25% and 97.5%, respectively. The removal efficiencies of heavy metals from actual samples (copper industry and the battery industry) in the optimum conditions were 82.25%, 69.95% and 91.23%, respectively. The results obtained showed the highest correlation with Langmuir isotherm model.
Conclusion: Based on the results obtained, the activated carbon produced from saffron leaves has a good capability in removal of the metal ions from the aqueous solutions. Considering the availability of saffron leaves in Khorasan, its cost-effectiveness, and high uptake capacity, it can be applied as a proper absorbent to remove the heavy metals from industrial wastewater.
Keywords: Adsorption, Heavy metal, Activated carbon, Saffron leaves

***Correspondence to:**
Mahshid Loloei
Email: mloloei@gmail.com

Introduction

Increasing pollution of municipal and industrial sewages by toxic compounds due to industry development and growth is a concerning issue. Heavy metals because of the nature of their non-degradability, sever toxicity, ability to be accumulated, and carcinogenicity not only endanger aquatic life, but also cause the acceptor waters to be inappropriate for various uses such as drinking (1). Discharging sewage of many industrial processes like plating, photography, nuclear power plants, and petrochemical industries into water resources causes water pollution. Heavy metals like lead and cadmium, even at low concentrations are serious threats to living organisms through their being stimulating, property aggregation ability, carcinogenicity, and mutagenesis (2). These metals are non-degradable and very resistant against biodegradation. The adverse effects of their presence in body can be diarrhea, abdominal pains, severe vomiting, fracture, sterilization, and they can damage the central nervous system, body immune systems, and also cause psychological disorders, possible damage to DNA, and cancer (3-8).

There are a variety of methods such as sedimentation, filtration, oxidation and reduction, ion exchange, and membrane separation for heavy metals removal. These methods are often ineffective or expensive in very low concentrations (3,4).

Adsorption is a process during which a soluble material accumulates on the surface of another substance (9). In fact, adsorption is the function of transferring from liquid phase to solid phase. Adsorption is an important phenomenon in many physical, chemical, and biological processes in the nature. Adsorption is also widely used in water and wastewater treatment (7). One of the most widely used adsorbents for this purpose is activated carbon. Its high cost of activation stages and its low regenerative capacity has limited the use of this material on a large scale. In recent years, using inexpensive adsorbents has attracted the attention of many researchers. These adsorbents are frequently found and are available, and their preparation costs are low (6). The use of bioadsorbents to remove metal ions from aqueous solutions is a cost-effective and environment-friendly method. Therefore in recent decades, it has attracted the attention of many researchers. Successful use of natural materials such as activated carbon produced from olive kernel in the removal of heavy metals like copper, lead and cadmium was experienced by Bohli *et al* (8) in 2013, in Tunisia.

Activated carbon produced from tassel to remove lead was one of the applied adsorbents used by Moyo *et al* (5). Also Hadoun *et al* (10) investigated the removal of cadmium from the aqueous solutions using activated carbon produced from palm stem in Algeria. *Yahaya* et al (11) investigated the removal of copper using activated carbon produced from rice husk. Amuda *et al* studied the heavy metals removal by charcoal made from coconut shell that resulted in a very effective absorbent from cheap row material (11). The study by Song *et al* (12) on the removal of lead by activated carbon made of coconut skin activated by potash had good results. Nale *et al* (13) performed studies of kinetics and copper absorption equilibrium from aqueous solutions on activated carbon produced from corn cob. Studies related to kinetics and cadmium removal equilibrium from aqueous solutions by activated carbon produced of apple skin were carried out by Sartape *et al* (14). Another study was conducted by Arivoli *et al* (15) titled "The dynamic of copper adsorption by low-cost activated carbon". Saffron with the scientific name of Crocus sativus, is a plant from the family of gladiola. There was 57,000 hectares of cultivated area in Razavi Khorasan which was equivalent to 77% total production of country in 2012.

The aim of this study was to investigate the removal efficiency of heavy metals (copper, cadmium and lead) with activated carbon prepared from leaves of saffron in the synthetic and real solutions as an available and inexpensive absorbent in the region. The effective parameters on absorption process such as contact time, pH, and initial concentration of metal ions were studied. Also the adsorption equilibriums were studied.

Methods

In this practical study, the efficacy of activated carbon prepared from saffron leaves for the removal of metal ions (copper, cadmium and lead) from the aqueous solutions was studied.

The chemical materials made by Merch company with high purity were used. The stock solutions of metal ions with concentration of 1000 mg/l were prepared. In all stages of the experiment, the 0.1 N normal solutions of NaOH and H_2SO_4 were used to adjust pH. pH meter (HANNA instruments HI 110 Model) was used to measure the pH of the solution

Adsorbent preparation

Sorbent preparation was performed as follows. Saffron leaves were harvested from the cultivated fields around Torbat Heydarie city located in Razavi Khorasan and collected in the suitable containers and moved to laboratory. The leaves were washed by distilled water, then dried at 60 °C, and were powered after crushing. In order to improve the adsorption capacity, 100 g of obtained powder ere mixed with a special volume of phosphoric acid with a mass ratio of 1:5, and this mixing alternatively continued for one hour to obtain a better contact of acid and saffron leaves. Then the modified powder was washed by distilled water for the removal of outputs. After removing the additional water, the obtained materials in a metal reactor in diameter of 50 mm and length of 100 mm were placed into an electric furnace for one hour in a temperature of 750 °C (16). This carbon was washed by distilled water until pH reached about 6.5 and then was dried in the oven for one hour at 100 °C, and then the two sieves with mesh sizes of 100 and 200 were used to separate the absorbent particles between 0.85 and 0.15 mm. Memert oven, which was made in Germany, and 1200 °C Electric Furnace were used to provide required temperatures.

Determining the characteristics of the adsorbent

In order to investigate the properties of the initial carbon and activated carbon prepared from saffron leaves, several experiments were conducted to determine the percentages of cellulose, lignin, volatile material, humidity, density, and iodine number (17). Morphological properties of activated carbon prepared from saffron leaves were studied by Scanning Electronic Microscope (SEM).

Adsorption tests

The effect of various parameters on the absorption process including the initial concentration of pollutants, the amount of adsorbent, contact time, and the optimum pH was studied. To determine the optimum pH, the value of 0.1 g activated carbon prepared from saffron leaves was poured in 100 ml of the synthetic solution with concentration of 30 ppm. Then experiment was conducted at contact times of 30, 45, 60, and 90 min at various pHs (3, 5, 7, and 9) separately, and then adsorbent was contacted with the metal ions of pollutant in the ambient temperature. Then the samples were filtered using filter paper in size of 0.45 μ and the remaining metal ions were measured by atomic absorption apparatus (YOUNGLTN ASS 8020 Model). The process was separately repeated for all the metal ions.

In the next step considering optimum pH determined,

the amounts of adsorbent of activated carbon (0.3, 0.6, 1, and 1.3 g), initial concentration of pollutants (20, 30, 50, and 40 mg/L), and the contact time (30, 45, 60, and 90 min) were separately tested for individual pollutants. The removal efficiency was calculated using the following equation:

$$Removal(\%)= (C_0-C_t)/C_0 \times 100 \quad (1)$$

Where C_0 is the initial concentration (mg/l), and C_t is metal ion concentration after each adsorption step.

Langmuir adsorption isotherm

The assumptions of Langmuir equation include the followings: a) maximum absorption occurs when the adsorbent surface is covered by a single molecular layer of soluble material. b) The absorption energy is fixed and identical at all the points. c) The molecules of adsorbed material cannot move in the adsorbent surface.

$$Q_0 = \frac{Q_{max} BC}{1+BC} \quad (2)$$

Where C is the concentration of soluble material in the steady state mg/L.

Q_{max} is the maximum absorption capacity (mg/g) and B is Langmuir equation constant (L/mg).

Freundlich adsorption isotherm

The Freundlich equation expresses adsorption on a heterogeneous surface in terms of adsorption, and it can be expressed as follows:

$$Q= KC_f^{1/n} \quad (3)$$

Where n is Freundlich intensity parameter, and K is Freundlich capacity factor.

The Freundlich equation is an empirical one, and it is applicable for interpreting the experimental data (7).

With respect to determining optimal conditions in synthetic samples, the efficiency of metals removal from the sewage of Copper Complex Industries was studied to provide copper ion and the battery-making for electronics power (for cadmium and lead ions) was sampled. After determining the characteristics of sewage [pH, concentrations of copper, lead, cadmium ions, Chemical Oxygen Demand (COD), Biochemical Oxygen Demand (BOD), and Total Dissolved Solids (TDS)], adsorption experiments were conducted by produced active carbon, and the removal efficiency was calculated (18).

Results

The results of studying the characteristics of activated carbon produced from saffron leaves are shown in the Table 1. The results showed that the density of activated carbon produced is lower than the other initial materials, and the amount of lignin is almost similar to the almond skin and walnut shell. The amount of cellulose is lower than pistachio bark and almond skin and is equal to walnut shell, but the value of the iodine number is less than these materials.

Figure 1 shows the results of the photos provided by the electron microscopy of coal and activated carbon prepared from saffron leaves.

In studying different pHs in the adsorption of metal ions, the optimum pH was 7. In the other pHs, the amount of adsorption was decreased.

According to efficiency results the absorption of copper and cadmium during contact time of 45 min was the highest with 83.34 % and 86.64 %, respectively. The lead adsorption was balanced at 90 min. At this time, the highest observed removal amount was 90.22%. Table 2 shows the results.

To investigate the amount of optimal absorbent, the adsorption experiments at optimum pH 7, the initial concentration of pollutants with 50 ppm, and the optimum contact times from the previous stage in the different values of adsorbents were tested and the results are shown in Table 3.

The results of adsorption experiments of heavy metals by activated carbon prepared from saffron leaves showed that in the optimum amount of adsorbent of 0.6 g and the equilibrium contact time of 45 min, the removal efficiency of cadmium ion is more than that of copper ion (82.52% against 75.56%). Removal efficiency of lead ion in the amount of adsorbent of 0.6 and 90 min was 95.55%. Increasing amount of adsorbent caused no significant change in absorption rate.

In the following research, to investigate the effect of adsorbent prepared on the real sample, samples of the effluents of two copper and battery-making industries were studied. The results related to study the raw wastewater quality of copper and battery-making industries are shown in the Table 4.

Testing optimized results on the actual samples related to the copper and cadmium ions showed that in optimum conditions (absorbent 0.6 g and the equilibrium contact time of 45 min) the removal efficiencies were equal to 68.12% and 78.95%, respectively. The experimental results related to the real lead sample showed that in the optimum contact time of 90 min and adsorbent amount

Table 1. The characteristics of activated carbon prepared from saffron leaves

Ingredients	Iodine number, mg/g	Percent of lignin	Percent cellulose	Density kg/m³	Percentage of total ash	Percentage of volatile material	Moisture (%)	References
Saffron leaves	501	30	34	160	7.84	1.05	5.4	This study
Almond Skin	830	27	39	470	1.5	-	-	Kaghzchi (17)
Walnut shell	806	33	34	457	6	-	-	Kaghzchi (17)
Pistachio bark	953	13	42	448	1.2	-	-	Kaghzchi (17)

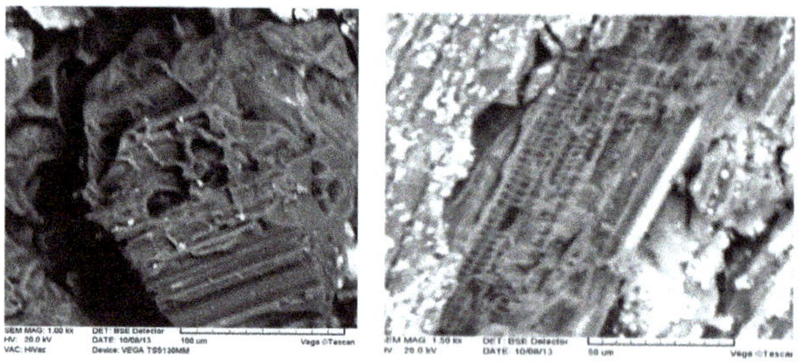

Figure 1. SEM image of charcoal (Left) prepared from saffron leaves without activating and activated carbon (Right).

of 0.6 g, the removal efficiency of this ion was 88.96%. To study the behavior of the adsorbent, Langmuir and Freundlich adsorption isotherms were plotted, and the results are shown in Figures 2 and 3. On the basis of the obtained correlation coefficients, it can be concluded that the adsorption of ions studied on prepared adsorbent given to the correlation coefficient higher than 0.99 follows Langmuir isotherm. Isothermal parameters have been shown in Table 5.

Table 2. The removal efficiency of the heavy metals (%) at different pHs and contact times (initial concentration 30 mg/L of pollutant and adsorbent dose 0.1 g).

Contact time(min)	Metal ion											
	Cd^{2+}				Cu^{2+}				Pb^{2+}			
	30	45	60	90	30	45	60	90	30	45	60	90
pH= 3	33.30	36.65	43.36	46.67	40.25	40.36	53.36	50.58	60.31	63.32	66.96	66.68
pH= 5	43.32	46.60	50.25	60.36	56.63	63.69	56.68	53.32	66.63	70.10	73.30	76.65
pH= 7	82.25	83.34	81.95	70.65	73.35	86.64	73.30	70.11	83.32	86.65	86.66	90.22
pH= 9	59.25	63.56	63.26	66.63	50.22	63.37	56.69	60.11	76.65	80.35	80.35	83.36

Table 3. The removal efficiency of heavy metals at different amounts of adsorbent (optimum contact time, optimum pH 7, initial concentration of 50 ppm)

Heavy metals	Optimum contact time (min)	The amount of adsorbent (g)	The final concentrations of heavy metals (ppm)	Absorption efficiency in synthetic solution (%)
Pb^{+2}	90	0.3	4.9	90.20
	90	0.6	2.22	95.55
	90	1	2.33	95.34
	90	1.3	2.27	95.45
Cu^{+2}	45	0.3	14.21	71.58
	45	0.6	12.22	75.56
	45	1	12.72	74.56
	45	1.3	12.37	75.25
Cd^{+2}	45	0.3	15.61	68.78
	45	0.6	8.75	82.50
	45	1	9.27	81.45
	45	1.3	9.21	81.58

Table 4. Characteristics of the sample of raw wastewater in the copper and battery-making industries

Type of industry	pH	Lead Concentration (ppm)	Cadmium concentration (ppm)	Copper concentration (ppm)	COD mg/L	BOD mg/L	TDS mg/L
Copper	4.21	1.4	0.4	5.88	185	60	260
Battery-making	5.9	53.56	20.32	2.8	350	180	1100

COD: Chemical Oxygen Demand; BOD: Biochemical Oxygen Demand; TDS: Total Dissolved Solids

Table 5. Adsorption isotherm parameters for Cu, Cd and Pb by activated carbon prepared from saffron leaves

Metal ion	Freundlich isotherms			Langmuir isotherm		
	R^2	1/n	K (mg/g)	R^2	B (L/g)	Q_{max} (mg/g)
Copper	0.96	0.476	1.74	0.99	1.90	62.96
Lead	0.96	0.476	1.50	0.99	1.44	79.6
Cadmium	0.98	0.44	1.77	0.99	16.66	68.75

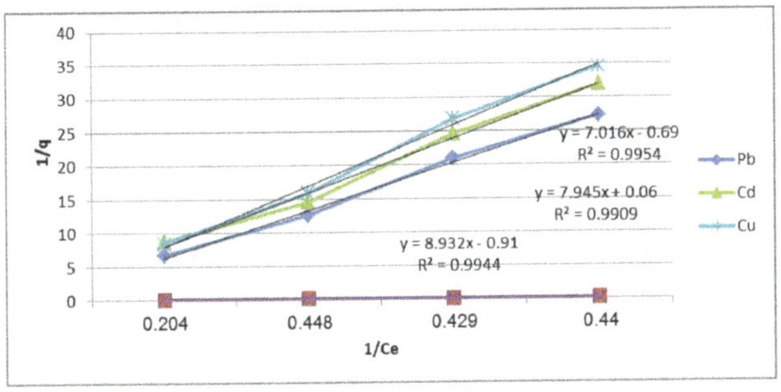

Figure 2. Langmuir adsorption isotherm of copper, cadmium, and lead

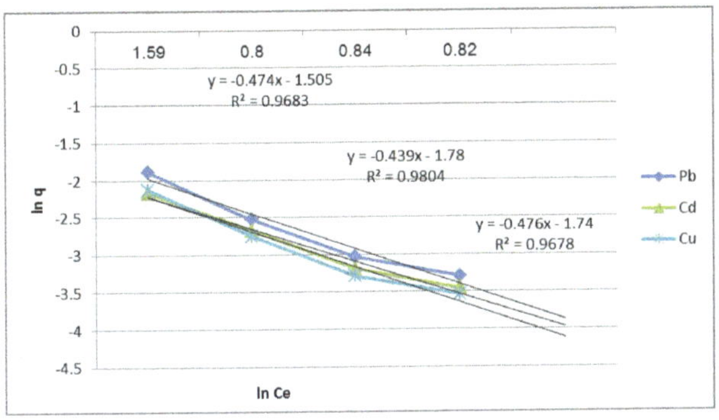

Figure 3. Freundlich adsorption isotherm of copper, cadmium, and lead

Discussion

The experimental results related to the prepared activated carbon shown that the way of activation stages have a significant impact on the quality of activated carbon prepared.

The effect of pH on adsorption efficiency of lead, cadmium, and copper by the activated carbon prepared from saffron leaves

pH is an important parameter in the adsorption process. In this study the effect of pH was tested by changing pH of solution in the range of 3-9 in concentration of 30 ppm from metal ions. Metal ions adsorption indicated more dependence from pH of solution (Table 2). Increasing solution pH increases the rate of adsorption because of electrostatic forces. This process continued until pH reached to 7 after that, increasing pH did not show positive effect on increasing absorption. This is because of reduced mobility of ions resulting from changing the properties and its load .The highest absorption was obtained in pH 7. In most of the studies, best pH for removal heavy metals was between 5-7. pH in terminal experiment was decreased by 1 value.

The results of this study were consistent with those of Amouei *et al*'s (19) research titled "Cadmium removal from canola plant", Madhava Rao *et al* (20) research in India about copper and cadmium removal from the aqueous solutions by activated carbon produced from Ceiba pentandra, and also and also with Venkatesan *et al* (21) about cadmium removal by activated carbon produced from Derris Indica wood. Nwabanne and Igbokwe (22) obtained some similar results related to the copper removal from aqueous solutions by activated carbon produced from various agricultural products in 2012.

The properties of the metal ion and also selectivity of the adsorbent are important factors in the adsorption process. In this study, the orders of ions absorption were observed Pb>Cd>Cu, respectively. This trend has also been the same in other studies (23). Pb ion occupies the adsorption places sooner than Cu and Cd due to its larger ionic radius. Some various trends have been also in the other studies (23).

The effect of adsorbent dose on the adsorption efficiency of copper, cadmium, and lead by activated carbon prepared from leaves of saffron

The dose of adsorbent is another important parameter in the adsorption process. The number of sites available for adsorption of metal ions depends on the amount of adsorbent used. In Table 3, it is observed that the adsorption of metal ions increases by increasing the amount of adsorbent to 0.6 g through holding the other parameters constant in the initial concentration of 50 mg/L. This increase is due to an increase in the surface area of adsorbent. At this value, the adsorbent surface is saturated with metal ions and after that the amount of adsorption reduces (24).

The results of this study regarding the effect of the adsorbent on the adsorption efficiency were consistent with Venkatesan *et al* research (21) related to the removal of cadmium by activated carbon produced from Derris Indica wood ,and also with the results of Madhava Rao *et al* research (20) on copper and cadmium removal from aqueous solutions by activated carbon prepared from Ceiba pentandra and were consistent with Amouei *et al* (19) studies about cadmium removal from water through activated carbon prepared from canola plant. In the study of Awwad and Salem about adsorption of copper and lead from aqueous solutions by modified adsorbent, the optimum amount of adsorbent was obtained 0.5 g (25).

The effect of contact time on adsorption efficiency of lead, cadmium, and copper by activated carbon produced from saffron leaves

The results related to ions adsorption of Cu (II) and Cd (II) on prepared adsorbent indicated that 45 min contact time was enough to reach equilibrium (Table 2). Adsorption does not change with an increase in contact time due to the saturation of adsorbent surface. Thus, this obtained contact time was used in other adsorption studies. The results indicated that this time is less than the contact time of these metal ions on some other adsorbents (25,26).

The results of this research on the effect of contact time were similar to those of Patnukao *et al* research (27) titled "Removal of metal ions (copper and lead) from synthetic wastewater by activated carbon produced from Eucalyptus Camaldulensis Dehnh shell related to copper metal". Also, Madhava Rao *et al* research (20) related to removal of copper and cadmium from aqueous solutions by activated carbon prepared from Povak tree skin was consistent with studies of Nale *et al* (13) on kinetics and equilibrium of lead adsorption from aqueous solutions on activated carbon produced from maize cobs (2012) with equilibrium contact time of 90 min. Additionally, these were associated with the other study by Arivoli *et al* (15) titled "Dynamic of copper adsorption by inexpensive activated carbon".

The isotherm study in the adsorption process of copper, lead, and cadmium from aqueous solutions by activated carbon prepared from saffron leaves

In the present study, the Freundlich and Langmuir isotherm models were studied to describe the relationship between the level of adsorption and the equilibrium concentration in liquid phase. This relationship and adsorption parameters for each model are shown in Figures 1, 2 and Table 5.

The amount of the correlation coefficient (R^2) shows that Langmuir model states a better relationship in this adsorption process. The maximum adsorption capacity for copper, lead, and cadmium ions is 62.92, 79.6, and 68.75 mg/g, respectively. These values represent high potential of the produced absorbent in the adsorption of metal ions studied from aqueous solutions because of its high adsorption capacity.

The results of this study on correspondence of adsorption isotherms are consistent with those of Saeedi *et al* (26) research related to cadmium removal by activated carbon produced from walnut and almond shell and Moreno-Piraján *et al* research (28) about the study of kinetic and removal of Mn, Ni, Cu, Fe ions from wastewater by activated carbon produced from coconut shell. Also, Nikazar and Noorbakhsh's (29) study on the removal of heavy metals Cd, Cr, and pb from aqueous solutions by activated carbon produced from agricultural wastewater (rice bran, wheat bran and straw) was consistent with these studies. Amouei *et al* (19) studied the Freundlich isotherm model related to cadmium adsorption using canola plant.

Comparing the absorption efficiency of heavy metals (copper, cadmium, and lead) from synthetic and real wastewater by activated carbon prepared from saffron leaves

Also in a research done by Elamin *et al* (30) about activated carbon produced from almond shell for the absorption of heavy metals of contaminated water, removal efficiencies of copper, and lead and cadmium in the synthetic model were 98%, 94%, and 49%, respectively and in the real model were 73%, 75%, and 20%, respectively.

The effect of initial concentration had an important effect on the absorption studies because removal efficiency decreased with rising initial concentration. Increasing the initial concentration of metal from 20 to 50 mg/L reduced the absorption efficiency of copper from 76.36% to 75.56% mg/L and those of lead absorption from 97.5% to 95.5% and cadmium absorption from 91.25% to 82.5%.

Conclusion

The results of experiments related to heavy metals absorption including copper, lead, and cadmium on activated carbon prepared from saffron leaves indicated a significant efficiency. The absorption level of Pb>Cd>Cu in the amount of adsorbent for all metals were 0.6 g, and the optimum contact times were 45, 45, and 90 min, respectively.

In these conditions the highest absorption efficiencies were observed 76.36%, 91.25%, and 97.5%, respectively. Also comparing the results of the study on synthetic and real models showed that the level of absorption in real wastewater is less than synthetic wastewater which is justifiable given analyzing the real wastewater of target industries and existence of other competing compounds, such as heavy metals and the other effective materials in absorption.

Due to the abundances of leaves and undesired use, saffron can be used as appropriate absorbent in the heavy metals removal from aqueous solutions.

Acknowledgments

This paper is the result of the students' thesis and it is conducted under the supervision of the Engineering Research Center for Environmental Health, Kerman University of Medical Sciences and sponsored by deputy of research and technology. Thereby, I thank them for their assistance to conduct this research.

Competing interests

The authors declare that they have no competing interests.

Authors' contributions

All authors participated equally in data acquisition, analysis and interpretation. All authors reviewed and approved the manuscript.

References

1. Ulmanu M, Marañón E, Fernández Y, Castrillón L, Anger I, Dumitriu D. Removal of copper and cadmium ions from diluted aqueous solutions by low cost and waste material adsorbents. Water Air Soil Pollut 2003; 142(1-4): 357-73.
2. Holan ZR, Volesky B. Biosorption of lead and nickel by biomass of marine algae. Biotechnol Bioeng 1994; 43(11): 1001-9.
3. Lee HS, Suh JH. Continuous biosorption of heavy metal ions by Ca-loaded laminaria japonica in fixed bed column. Korean J Chem Eng 2000; 17(4): 477-9.
4. Monteiro A, Boaventura R, Dinis MA. Treatment Aguas De Residuais: O Papel Das Microalgas. Revista from Faculdade de Ciencia and Technology 2004; 1: 41-54.
5. Moyo M, Chikazaza L, Nyamunda BC, Guyo U. Adsorption batch studies on the removal of Pb (II) using maize tassel based activated carbon. J Chem 2013; (2013): 1-8.
6. Sharma YC. Thermodynamics of removal of cadmium by adsorption on an indigenous clay. Chem Eng J 2008; 145(1): 64-8.
7. Weber WJ. Physicochemical processes for water quality control. New York: Wiley Interscience; 1972.
8. Bohli T, Villaescusa I, Ouederni A. Comparative study of bivalent cationic metals adsorption Pb (II), Cd (II), Ni (II) and Cu (II) on olive stones chemically activated carbon. J Chem Eng Process Technol 2013; 4(4): 1-7.
9. Carey RO, Migliaccio KW. Contribution of wastewater treatment plant effluents to nutrient dynamics in aquatic systems: a review. Environ Manage 2009; 44(2): 205-17.
10. Hadoun H, Belmedani M, Sadaoui Z, Toumert I. Removal of cadmium from aqueous solution by adsorption onto activated carbon prepared from date stems. J Chem Chem Eng 2013; 7: 979-84.
11. Amuda OS, Giwa AA, Bello IA. Removal of heavy metal from industrial wastewater using modified activated coconut shell carbon. Biochemical Engineering Journal 2007; 36: 174-81.
12. Song C, Wu S, Cheng M, Tao P, Shao M, Gao G. Adsorption studies of coconut shell carbons prepared by KOH activation for removal of Lead (II) from aqueous solutions. Sustainability 2014; 6(1): 86-98.
13. Nale B, Kagbu J, Uzairu A, Nwankwere E, Saidu S, Musa H. Kinetic and equilibrium studies of the adsorption of Lead (II) and Nickel (II) ions from aqueous solutions on activated carbon prepared from maize cob. Der Chemica Sinica 2012; 3(2): 302-12.
14. Sartape AS, Mandhare AM, Salvi PP, Pawar DK, Kolekar SS. Kinetic and equilibrium studies of the adsorption of Cd (II) from aqueous solutions by wood apple shell activated carbon. Desalination and Water Treatment 2013; 51(22-24): 4638-50.
15. Arivoli S, Nandhakumar V, Saravanan S, Nagarajan S. Adsorption dynamics of copper ion by low cost activated carbon. Arabian Journal of Science and Engineering 2009; 34: 1-12.
16. Owlad M, Aroua MK, Daud WA, Baroutian S. Removal of hexavalent chromium-contaminated water and wastewater: a review. Water Air Soil Pollut 2009; 200(1-4): 59-77.
17. Yenisoy-Karakas S, Aygun A, Gunes M, Tahtasakal E. Physical and chemical characteristics of polymer-based spherical activated carbon and its ability to adsorb organics. Carbon 2004; 42(3): 477-84.
18. APHA, AWWA, WEF. Standard methods for the examination of water and wastewater. 20th edition. Washington DC: American Public Health Association, American Water Work Association, Water Environment federation; 1998.
19. Amouei A, Ehrampoush MH, Ghaneian MT, Asgharzadeh F, Mousapour A, Parsian H. Removing cadmium from aqueous solutions by the Canola residuals. J Mazand Univ Med Sci 2014; 23(110): 153-64.
20. Madhava Rao M, Ramesh A, Purna Chandra Rao G, Seshaiah K. Removal of copper and cadmium from the aqueous solutions by activated carbon derived from Ceiba pentandra hulls. Journal of Hazardous Materials 2006; 129(1-3): 123-9.
21. Venkatesan G, Senthilnathan U. Adsorption batch studies on the removal of cadmium using wood of derris Indica based activated carbon. Research Journal of Chemistry and Environment 2013; 17(5): 19-24.
22. Nwabanne J, Igbokwe P. Mechanism of copper (II) removal from aqueous solution using activated carbon prepared from different agricultural materials. International Journal of Multidisciplinary Sciences and Engineering 2012; 3(7): 46-52.
23. Kazemipour M, Ansari M, Tajrobehkar S, Majdzadeh M, Kermani HR. Removal of lead, cadmium, zinc, and copper from industrial wastewater by carbon developed from walnut, hazelnut, almond, pistachio shell, and apricot stone. Journal of Hazardous Materials 2008; 150(2): 322-7.
24. El-Sherif IY, Ashmawy A, Badr S. Biosorption of cadmium and nickel by nile water algae. Journal of

Applied Sciences Research 2008; 4(4): 391-6.
25. Awwad AM, Salem NM. Biosorption of copper (II) and lead (II) ions from aqueous solutions by modified loquat (Eriobotrya japonica) leaves (MLL). J Chem Eng Mater Sci 2012; 3(1): 7-17.
26. Saeedi M, Jamshidi A, Abessi A. Removal of dissolved cadmium by adsorption onto walnut and almond shell charcoal: comparison with Granular Activated Carbon (GAC). Water and Wastewater 2009; 20(70): 16-22.
27. Patnukao P, Kongsuwan A, Pavasant P. Batch studies of adsorption of copper and lead on activated carbon from Eucalyptus camaldulensis dehn. bark. J Environ Sci (China) 2008; 20(9): 1028-34.
28. Moreno-Piraján JC, Garcia-Cuello VS, Giraldo L. The removal and kinetic study of Mn, Fe, Ni and Cu ions from wastewater onto activated carbon from coconut shells. Adsorption 2011; 17(3): 505-14.
29. Nikazar M, Noorbakhsh N. Removal of heavy metals ((Cr (VI), Pb (II), Cd (II) from aqueous solution by active carbon prepared from agricultural waste (rice bran, wheat bran, straw). Science and Technology Environment 2006; 8(1): 34-43.
30. Elamin A, Reddy M, Rehrah D. Activated carbon from almond shells to adsorb the heavy metals from contaminated water. Int J Chem Environ & Tech 2013; 1(3): 1-8.

33

Biodegradation of glyphosate herbicide by *Salinicoccus* spp isolated from Qom Hoze-soltan lake, Iran

Yaser Sharifi[1], Ahmad Ali Pourbabaei[2], Ali Javadi[3*], Mohammad Hossein Abdolmohammadi[4], Mehri Saffari[5], Abbas Morovvati[2]

[1]MSc, Department of Microbiology, Qom Branch, Islamic Azad University, Qom, Iran
[2]Assistant Professor, Department of Soil Science, University of Tehran, Tehran, Iran
[3]PhD Student, Department of Pathobiology, School of Public Health, Tehran University of Medical Sciences, Tehran, Iran
[4]Assistant Professor, Research Center for Environmental Pollutants, Qom University of Medical Sciences, Qom, Iran
[5]Associate Professor, Department of Agronomy and Plant Breeding, Faculty of Agriculture, Shahid Bahonar University, Kerman, Iran

Abstract
Background: Glyphosate (N-phosphonomethyl Glycine) is an organophosphorus pesticide with dangerous effects on the environment. In this study, the biodegradation of glyphosate herbicide by halophilic bacteria isolated from Qom Hoze-Soltan Lake has been investigated.
Methods: After sampling and bacterial isolation, native halophilic strains grown in the presence of glyphosate at a wavelength of 660 nm and also the disappearance of the glyphosate in the plates at a wavelength of 220 nm were determined and the dominant bacteria were isolated. Biochemical, molecular (according to the 16S rRNA sequence), antibiotic, and the Minimum Inhibitory Concentration (MIC) test was performed for the dominant bacteria. Analysis of the remaining glyphosate herbicide was performed by HPLC analysis after derivation with FMOC-Cl.
Results: According to the results of the biochemical, antibiotic and molecular 16S rRNA tests, the native halophilic isolates with the ability to biodegrade glyphosate were gram positive cocci very similar to *Salinicoccus* spp. The results of HPLC showed that *Salinicoccus* spp is able to biodegrade glyphosate herbicide.
Conclusion: The native bacteria in Qom Hoze-soltan lake, Iran can be used for biodegradation of glyphosate herbicide.
Keywords: Glyphosate, Biodegradation, Salinicoccus spp

***Correspondence to:**
Ali Javadi
Email: arm1358@yahoo.com

Introduction

The increase in human population and therefore increase in the demand for agricultural products has led humans to search for more efficient methods for increasing agricultural products. Weed control is one of these methods. Nowadays, humans control weeds by mechanical or chemical methods. One of the chemical methods is using herbicides. The sales of herbicides in 2006 were about 3 billion liters. One of these herbicides is glyphosate (N-phosphonomethyl Glycine), commercially known as roundup. Glyphosate broad-spectrum and nonselective systemic herbicide, is described by the possession of a stable and covalent Carbon-to-Phosphorus (COP) bond. Glyphosate is utilized extensively for control of plants including grass, sedge, broad-leaved weeds and woody plants. It can be used on non-cropland as well as on a great variety of crops. Demand for glyphosate has increased substantially in the world. Ho_4 has been reported a 15-fold increase in usage of glyphosate on major crops between 1994 and 2005. Glyphosate itself is an acid, but it is commonly used in salt form, most commonly isopropyl-amine salt (1,2). This herbicide is from the phosphoric acid group, and blocks the EPSPS enzyme by disturbing the plant's synthesis of amino acids and enzyme activity, and blocks its shikimate pathways (1). Considering the fact that most of the agricultural soil in Iran is saline soil, the environmental problems derived from harmful chemicals especially organophosphorus chemicals in saline environments have been known for long, but our information about the contaminants of these environments is still little, because the halophilic microorganisms that degrade these toxic chemicals have not yet been evaluated. Due to the wide range of used pesticides, it is difficult to produce a single method for the removal of pesticide from water and wastewater. Thus, there are several treatment processes for the removal of pesticides – e.g. biodegradation, photodegradation, oxidation (with air, chlorine, permanganate or ozone), flocculation and filtration, adsorption and membrane techniques. As a general rule, biological treatment is more economical than physicochemical remediation methods as it can be cost-effective and achieve the complete degradation of organic pollutants (3).

Microorganisms that degrade glyphosate act in two ways. One path leads to the intermediate formation of sarcosine and glycine, and the other path leads to the formation of AMPA or 2-amino-3(5-methyl-3-oxo-1,2-oxazol-4-yl) propanoic acid (4,5). Halophilic microorganisms, are the ones that are capable of living in environments with high and low temperatures, with acidic and alkaline pH, high hydrostatic pressure, and high salt concentrations (6). In Iran there are many lakes and saline ecosystems in which the concentration of sodium and chloride ions are high. One of these salinas is the Hoze-Soltan lake in Qom. The salt march and arable soils around this lake make it one of the most important and rich sources of halophilic bacteria (7).

The aim of this study was to evaluate the degradation glyphosate herbicide by halophilic bacteria from the environmental soil samples collected from 5 different districts around the lake.

Methods

Isolating halophilic bacteria

The medium for isolating halophilic bacteria includes; 51 g/l NaCl, 0.026 g/l NaBr, 15 g/l Agar-agar, 9.7 g/l $MgSO_4.7H_2O$, 5 g/l Yeast-extract, 5 g/l Polypeptone, 2 g/l KCl, 0.06 g/l $NaHCO_3$, 10 g/l Glucose, 7 g/l $MgCl_2.6H_2O$, 3.6 g/l $CaCl_2$, and 1000 ml distill water (3).

In order to isolate the halophilic microorganisms, Broth and Agar medium were used. The concentration of salt in the environment was between 5% to 10% and the pH of the water; saline soil, and salt sedimentsrange between 6.5 and 8.2. Major chemical composition of the soil, brine, mud, and salt consists of NaCl, KCl, $MgSO_4$, $MgCl_2$, and Na_2SO_4 and the amount of herbicide used is 500 ppm which is equal to the that of this herbicide used in soil (3,8). The important fact is that instead of glucose, the glyphosate herbicide was used in this medium, in other words glyphosate was used as the source of carbon in this medium. This herbicide was added after autoclaving and filtering to the medium. About 1 gram of soil in 250 ml Erlenmeyer flask containing 100 ml of culture medium and 1% glyphosate was added and incubated at 34°C shaking at 150 rpm for 7 days. Then it was inoculated and incubated in the agar medium at 30°C for 48 hours. After incubation (in 30°C for 48 hours), the bacteria were detected with diagnostic tests. Eventually the isolating and purifying processes were done.

Diagnosing halophilic bacteria

After gram staining the bacteria and spores staining, the initial identification and biochemical tests including motivation tests, oxidation tests, catalase tests, gelatin-starch-caseine hydrolysis tests, Tween 80 hydrolysis tests, Bile Esculin hydrolysis tests, Nitrate reduction test, H2S production, acid production from sugar (glucose, lactose, raffinose, arabinose, mannitol) and tolerance and sensitivity to antibiotic tests including chloramphenicol, penicillin G, tetracycline, nalidixic acid, cephalothin, ampicilin, rifampin, erythromycin, and streptomycin were performed (9).

Determining herbicide MIC

In order to determine the sensitivity of the toxin and bacteria, initially a thick solution (4500 ppm) of the glyphosate herbicide was made. Then in sterile tubes containing the Mueller Hinton Broth medium with 10% salt, 1.25 ml of herbicide was added and the solution was prepared. Then 0.01 ml of the bacteria under study equal to 0.5 according standard microbial test was added to the solutions and was placed in an incubator in 30°C. After 48 hours the samples were checked for turbidity and the MIC was determined (10).

Evaluating the logarithmic growth of bacteria in the presence of herbicide

In order to evaluate the 10 isolated bacteria's degradation ability, initially specific sterile mediums including NaCl 10% were made and the herbicide was added and then bacteria equal to 0.5 McFarland was injected. One flask was used as blank for the spectrophotometer and another flask with salt and herbicide was used as control.

The flasks were placed in a shaker incubator in 30°C and 150 rpm, and after 48 hours, their absorption was measured by the spectrophotometer in 660 nm wave lengths for evaluating growth and in 220 nm for evaluating degradation of the herbicide (9,10). The best isolates with maximum absorption at 660 nm and minimum absorption at 220 nm were chosen.

In order to choose the best isolates based on optimum growth in the presence of herbicide, their growth during different hours of incubation in wave lengths of 660 nm were measured (Figure 1).

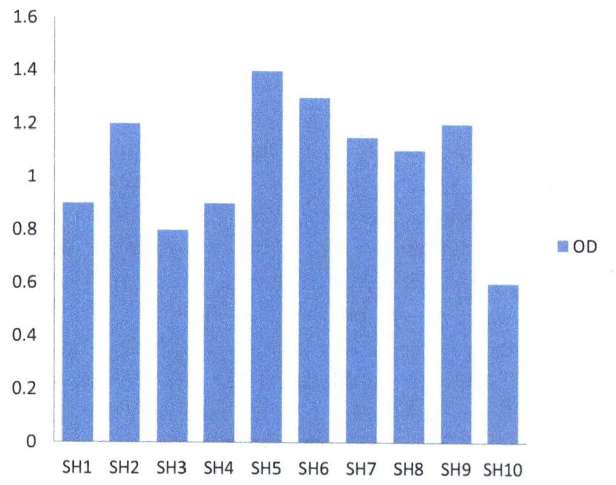

Figure 1. Evaluating the growth capability of halophilic isolates in the presence of glyphosate herbicide.

Analysis of glyphosate degradation by Thin Layer Chromatography (TLC)

In order to do this experiment, cellulose chromatography paper and solutions of ethanol, water, ammonium hydroxide (17 molar), trichloroacetic acid and acetic acid (15 molar) with proportions of (2:3.5:2.5:35:55 v/w/v/v/v) were used (11,12).

After 48 hours the best isolated grown bacteria were taken from the top of the solution in the flask and were placed on chromatography paper. Also glyphosate herbicide was used as control and was placed on chromatography paper. Then, the paper was placed in a dish including a prepared solvent. After a while the paper was viewed by UV light in 220 nanometers (6).

Analysis of glyphosate herbicide by HPLC

The material needed for HPLC were glyphosate, acetonitrile (HPLC grade), potassium dihydrogen phosphate, disodium tetraborate decahydrate, HCL 32%, KOH 4 M, FMOC-CL (9-Fluorenylmethyl)-chloroformate, ethyl acetate (HPLC grade), the HPLC device, and ultra pure water (9,13).

The preparation method for injecting the samples to HPLC

After 48 hours, the best grown isolates in the shaker incubator were taken from the top of the solution in the flask and were centrifuged for 10 minutes at twice in 12,000 rpm. Then the top solution was filtered through a Millipore filter. After making sure that the solution was clear, it was concentrated by the rotary device in 40°C. Also one sample was used as control (9).

For preparing the 1.5% phosphate buffer, the amount of 7.5 grams of KH_2PO_4 was dissolved in 500 ml of ultra pure water. The borate buffer 0.05 M was made by dissolving 1.9 grams of disodium tetraborate decahydrate in 100 ml of ultra pure water. 10 mg of FMOC-Cl was dissolved in 10 mm of acetonitrile in order to prepare 1000 ppm FMOC-Cl (9).

The pre-column derivation method before injecting into the HPLC

The amount of 3 ml of the specified sample (clear and concentrated) with 0.5 ml of 0.05 M Borate Buffer and 0.5 ml of 1000 ppm FMOC-Cl solution was poured in a vial and was placed for one hour in the room temperature. Then in order to eliminate the extra derivative, it was washed by 2 ml ethyl acetate and the aqueous phase was injected into the HPLC (9).

Calibrating the HPLC

The column used in this device was a C18 (4.6 mm×250 mm) column (14). The mobile phase used included acetonitrile and 1.5% phosphate buffer with pH=5.8 proportionate to 45/55. The type of detector used was florescent. The flow rate was 1 ml/min, and the amount of sample injected was 50 μL, ex λ was at 260 nm and em λ was 310 nm. Then the sample was injected into the HPLC (9,15).

The DNA extraction process from the bacteria was performed by the Bioneer Extraction Kit. In order to confirm the extraction of DNA, electrophoresis was used. Then in order to do PCR these listed primers were used (7).

8F: AGAGTTTGATMLTGGCTCAG

1541R: AAGGAGGTGATMLAGMLGCA

The PCR reaction started with the initial melting temperature of 95°C for 5 minutes and continued with 10 cycles in 93°C for 1 minute, 63°C for 1minute, 72°C for 1 minute, and finished with 20 cycles in 93°C for 1 minute, 67°C for 1 minute, 72°C for 1 minute, and eventually 72°C for 5 minutes (6).

Results

Results from bacteria logarithmic growth and toxin degradation

Diagnostic tests revealed that bacteria are gram-positive, catalase-positive, oxidase-positive, non-sporeforming bacteria, and non-motile and has the ability to grow in salt, 1% to 15%. The SH5, SH6, and SH9 isolates from the 10 halophilic native bacteria showed good activity in degrading glyphosate herbicide which is valuable, and the SH5 isolate had the highest growth rate among the isolates taken from region 5 (soil beside plants).

As it can been seen in Figure 2 the SH5, SH6, and SH9 isolates have shown a better activity in comparison to the other isolates and decreased the amount of herbicide. The SH5 isolate in comparison to the other isolates decreased the herbicide more and had better capability in degrading glyphosate herbicide.

Eventually 3 isolates from the 10 isolates, had a higher activity in degrading the glyphosate herbicide in comparison to the other isolates. In order to choose the best isolates, their growth in different hours during incubation was evaluated.

The SH5 isolate had a better function in regard to growth and degrading the glyphosate herbicide. Figure 3 shows that the isolates taken from soil in the presence of this herbicide in the first 20 hours after the inoculation of bacteria are in lag phase and show little growth. After 36 to 48 hours, they grow abruptly and fast, and this accelerated growth continues with less speed to 120 hours later. Eventually their increased growth stops and bacteria enter a stationary phase.

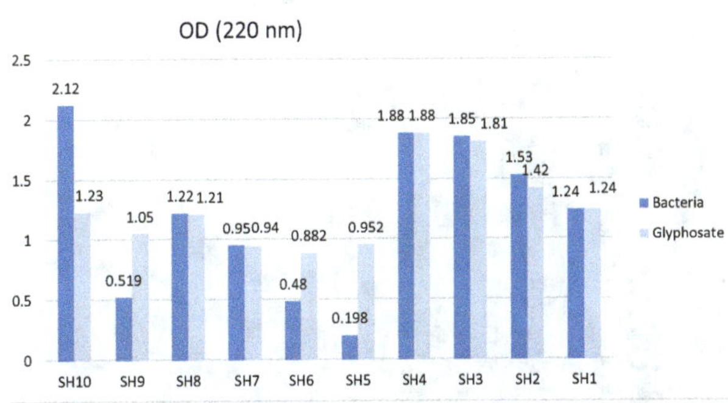

Figure 2. Evaluating the capability of halophilic isolates in degrading the glyphosate herbicide in comparison to control

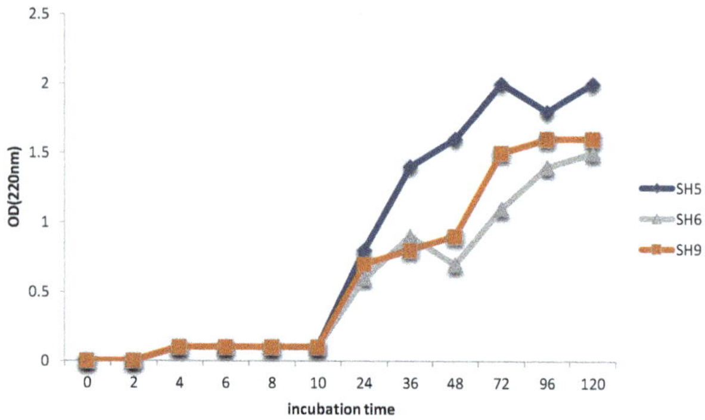

Figure 3. Comparing the growth of 3 dominant halophilic isolates in degrading the glyphosate herbicide.

Determining the MIC of the dominant SH5 bacteria

After experimenting, we found out that the SH5 isolate can tolerate the glyphosate herbicide up to 2250 ppm after 48 hours incubation.

Thin layer chromatography

The SH5 isolate is capable of degrading the glyphosate herbicide after 48 hours incubation. In the picture below, the result of the experiment can be seen. The right column (column 2) is the control (glyphosate herbicide), and its band can be seen. The left column (column 1) is the 48-hour result of the SH5 isolate, and no band can be seen (Figure 4).

The HPLC analysis

As it can be seen in Figure 5, initially a big peak that lasts between 3 to 4 minutes and is related to FMOC-OH was seen. Then, other peaks were seen at 7 and 9.5 minutes. And eventually the peak related to glyphosate herbicide was seen at 16.567 minutes.

In Figure 6, initially a big peak between 3 to 4 minutes can be seen which is related to FMOC-OH. Then another peak at 6.247 minutes can be seen which is related to

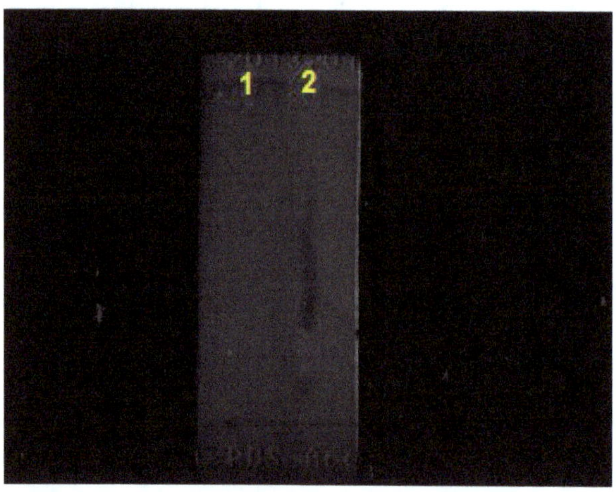

Figure 4. The chromatography result of TLC from the 48-hour sample of the SH5 isolate and glyphosate herbicide

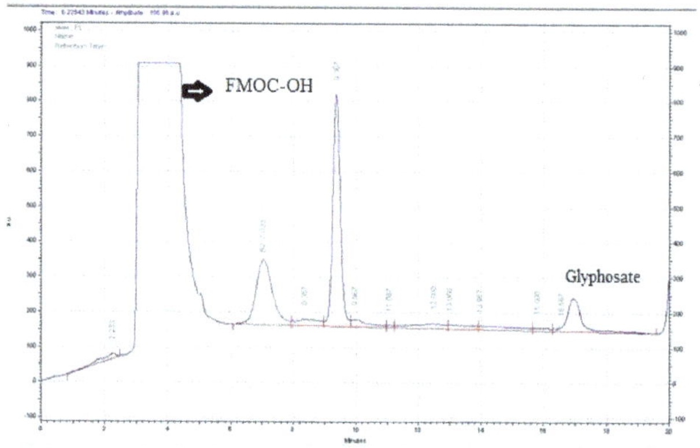

Figure 5. The chromatography of glyphosate herbicide from HPLC after derivation by FMOC-Cl.

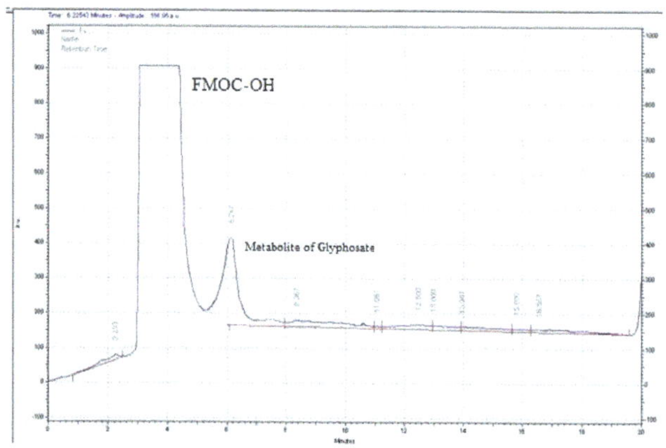

Figure 6. The chromatography of treated glyphosate herbicide with the dominant isolated by HPLC after derivation by FMOC-CL

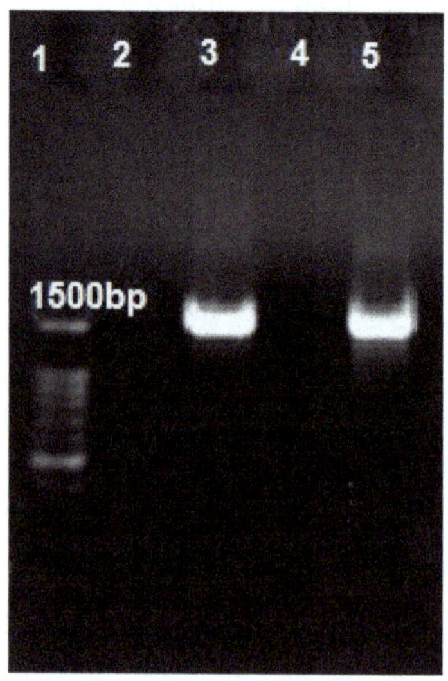

Figure 7. The electrophoresis gel from PCR in the gel displaying device (Column 1: marker, Column 2 space, Column 3: the specified sample which includes 2 microliters of DNA, Column 4 : space, Column 5 :the specified sample that includes 3 microliters of DNA)

the metabolite extracted from the 48-hour concentrated and derived sample (SH5 isolate), and as it can be seen at 16.567 minutes, the peak related to glyphosate herbicide cannot be seen.

The PCR experiment of 16S rRNA gene

The band at 1500 bp in the PCR reaction shows the proliferation of 16SrRNA piece.

Molecular analysis

The band from proliferation of the 16S rRNA gene in PCR was sent to Iran Pasteur Institute for determination. Evaluation and comparison of the sequence of 16S rRNA from bacteria isolated from the salty soil of Hoze-Soltan lake, with the available sequences at the NBCI information bank showed that the bacteria isolated was strain QW6 *Salinicoccus* sp. (DQ767692) (Figure 7).

Discussion

Herbicides are chemicals that are used for weed control. When herbicides are added to soil, the consequences of their presence might be critical. Their long presence in soil can lead to elimination of the beneficial microorganism in soil. Therefore their biodegradation is important and is the best alternative for preventing their accumulation and environmental stability. Now, we can achieve this goal by isolating bacteria that can degrade this herbicide. Usually microbial ways for eliminating glyphosates are more effective than chemical ways, because herbicides have a strong carbon-phosphorus bond that can be degraded by these bacteria (11).

According to the result of these experiments, the dominant halophilic bacteria can be effective in degrading this herbicide up to 2250 ppm, but higher concentrations of the herbicide have a prohibiting effect, and the best growth is seen in 1080 ppm.

Monke *et al* in 2010 evaluated the effect of different concentrations of the glyphosate herbicide in non-saline environments and in regular conditions in the *Acetobacter* sp and *P. fluorescens* bacteria and found out that the best growth was in concentrations equal to 7200 ppm, and these two bacteria could tolerate herbicides up to 10,000 ppm (16).

Ermakova *et al* in 2010 claimed that none of the two *Achromobacter* sp and *Ochrobactrum anthropi* bacteria could use glyphosate as a source of carbon and phosphorus. Both bacteria grew in an environment that the herbicide and methyl phosphonic were added as a source of phosphorus; and were able to break the C-P bond in glyphosate (4).

Researchers have been able to eliminate the dichlorvos herbicide from saline environments by halophilic bacteria. Four halophilic isolates from the Techirghiol lake in Romania were able to affect glyphosates.

Researcher observed that the semi-halophilic bacteria such as *Chromohalobacter marismortui* can degrade methy-, ethyl-, 3-aminopropyl and 4-aminobutyl- phosphonate which is an organophosphorus compound. The optimum concentration of salt used in this environment was 10%, and they were able to grow in 2% to 25% concentration of salt and pH=7.2 (13).

Other bacteria that have been identified in degrading glyphosates are *Arthrobacter atrocyaneus* and *flavobacterium* sp (1,5). Researchers think that the bacteria in soil are the only organisms that degrade glyphosate (14). Also *Pseudomonas* sp isolate LBr (15) *Acetobacter atrocyaneus* (13), and *Flavobacterium* sp bacteria (1) were able to degrade the glyphosate herbicide. Adelowo *et al* discovered this first fungal degradation of glyphosate by penicillium citrinum (17).

The results from HPLC with fluorescent detector in this research after extraction, concentration, and derivation by FMOC-Cl showed a big peak which is specific to FMOC-OH at 3 minutes that lasted for 4 minutes and the peak for glyphosate herbicide was at 16.567 minutes and the peak for the metabolites of degradation was seen at 6.247 minutes.

In 2008, researchers able to obtain the detector peak of glyphosate herbicide at 10.013 minutes and AMPA (the main metabolite of the glyphosate herbicide) at 6.3 minutes after deriving the glyphosate herbicide and AMPA by FMOC-Cl and by the florescent HPLC (18).

Bot *et al* in 2002 observed one big peak at 3 minutes which lasted for 4 minutes and was related to FMOC- OH, a peak related to glyphosate herbicide at 16.344 minutes, and a peak related to AMPA (the main metabolite of the glyphosate herbicide) at 6.05 minutes after deriving the glyphosate herbicide and AMPA by FMOC-Cl and by the fluorescent detector HPLC (2).

Conclusion

Halophilic bacteria isolated from Qom Hoze Soltan lake can grow in the presence of herbicide and can metabolize this environmental contaminant.

Acknowledgments

The authors would like to thank the research council of Qom Islamic Azad University.

Competing interests

The authors declare that they have no competing interests.

Authors' contributions

All authors were involved in study design, data collection, and article approval.

References

1. Kafilzadeh F, Javid H, Kargar M. Isolation of halophilic and halotolerant microorganisms from the Bakhtegan

lake and the effect of physicochemical factors on their frequency. Water and Wastewater 2007; 18(3): 81-7. [in Persian]

2. Bot BL, Colliaux K, Pelle D, Briens C, Seux R, Clement M. Optimization and performance evaluation of the analysis of glyphosate and AMPA in water by HPLC with fluorescence detection. Chromatographia 2002; 56(3-4): 161-4.
3. Rahban R, Amozegar M. Biodiversity of halophilic bacteria producing hydrolytic enzymes in the Hoze Slotan lake. Environmental Science and Technology 2010; 11(4): 1-17. [in Persian]
4. Ermakova IT, Kiseleva NI, Shushkova T, Zharikov M, Zharikov GA, Leontievsky AA. Bioremediation of glyphosate-contaminated soils. Appl Microbiol Biotechnol 2010; 88(2): 585-94.
5. Pipke R, Amrhein N, Jacob GS, Schaefer J, Kishore GM. Metabolism of glyphosate in an Arthrobacter sp. GLP-1. Eur J Biochem 1987; 165(2): 267-73..
6. Partoazar M, Keramati P. Soil microbial activity and biodegradation of the herbicide glyphosate, university of Tehran. 4th Conference of Environmental Engineering, Civilica, Tehran, Iran, 2011. p. 7-12. [in Persian]
7. Oncescu T, Oancea P, Enache M, Popescu G, Dumitru L, Kamekura M. Halophilic bacteria are able to decontaminate dichlorvos, a pesticide, from saline environments. Cent Eur J Biol 2007; 2(4): 563-73.
8. Duke SO. Glyphosate degradation in glyphosate-resistant and -susceptible crops and weeds. J Agric Food Chem 2011; 59(11): 5835-41.
9. Pipkin BW, Gorsline DS, Casey RE. Laboratory Exercises in oceanography. San Francisco: WH Freeman; 1997.
10. Hayes VE, Ternan NG, McMullan G. Organophosphonate metabolism by a moderately halophilic bacterial isolate. FEMS Microbiol Lett 2000; 186(2): 171-5.
11. Alexa E, Hafner M, Negrea M, Lazureanu A. HPLC and GC determination of glyphosate and aminomethylphosphonic acid (AMPA) in water samples. 43rd Croatian and 3rd International Symposium on Agriculture. Opatija, Croatia; 2008. p. 100- 5.
12. Jacob GS, Garbow JR, Hallas LE, Kimack NM, Kishore GM, Schaefer J. Metabolism of glyphosate in Pseudomonas sp. strain LBr. Appl Environ Microbiol 1988; 54(12): 2953-8.
13. Balthazor TM, Hallas LE. Glyphosate-degrading microorganisms from industrial activated sludge. Appl Environ Microbiol 1986; 51(2): 432-4.
14. Singh BK, Walker A. Microbial degradation of organophosphorus compounds. FEMS Microbiol Rev 2006; 30(3): 428-71.
15. Dick RE, Quinn JP. Glyphosate-degrading isolates from environmental samples: occurrence and pathways of degradation. Appl Microbiol Biotechnol 1995; 43(3): 545-50.
16. Moneke AN, Okpala GN, Anyanwu CU. Biodegradation of glyphosate herbicide in vitro using bacterial isolates from four rice fields. African Journal of Biotechnology 2010; 9 (26): 4067-74.
17. Adelowo FE, Olu-Arotiowa OA, Amuda OS. Biodegradation of Glyphosate by Fungi Species. Advances in Bioscience and Bioengineering. 2014: 2(1): 104-18.
18. Amrhein N, Deus B, Gehrke P, Steinrucken HC. The site of the inhibition of the shikimate pathway by glyphosate: ii. interference of glyphosate with chorismate formation in vivo and in vitro. Plant physiology. 1980; 66(5): 830-4.

Humic acid removal from aqueous solutions by peroxi-electrocoagulation process

Ahmad Reza Yazdanbakhsh[1], Majid Kermani[2], Sanaz Komasi[3], Ehsan Aghayani[4], Amir Sheikhmohammadi[5*]

[1]Associate Professor, Department of Environmental Health Engineering, Shahid Beheshti University of Medical Sciences, Tehran, Iran
[2]Assistant Professor, Department of Environmental Health Engineering, Iran University of Medical Sciences, Tehran, Iran
[3]MSc of Environmental Engineering, Department of Environmental Engineering, Islamic Azad University, West Tehran Branch, Tehran, Iran
[4]PhD Student, Department of Environmental Health Engineering, Tarbiat Modares University of Medical Sciences, Tehran, Iran
[5]PhD Student, Department of Environmental Health Engineering, Shahid Beheshti University of Medical Sciences, Tehran, Iran

Abstract
Background: Natural organic matter is the cause of many problems associated with water treatment such as the presence of disinfection by-products (DBPs) and membrane fouling during water filtration. In this study, the performance of the peroxi-electrocoagulation process (PEP) was investigated for the removal of humic acids (HAs) from aqueous solutions.
Methods: PEP was carried out for the removal of HA using a plexiglas reactor with a volume of 2 L and fitted with iron electrodes and a direct current supply (DC). Samples were taken at various amounts of pH (2-4), current density (1 and 2A/cm^2), hydrogen peroxide (50-150 mg/L) and reaction time (5-20 minutes) and then filtered to remove sludge formed during reaction. Finally, the HA concentration was measured by UV absorbance at 254 nm (UV_{254}).
Results: Results indicated that increasing the concentration of H_2O_2 from 50 to 150 mg/L increased HA removal efficiency from 83% to 94.5%. The highest removal efficiency was observed at pH 3.0; by increasing the pH to the alkaline range, the efficiency of the process was reduced. It was found that HA removal efficiency was high in current density 1A/cm^2. Increasing current density up to 1 A cm^{-2} caused a decrease in removal efficiency. Results of this study showed that under the optimum operating range for the process ([current density] = 1A/cm^2, [hydrogen peroxide concentration] = 150 mg/L, [reaction time]= 20 minutes and [pH]= 3.0), HA removal efficiency reached 98%.
Conclusion: It can be concluded that PEP has the potential to be utilized for cost-effective removal of HA from aqueous solutions.
Keywords: Humic acid, Peroxi-electrocoagulation, Iron electrode, UV_{254}, Water solutions

***Correspondence to:**
Amir Sheikhmohammadi
Email: asheikh1359@gmail.com

Introduction

Humic acid (HA) is one of the major components of humic substances which arise from the microbial degradation of biomolecules. Natural organic materials (NOM) such as HA enter into water from natural and artificial sources. They pose a variety of problems in treatment operations and distribution systems because of their specific attributes including an unpleasant smell and taste, a yellow to brown color, reaction with chlorine, and the formation disinfection by-products (DBPs), eg, trihalomethanes (THMs). These exhibit mutagenic properties during the chlorination step in drinking water production or water treatment.

The guideline for DBPs in drinking water announced by the World Health Organization state that DBPs should not exceed 100 µg/L (1-3). Consequently, the removal of HA from surface water or wastewater is important because of health and environmental concerns. HA may account for up to 90% of NOM. It is not possible to completely remove NOM in conventional water treatment plants (4,5). Different treatment technologies have been used in practice to improve NOM removal. These methods included ion exchange, sorption, membrane processes (such as reverse osmosis), and ultra-filtration, but they either provide only a partial solution or are expensive. Coagulation is a key process which may be carried out in the conventional mode (chemical) or by peroxi-electrocoagulation process (PEP) (6). Thus, PEP has been suggested as an alternative to conventional coagulation because it provides better removal capabilities, produces less sludge, and has a more readily filterable, minimal startup time (7-9).

Some limitations of the PEP are the periodical replacement of sacrificial anodes, minimum solution conductivity, the formation of toxic chlorinated organic compounds from effluent containing chlorides, the formation of an impermeable oxide film on the cathode, and resistance to the flow of electric current, which increases the cost of electricity thus increasing operational costs (10).

Stages in the PEP process include anode dissolution, formation of OH^- ions and H_2 at the cathode, electrolytic reactions at electrode surfaces, adsorption of coagulant on colloidal pollutants, and removal of colloids by sedimentation or flotation. Reactions carried out in the cathode and anode for the production of metal hydroxides include:

Mechanism 1: Anode:

$$4Fe_{(s)} \rightarrow 4Fe^{2+}_{(aq)} + 8e^- \quad (1)$$

$$4Fe^{2+}_{(aq)} + 10H_2O_{(l)} + O_{2(aq)} \rightarrow 4Fe(OH)_{3(s)} + 8H^+_{(aq)} \quad (2)$$

Cathode:

$$8H^+_{(aq)} + 8e^- \rightarrow 4H_{2(g)} \quad (3)$$

Overall:

$$4Fe_{(s)} + 10\,H_2O_{(l)} + O_{2(aq)} \rightarrow 4Fe(OH)_{3(s)} + 4H_{2(g)} \quad (4)$$

In recent years, it has been recommended to combine electrocoagulation with hydrogen peroxide to increase the power of the electrocoagulation process. This method is based on the generation of a powerful oxidant (the hydroxyl radical [$^{\bullet}OH$]), because the OH radical attacks the organic substrates present in the water and wastewater and then degrades them (11-15). During the electrocoagulation process, Fe^{2+} is the common ion generated at the anode; in contrast, OH^- ions are produced at the cathode (16-19). By adding hydrogen peroxide into the PEP reactor, Fenton reactions are carried out in accordance with the following:

$$Fe^{2+} + H_2O_2 \rightarrow Fe^{3+} + OH^- + {}^{\bullet}OH \quad (5)$$

$$Fe^{3+} + H_2O_2 \leftrightarrow Fe\text{-}OOH^{2+} + H^+ \leftrightarrow Fe^{2+} + HO_2^{\bullet} + H^+ \quad (6)$$

Vasudevan (20) studied the removal of phenol from water by the PEP. Their results showed that phenol was removed by PEP at 92% efficiency. Evrim Yüksel et al (21) achieved a removal efficiency of 81.6% in the removal of sodium dodecyl sulfate from synthetic wastewater by the peroxi-electrocoagulation method. Vasudevan and Lakshmi (22) also studied the removal of boron from water by electrochemical processes and investigated various operating parameters such as initial boron ion concentration, initial pH, current density, and temperature. Their results showed a removal efficiency of 93.2% under optimum operating conditions. Kamaraj et al (23) studied the adsorption of 2,4-dichlorophenoxyacetic acid (2,4-D) from water by in situ generated metal hydroxides using sacrificial anodes. The results showed that the maximum removal efficiency of 91.0% was achieved with iron as the anode. The current study examined the possibility of HA removal from aqueous solutions by PEP and evaluated the influence of operation parameters such as initial pH, current density, amount of hydrogen peroxide, and reaction time on HA removal efficiency.

Methods

Material

All chemical reagents used in bench-scale tests were analytical grade. The materials used in this study included sulfuric acid (96%) and NaOH (98%) for pH adjustment and technical grade hydrogen peroxide (30% w/w and density of 1.13 kg/L), purchased from the Merck company.

Set-up and Procedure

A stock solution of HA was prepared by dissolving HA powder in 100 mL NaOH (0.1N). The prepared solution was kept for a day, and then its volume was increased to 1 L with distilled water. The solution was filtered using a Whatman filter, which was then placed in an oven at a temperature of 103°C-105°C. The difference between the primary and secondary weight of the filter was determined to be 314.5 mg/L. Working solutions (4, 8, and 10 mg/L) were prepared by diluting the stock solution in deionized water.

The batch experimental setup is schematically shown in Figure 1. Water was electrochemically oxidized in an undivided cell reactor equipped with a magnetic stirrer using a constant speed of 200 rpm in order to get a correct homogenization of the wastewater-floc mixture. The reactor consisted of an EC cell, a DC power supply, and monopolar electrodes in parallel connections. All experiments were run under isoperibolic conditions and at a temperature of 20°C. The reaction was timed starting when the DC power supply was switched on. Two flat plates with smooth surfaces were connected as cathodes and 2 as anodes. Each electrode measured 4 cm × 3 cm, and the distance between the iron electrodes was 1 cm. To remove the influence mass transfer rate of pollutants to the electrodes (iron salts produce electrode passivation and cause a 50% increase in treatment time and power requirements), high mixing was ensured by a magnetic stirrer. To maintain

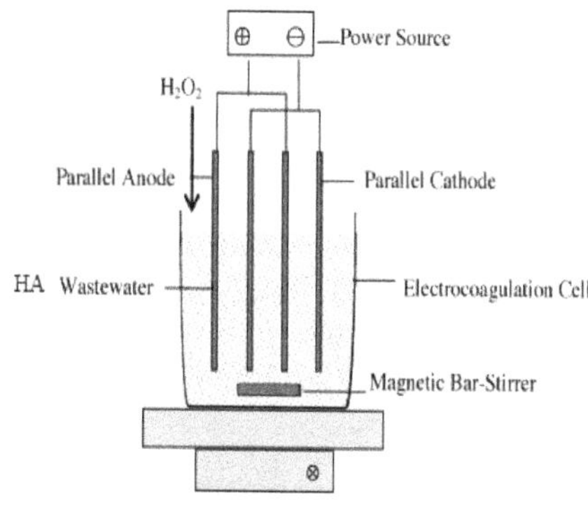

Figure 1. A schematic diagram of the electrochemical reactor.

the same experimental conditions, the Fe electrodes were polished with grinding papers and then rinsed with soapy water and deionized water after each experiment.

The effects of the main operational variables (including solution pH [2-4], current density [1 and 2 A/cm^2], reaction time [5–20 minutes], and H_2O_2 [50-150 mg/L]) on the electrochemical process in treating HA were investigated in various runs. At the beginning of a run, the HA solution was fed into the reactor; then the electrodes were connected to the DC power supply and the reaction was started while the cell content was gently stirred (200 rpm). H_2O_2 was added at desired rates to the reactor for enhanced pollutant removal.

Analytic Procedure

The HA samples were measured by HACH spectrophotometer (DR 5000) at a wavelength of 254 nm after filtration through a Millipore membrane filter with a 0.45 μm pore size. Experiments with 3 replications were conducted according to the standard methods for examination of water and wastewater (24). Data was analyzed using Excel software.

Results

To determine the optimal amount of H_2O_2, concentrations in the range of 50 to 150 mg/L were investigated, and the results are presented in Figure 2. It was observed that increasing the concentration of H_2O_2 increased the removal of HA. For example, in the initial HA concentration of 4 mg/L, increasing the H_2O_2 concentration from 50 to 150 mg/L increased HA removal efficiency from 83% to 94.5% at pH 3.0 and current density 1A after 20 minutes.

pH plays a significant role in the performance of the Fenton process. Various studies have shown that an acidic pH of 2-4 is the best range for the Fenton reaction; therefore, the performance of PEP for the removal of HA was investigated in a pH range of 2-4 (Figure 3). The highest removal efficiency was observed at pH 3.0; increasing pH to the alkaline range reduced the efficiency of the process.

The results of the influence of the current density on the HA removal are presented in Figure 4. It was found that the HA removal efficiency was high in current density 1A/cm^2. Increasing current density up to 1A/cm^2 caused a decrease in removal efficiency. The minimum energy consumption, was 10 kWh (kg HA)$^{-1}$ at current density 1 1A/cm^2 for a 20 minutes reaction time.

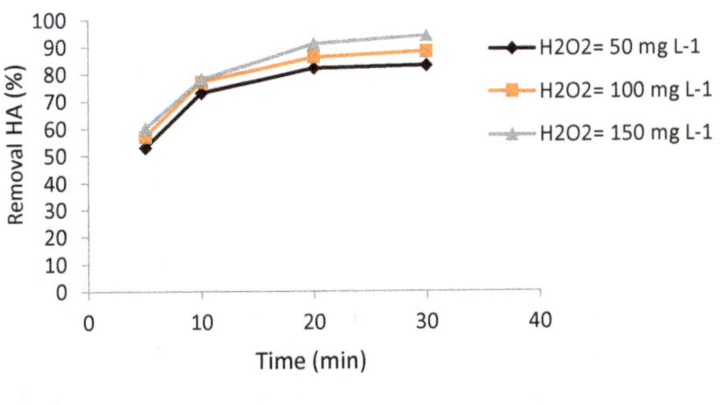

Figure 2. Effect of hydrogen peroxide on HA removal efficiency (peroxi-electrocoagulation process [PEP]; initial HA, 4 mg/L; pH, 3; current density, 1A/cm^2; distance between plates, 1 cm).

As shown in Figure 5, early on, the pollutant decomposition rate was very high, and increasing reactive time did not significantly affect the removal of HA. The effects of initial HA on removal efficiency are shown in Figure 6. Results of this study confirm that increasing the HA concentration increases the efficiency of the electrochemical process.

Discussion

Results of the current study indicated that increasing the H_2O_2 concentration increased HA removal efficiency. Determining the optimal amount of hydrogen peroxide in PEP is very important and necessary because of: (*a*) the high cost of hydrogen peroxide in high concentrations; (*b*) reduced production of hydroxyl radical exceeding H_2O_2

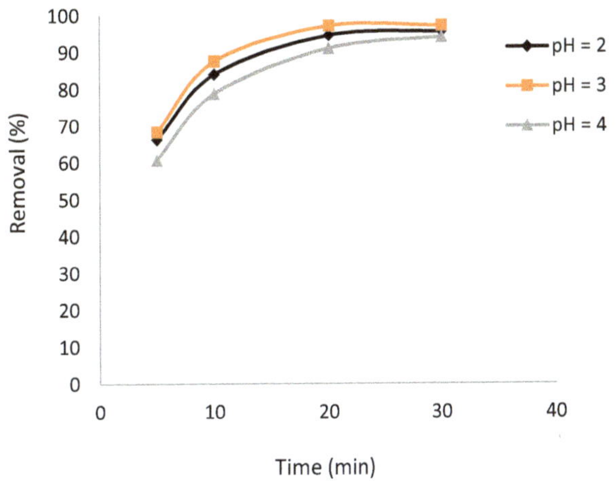

Figure 3. Effect of initial pH on HA removal efficiency (peroxi-electrocoagulation process [PEP]; initial HA, 4 mg/L; hydrogen peroxide, 150 mg/L; current density, 1A/cm^2; distance between plates, 1 cm).

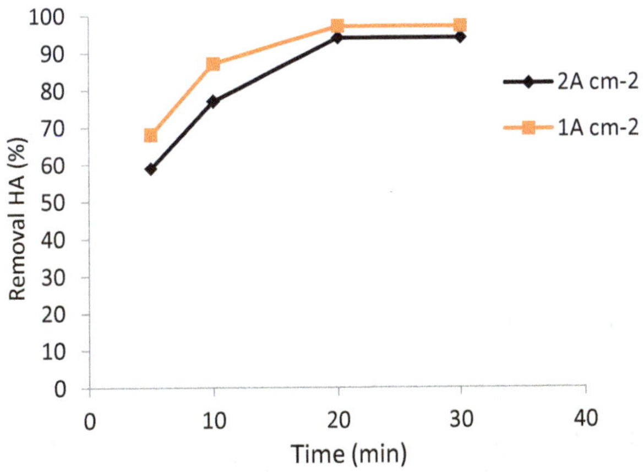

Figure 4. Effect of current densityon HA removal (initial HA, 4 mg/L; pH, 3; H_2O_2, 150 mg/L; distance between plates, 1 cm).

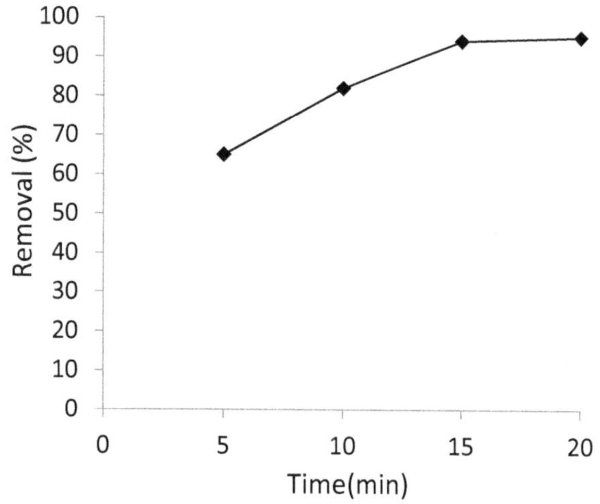

Figure 5. Effect of reaction time on HA removal efficiency (peroxi-electrocoagulation process [PEP]; initial HA, 4 mg/L; hydrogen peroxide, 150 mg/L; pH, 3; current density, 1A/cm^2; distance between plates, 1 cm).

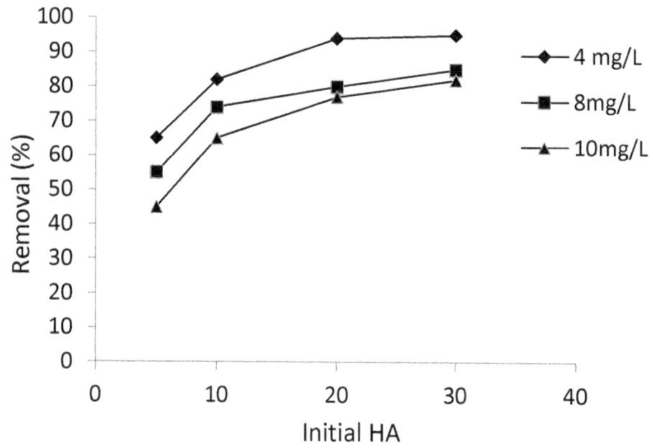

Figure 6. Effect of initial HA (peroxi-electrocoagulation process [PEP]; hydrogen peroxide,150 mg/L; Initial HA, 4-10 mg/L; pH, 3; current density, 1A/cm^2; distance between plates, 1 cm).

(H_2O_2 acts as a scavenger of the OH according to reaction 7); and (*c*) increased chemical oxygen demand by residual H_2O_2 (15,16,25,26).

$$H_2O_2 + {}^{\bullet}OH \rightarrow H_2O + HO_2^{\bullet} \quad (7)$$

It can be concluded that the removal of HA increases when the concentration of hydrogen peroxide is increased. Mahesh et al (26) examined the effects of different concentrations of hydrogen peroxide on the reduction of humic substances from leachate using the Fenton oxidation process and chemical coagulation. They concluded that the removal of humic substances increases when the concentration of hydrogen peroxide is increased to a certain concentration due to the production of hydroxyl radicals. Increasing the hydrogen peroxide concentration over this amount caused a reduction in removal efficiency. They also determined that the decreased removal efficiency in excessive amounts of hydrogen peroxide can be caused by the production of OOH radicals that consume the OH. Farhadi et al (27) used PEP for COD removal from pharmaceutical wastewater. Their results showed that the maximum removal rate was nearly 42.2% for the optimum level of 300 mg/L H_2O_2 after 20 minutes of electrolysis time for the voltage of 40 V.

The decrease in removal efficiency in alkaline pH is probably due to the formation of ferric species and decreased production of ferrous ions, both of which reduce the production of hydroxyl radicals and so decrease the efficiency of removal. A decrease in the efficiency of HA removal at pH <3 could be explained by the following:

1. $Fe(OH)^{2+}$, $Fe(OH)_2^{+}$, and $Fe_2(OH)_2^{4+}$ were produced, which react more slowly with H_2O_2.
2. The scavenging effect of OH by H^+ becomes significant at very low ranges of pH (at lower pH the protons in the solution are reduced to H_2 at the cathode, and the ions of H^+ may inhibit the generation of hydroxyl and perhydroxyl radicals) (28).

$${}^{\bullet}OH + H^+ + e^- \rightarrow H_2O \quad (8)$$

Farhadi et al (27) used PEP for COD removal from pharmaceutical wastewater. The optimum pH for this process was determined to be 3.0. Su et al (29) used electro-Fenton processes for the degradation of acetaminophen (ACTP). The experimental results showed that the electro-Fenton processes had maximum ACTP degradation efficiencies of 100%. ACTP degradation efficiency increased 74% at pH 4 in the electro-Fenton process. Cheng et al (30) used the electro-Fenton process with a Ce/SnO_2–Sb-coated titanium anode for the mineralization of metronidazole. A decrease in pH from 7.0 to 2.0 increased removal efficiency from 10% to 37%.The optimum pH was found to be about 2.0.

Current density is an important factor in the electrochemical processes because of its effects on the coagulant dosage rate, bubble production rate, size and growth of the flocs. Increasing the current density increased HA removal. This is in accordance with Faraday's law; with an increase in current density and reaction time, the anodic dissolution rate increases that will give rise to Fe^{2+} being released from the anode as in equation 9 (31,32).

$$C_{Fe} = \frac{M_w I t_{EC}}{ZFV} \quad (9)$$

where C_{Fe}, Z, F, V, and M_w are the theoretical concentration of Fe^{2+} (g/m^3), the chemical equivalence, Faraday's constant (96,487 C/mol), reactor volume (m^3), and molecular weight of iron (g/mol), respectively. The increase of removal efficiency upon increasing current density is the result of the extent of anodic dissolution of iron, increased hydroxyl radical generation, increased bubble generation rate, and decreased bubble size. These trends are beneficial in terms of high pollutant removal efficiency by H_2 flotation (33). Increasing current density up to 1A/cm^2 caused a decrease in the efficiency of removal. This decrease could be due to the decomposition of hydrogen peroxide in higher current densities. Wang (34) studied COD removal from real dyeing wastewater by electro-Fenton technology using an activated carbon fiber cathode. In this study, 75% COD removal was achieved under the optimum conditions of current density= 32 mA/cm^2, pH = 3.0, Fe^{2+}= 2 mM/L, and T= 20°C (34). Vasudevan et al (35) studied the removal of copper by electrochemically-assisted coagulation. Their results showed that the optimum removal efficiency of 96.6% was achieved at a current density of 0.05 A/dm^2 and a pH of 7.0. Babuponnusami and Muthukumar (36) used the electro-Fenton process for the advanced oxidation of phenol. Their results showed 62.5% phenol degradation for the EF process at 16 mA/cm^2 in 60 minutes. Increasing current density from 0 to 16 mA/cm^2 offered faster phenol degradation and COD removal. The important economical parameter in PEP is electrical energy consumption which is the major operating cost of the electrochemical process. The minimum amount of energy consumption was 10 kWh (kg HA)$^{-1}$ at a current density of 1A/cm^2 for a 20 minutes reaction time that was calculated using the following equation:

$$E = UIt_{EC} \tag{10}$$

where E is the electrical energy in Wh, U= the cell voltage in volt (V), I= the current in ampere (A), and t_{EC} is the time of EC process per hour.

Reactive time influences the treatment efficiency of PEP. To explore the effect of operating time, the optimal conditions of these processes were used, and all processes were started simultaneously. Early on, the pollutant decomposition rate was very high, possibly due to the appropriate amounts of Fe (II) and hydrogen peroxide used to produce hydroxyl radicals. It was observed the percentage of HA removal was higher for PEP at 20 minutes, pH= 3.0, and current density 1A/cm^2. The decrease of HA as a function of elapsed time might be caused by the production of Fe^{2+} or Fe^{3+} ions from iron and the formation of OH, because by adding H_2O_2 into the system, hydrogen peroxide is catalyzed by ferrous ion to produce hydroxyl radicals, and a reaction is propagated from ferrous ion regeneration mainly by the reduction of the produced ferric species with hydrogen peroxide. Therefore, the dosage of H_2O_2 could enhance the performance of these processes. Ruppert et al (37) investigated the mineralization of several organic matters by hydroxyl radicals. They reported that organic material only affected the behavior of ferrous ions. Ferrous ions compete with organic material for the use of hydroxyl radicals. At low concentrations of organic material, ferrous ions react with hydroxyl radicals and reduce the amount of them in the environment. In the absence of organic compounds, hydrogen peroxide is decomposed slowly by ferric ions. Excessive amounts of organic matter prevent the reaction between ferrous ions and hydroxyl radicals with the increase in reactivity between ferrous ions and hydrogen peroxide.

Conclusion

The PEP was tested on HA synthetic wastewater, and the effects of operational parameters such as pH, amount of hydrogen peroxide, current density, and reaction time on HA removal efficiency were investigated. The HA removal efficiency that was achieved using PEP was 98% for the initial HA concentration of 4 mg/L. The ferric hydroxide and hydroxyl radical generated in the cell can decrease the HA present in the wastewater. The optimal conditions for the process were determined to be current density = 1A/cm^2, hydrogen peroxide concentration= 150 mg/L, reaction time= 20 minutes, mean energy consumption= 10 kWh (kg HA)$^{-1}$, and pH=3.0. Finally, given the results ultimately obtained in this research, it became clear that the process is technologically feasible.

Competing interests

The authors have declared that no competing interests exist.

Authors' contributions

All authors contributed equally, and all authors participated in the data acquisition, analysis, and interpretation. All authors critically reviewed, refined, and approved the manuscript.

References

1. Jacangelo JG, Demarco J, Owen DM, Randtke SJ. Selected processes for removing NOM: an overview. J Am Water Works Assoc 1995; 87(1): 64-77.
2. Katsumata H, Sada M, Kaneco S, Suzuki T, Ohta K, Yobiko Y. Humic acid degradation in aqueous solution by the photo-Fenton process. Chem Eng J 2008; 137(2): 225-30.
3. Magdaleno GB, Coichev N. Chemiluminescent determination of humic substances based on the oxidation by peroxymonosulfate. Anal Chim Acta 2005; 552(1-2): 141–46.
4. Panyapinyopol B, Marhaba TF, Kanokkantapong V, Pavasant P. Characterization of precursors to trihalomerthanes formation in Bangkok source water. J Hazard Mater 2005; 120(1-3): 229-36.
5. Yoon Y, Lueptow RM. Removal of organic contaminants by RO and NF membranes. J Memb Sci 2005; 261(1-2): 76-86.
6. Abdelwahab O, Amin NK, El-Ashtoukhy ES. Electrochemical removal of phenol from oil refinery wastewater. J Hazard Mater 2009; 163(2-3): 711–6.
7. Apaydin O, Kurt U, Gonullu MT. An investigation on the treatment of tannery wastewater by electrocoagulation. Global Nest Journal 2009; 11(4): 546-55.
8. Enric B, Ignasi S, Mehmet A. Electro-Fenton process

and related electrochemical technologies based on Fenton's reaction chemistry. Chem Rev 2009; 109(12): 6570-631.
9. Cho JH, Lee JE, Ra CS. Effects of electric voltage and sodium chloride level on electrolysis of swine wastewater. J Hazard Mater 2010; 180(1-3): 535-41.
10. Chou W-L, Wang C-T, Huang K-Y. Investigation of process parameters for the removal of polyvinyl alcohol from aqueous solution by iron electrocoagulation. Desalination 2010; 251(1-3): 12-19.
11. Kabdasl I, Vardar B, Arslan-Alaton I, Tunay O. Effect of dye auxiliaries on color and COD removal from simulated reactive dye bath effluent by electrocoagulation. Chem Eng J 2009; 148(1): 89–98.
12. Kurt U, Apaydin O, Gonullu MT. Reduction of COD in wastewater from an organized tannery industrial region by Electro-Fenton process. J Hazard Mater 2007; 143(1-2): 33-40.
13. Nidheesh PV, Gandhimathi R. Trends in electro-Fenton process for water and wastewater treatment: an overview. Desalination 2012; 229: 1-15.
14. Bagga A, Chellam S, Clifford DA. Evaluation of iron chemical coagulation and electrocoagulation pretreatment for surface water microfiltration. J Memb Sci 2008; 309(1-2): 82-93.
15. Ben Sasson M, Adin A. Fouling mitigation by iron-based electroflocculation in microfiltration: mechanisms and energy minimization. Water Res 2010; 44(13): 3973-81.
16. Gao P, Chen X, Shen F, Chen V. Removal of chromium(VI) from wastewater by combined electrocoagulation - electroflotation without a filter. Sep Purif Technol 2005; 43(2): 117-23.
17. Harif T, Hai M, Adin A. Electroflocculation as potential pretreatment in colloid ultrafiltration. Water Supply 2006; 6(1): 69-78.
18. Harif T, Adin A. Characteristics of aggregates formed by electroflocculation of a colloidal suspension. Water Res. 2007; 41(13): 2951-61.
19. Holt PK, Barton GW, Wark M, Mitchell CA. A quantitative comparison between chemical dosing and electrocoagulation. Colloids Surf A Physicochem Eng Asp 2002; 211(2–3): 233-48.
20. Vasudevan S. An efficient removal of phenol from water by peroxi-electrocoagulation processes. Journal of Water Process Engineering 2014; 2: 53-7.
21. Yüksel E, Şengil İA, Özacar M. The removal of sodium dodecyl sulfate in synthetic wastewater by peroxi-electrocoagulation method. Chem Eng J 2009; 152(2-3): 347-53.
22. Vasudevan S, Lakshmi J. Electrochemical removal of boron from water: adsorption and thermodynamic studies. Can J Chem Eng 2012; 90(4): 1017-26.
23. Kamaraj R, Davidson DJ, Sozhan G, Vasudevan S. Adsorption of 2,4-dichlorophenoxyacetic acid (2,4-D) from water by in situ generated metal hydroxides using sacrificial anodes. Journal of the Taiwan Institute of Chemical Engineers 2014; 45(6): 2943-9.
24. APHA, AWWA, WPCF. Standard Methods for the Examination of Water and Wastewater. 21st ed. Washington, DC: American Public Health Association; 2005.
25. Jiang J-Q, Graham N, André C, Kelsall GH, Brandon N. Laboratory study of electro-coagulation–flotation for water treatment. Water Res 2002; 36(16): 4064-78.
26. Mahesh S, Prasad B, Mall ID, Mishra IM. Electrochemical degradation of pulp and paper mill wastewater. Part 1. COD and color removal. Ind Eng Chem Res 2006; 45(8): 2830-9.
27. Farhadi S, Aminzadeh B, Torabian A, Khatibikamal V, Fard MA. Comparison of COD removal from pharmaceutical wastewater by electrocoagulation, photoelectrocoagulation, peroxi-electrocoagulation and peroxi-photoelectrocoagulation processes. J Hazard Mater 2012; 219-220: 35-42.
28. Vasudevan S, Lakshmi J, Jayaraj J, Ganapathy S. Remediation of phosphate-contaminated water by electrocoagulation with aluminum, aluminum alloy and mild steel anodes. J Hazard Mater 2009; 164(2-3): 1480-86.
29. Su C-C, Chang A-T, Bellotindos LM, Lu M-C. Degradation of acetaminophen by Fenton and electro-Fenton processes in aerator reactor. Sep Purif Technol 2012; 99: 8-13.
30. Cheng W, Yang M, Xie Y, Liang B, Fang Z, Tsang EP. Enhancement of mineralization of metronidazole by the electro-Fenton process with a Ce/SnO2–Sb coated titanium anode. Chem Eng J 2013; 220: 214-20.
31. Wu Y, Zhou S, Qin F, Peng H, Lai Y, Lin Y. Removal of humic substances from landfill leachate by Fenton oxidation and coagulation. Process Saf Environ Prot 2010; 88(4): 276-84.
32. Meunier N, Drogui P, Montané C, Hausler R, Mercier G, Blais JF. Comparison between electrocoagulation and chemical precipitation for metals removal from acidic soil leachate. J Hazard Mater 2006; 137(1): 581-90.
33. Saleem M, Bukhari A, Akram MN. Electrocoagulation for the treatment of wastewater for reuse in irrigation and plantation. Journal of Basic and Applied Sciences 2011; 7(1): 11-20
34. Wang S. A comparative study of Fenton and Fenton-like reaction kinetics in decolourisation of wastewater. Dyes Pigments 2008; 76(3): 714-20.
35. Vasudevan S, Lakshmi J, Kamaraj R, Sozhan G. A critical study on the removal of copper by an electrochemically assisted coagulation: equilibrium, kinetics, and thermodynamics. Asia-Pacific Journal of Chemical Engineering 2012; 8(1): 162-71.
36. Babuponnusami A, Muthukumar K. Advanced oxidation of phenol: a comparison between Fenton, electro-Fenton, sono-electro-Fenton and photo-electro-Fenton processes. Chem Eng J 2012; 183: 1-9.
37. Ruppert G, Bauer R, Heisler G. The photo-Fenton reaction — an effective photochemical wastewater treatment process. J Photochem Photobiol A Chem 1993; 73(1): 75-8.

Strategic management of solid waste in Tehran

Monireh Majlessi[1], Aida Vaezi[2*], Mohsen Mehdipour Rabori[3]

[1]Associate Professor, Department of Environmental Health Engineering, School of Public Health, Shahid Beheshti University of Medical Science, Tehran, Iran

[2]MA of Environmental Science, Islamic Azad University, Science and Research Branch, Tehran, Iran

[3]PhD Student of Environmental Health in SBMU, Member of Environmental Health Engineering Research Center, Kerman University of Medical Sciences, Kerman, Iran

Abstract

Background: Successful waste management programs are linked to internal factors, SW (strength and weakness points), and external factors, OT (opportunities and threats), and at the macro level are grounds for sustainable development. Studies may be related to David's study which presented a method to quantify strength, weakness, opportunity, threats (SWOT) analysis.

Methods: In this study, designed to investigate recycling and managing dry residues in District 1, threat factors were studied and internal factors evaluation (IFE) and external factors evaluation (EFE) matrixes were scored. Tehran Municipality District 1 has 10 subdistricts and 26 neighborhoods. The dry residues from Municipality District 1 that currently weigh approximately 2678 tons per day.

Results: Results showed that WO strategies for improving weaknesses and employing opportunities available in District 1 are ideal. After constructing the Quantitative Strategic Planning Matrix (QSPM), WO strategies were prioritized.

Conclusion: The evaluation matrix of internal and external factors in the city of Tehran indicated that waste management has weak internal factors. Meanwhile, evaluation points of external factors showed that, in the current situation, SWOT could achieve good results. Waste management systems are involved with different multi-disciplinary factors; therefore, trends in the development of waste treatment technologies have been led by various social, economic, and environmental drivers in Tehran.

Keywords: Solid waste management, SWOT, Strategic management

***Correspondence to:**
Aida Vaezi
Email: vaezei.ac@gmail.com

Introduction

Management, planning, and efforts to find optimal solutions for improving urban residue problems are inevitable, and city authorities seek optimal procedures to remedy urban problems and issues (1). Successful waste management programs are linked to internal factors (strength and weakness points) and external factors (opportunities and threats), and at the macro level are grounds for sustainable development (2). Studies on such subjects may be related to David's study in which the author presented a method to quantify SWOT. David (3) formed the matrix of internal & external factors and matrix-profile competition, but allocating a score to main factors having to be done mentally was a shortcoming of this method. Halla (4) studied the city of Dar al-Salam in Tanzania to analyze internal and external factors for urban management planning. Observations were made along with the participation and documented investigations in accordance with the available data.

Among the most important issues considered in this design are the collection, transfer, and disposal of environmentally friendly urban residues. Among other studies in this regard, the work of Abedin-Zadeh et al (2) can be noted. In this study, internal and external factors affecting waste management in the city of Tehran were identified, and analysis and strategy formulation using Quantitative Strategic Planning Matrix (QSPM) was performed. From other research papers, that of Zarei et al (5) can be noted, which attempted to study solid waste management in the city of Minab. Based on their results, WT strategies based on weaknesses and threats were chosen. Tehran Municipality District 1 has 10 regions and 26 neighborhoods. Currently, dry residues weighing approximately 2678 tons per day are collected from door fronts by a contractor company and 24 pick-up trucks. Seventeen recycling units have been established at the regional level so that residents can deliver their dry residues, which weigh about 103 tons per day, in person. The current study examined the strengths, weaknesses, opportunities, and threats of recycling and waste management of Tehran's dry residues in 2011 and prioritized relevant strategies.

Methods

Library information on recycling and urban waste management was collected by studying conducted internal and external research:

1. Data about regional waste from the waste management organization was collected, and
2. The internal and external factors evaluation (EFE) matrix and Quantitative Strategic Planning Matrix (QSPM) were created as described below.

After reviewing the internal and external factors, the most important items were listed. A number was then allocated to each coefficient: 0 (unimportant) to 1(very important). The number allocated to each coefficient is expressive of its significance. The sum of these coefficients had to equal one. Scores from 1 to 4 were allocated to each factor. A score of 1 showed fundamental weakness, 2 showed little weakness, 3 indicated strength, and 4 indicated high strength for the factor in question. The coefficient of each factor was then multiplied by the score, and so the overall scores for each factor and the final score was determined (4). To create the QSPM matrix, the first and second stages of the analysis framework (the evaluation matrix of internal and external factors) were used to objectively determine implementable strategies. In the QSPM matrix, important internal and external factors that influence design were considered. In this matrix, each factor was allocated an attractiveness score, which showed the attractions and the ability to deal effectively with the strategy of internal and external factors (5).

Results

Internal and External Factors Evaluation Matrix

After determining the strengths, weaknesses, opportunities, and threats of an organization in the area of Tehran, the internal and external factors matrix of the waste management system were set up in Tables 1, 2, 3, and 4 as follows:

Weights of dry residues from Tehran in the years 2007, 2009, and 2011 (kg) are shown in Table 5.

The final score for the internal factors evaluation (IFE) matrix is less than 2.5; therefore,the organization is weak at internal factors.

The final score for the EFE matrix final is 2.5; therefore, there are more organizational opportunities than threats, and the organization can take advantage of these opportunities to improve the trend of its activities.

Internal and External Matrix

To form this matrix, the scores created by the evaluation matrixes of internal and external factors already obtained are inserted in the horizontal and vertical dimensions of the matrix. Since the internal and external factor scores rate the situation of the organization as conservative (Figure 1), a conservative strategy (WO) is recommended. Since the organization is in a conservative position, strategies used are:

- WO_1: Development and promotion of recycling industries through financial support and marketing for

Table 1. Matrix of internal factors, recycling and management of dry residues from District 1

Descriptions	Weighted Score	Current Weight Score	Normalized weight	Internal Strategy Factors (Strong Points)
Waste separation scheme was conducted in District 1, but lacks proper quality.	0.12	3	0.04	1. Waste separation project in District 1
In some families, educated women have been effective in waste separation and recycling programs, but not enough.	0.15	3	0.05	2. Educated housewife awareness
Waste production volume is reduced through source separation and recycling.	0.12	3	0.04	3. Reduction of size and weight of residues
Using reflective clothing and uniforms has been effective in reducing accidents, especially at night.	0.08	4	0.04	4. Reflective clothing worn by municipal officers
Locating dry plastic residues into blue or black tanks at the regional level.	0.09	3	0.04	5. Locating dry residue tanks in District 1
The training of target groups by educators promotes citizen awareness and increases public participation.	0.21	3	0.07	6. Face to face training in source separation and recycling by educators in District 1
Existence of experienced experts in the field of urban services of municipal services and training is potentially possible.	0.24	4	0.06	7. Existence of specialists and experts in recycling and waste management
Employment opportunities are created through the creation of recycling industries and lateral affairs such as collection and recycling.	0.18	3	0.06	8. Employment opportunities through recycling industries
Studies and research to improve the system of collection, recycling, and disposal sites will be conducted.	0.28	4	0.07	9. Conducting research and studies in the field of waste management
The morning collection of dry residues by patrolling pick-up trucks plays an important role in enhancing cooperation and public participation.	0.12	3	0.04	10. Morning collection of dry residues by recycling office agents

Table 2. IFE matrix of recycling and waste management of District 1

Description	Weighted Score	Current Weight Score	Normalized Weight	Internal Strategy Factor (Weaknesses)
Municipal officers stand at the rear of the waste-carrying car and lack personal protective equipment such as gloves and mask which causes high risk, and conducted trainings are insufficient.	0.05	1	0.05	1. Failure of municipal officers to observe safety rules
Shortages in collection machinery exist, but essential measurements are being made in this respect.	0.1	2	0.05	2. Lack of adequate machinery for waste collection in District 1
Consumption patterns change and the willingness of citizens toward consumerism has increased waste volume; effective measures have not been made in this regard.	0.08	2	0.04	3. Changing consumption patterns and increasing volume of waste (consumerism)
The separation of waste from its origin is not performed principally; the necessary actions have not yet been taken.	0.06	1	0.06	4. Lack of segregation of waste at origin
Even if waste is to be separated at its point of origin, it will not be done during collection.	0.04	1	0.06	5. Porting mixed wastes by municipal officers
Citizens do not separate waste and the washing by agents is unprincipled, causing the vessel to be smelly.	0.04	1	0.04	6. Odors eliminated from waste tanks
Recycling industries require financing and face a lack of credit and investment risks.	0.12	2	0.06	7. Lack of financial resources; lack of independent funding defined in the recycling and waste management industries.
Creation of traffic and noise during waste loading and collection results in residents' unhappiness.	0.08	2	0.04	8. Road blocking and creation of traffic in District 1
Comprehensive information on all areas of the district has been targeted.	0.07	1	0.07	9. Lack of sufficient information to distinguish the origin of the waste
Non-compliance with waste collection schedule by officers has resulted in complaints from residents.	0.08	2	0.04	10. Noncompliance with the schedule of waste collection by officers
	2.42		1	Total internal factors

Abbreviation: IFE, internal factors evaluation.

Table 3. Recycling and waste management system of external evaluation matrix in District 1

Description	Weighted Score	Current Weight Score	Normalized Weight	External Strategy Factor (Opportunities)
Environmental laws and regulations are a suitable way to control the waste management process.	0.15	3	0.05	1. Environmental laws and regulations
Existence of traffic rules in order to reduce accidents during transportation of waste can be effective.	0.16	4	0.04	2. Traffic rules
Bread waste must be isolated and separated because of religious beliefs and optimal consumption.	0.12	3	0.04	3. Religious beliefs
The presence of NGOs can greatly help the management of waste materials.	0.24	4	0.06	4. NGOs presence in the district and their relationships with other NGOs
Given the importance of recycling policies and upstream financial support, there is a good opportunity to attract funding and implement projects.	0.15	3	0.05	5. Acceptance and support of separation from the source by institutions and classes
Technology improvements in all aspects of waste management have not been carried out; in this respect, the experiences of other countries should be used.	0.15	3	0.05	6. Improving technology in waste collection
Potential and existing capacities have not been well utilized.	0.12	3	0.04	7. Presence of recycling industries
Greater possibilities for the participation of the private sector, public sector cuts, and attraction of private investors in this sector exist.	0.24	4	0.06	8. Presence of efficient and experienced contractors, and welcome from the private sector
Taking advantage of TV channels, especially provincial ones, and newspapers play an important role in informing citizens.	0.28	4	0.07	9. Use of advertising media to encourage waste separation and waste removal schedule implementation
The mentioned costs have been reduced to collecting and disposing of waste, and less need exists for waste disposal land.	0.15	3	0.05	10. Saving money in collection and deposal of wastes expenditures

Abbreviation: NGO; nongovernmental organization.

Table 4. Matrix of external evaluation in waste management for the dry residues recycling and management systems of District 1

Description	Weighted Score	Current Weight Score	Normalized weight	External strategy factor (Threats)
Paying salaries monthly leads to dissatisfaction, and the discontent of the people will influence both sides.	0.05	1	0.05	1. Obtain monthly salary from area residents 1
Many municipal activities take place at night, increasing the risk of accidents.	0.08	2	0.04	2. Traffic accidents due to non-compliance with traffic laws
Unauthorized or unlawful factors in processing industry and the absence of a formal market are issues.	0.05	1	0.05	3. Existence of black market and non-fixed prices
Population growth in the region increases waste volume and worn textures that prevent mechanized machines from moving easily.	0.08	2	0.04	4. Worn population structure and texture in some locales
Existing legislation on the environment (waste management) is not supported by implementation.	0.1	2	0.05	5. Lack of enforcement of environmental laws
A lack of coordination exists among various organizations and institutions such as the judiciary, environmental organizations, universities, and television.	0.12	2	0.06	6. Lack of external coordination of waste management
Advanced and up-to-date techniques for recovery of waste exist in the world but are not used or are used in inappropriate consumption ways.	0.14	2	0.07	7. Best techniques not used for waste recycling
Popular belief dictates that recycled containers are unhealthy; therefore, people do not use them.	0.1	2	0.05	8. Lack of a culture of using recycled goods
Mischievous animals cause bags to rupture the dispersion of waste. An animal removal plan is being conducted through health department cooperation.	0.08	2	0.04	9. Existence of stray animals and vermin in the region
The decay of automobiles leads to the distribution of environmental pollution and waste in the region.	0.08	2	0.04	10. State of decay of cars and vehicles, and falling of residual waste from their rear.
	2.64		1	Total internal and external factors

Table 5. Weight of dry residues in the years 2007, 2009, and 2011 (kg)

Year	District No.	Dry Bread	Plastic Types	Paper and Cardboard	Ferrous Metals (Light and Heavy)	Colored metals(Copper, Zinc, Aluminum, Brass)	Metals Types	PET	Textiles	Glass	Burial waste	Weights of Collected Dry Waste
2007	1	785730	948263	926113	-	-	562860	332735	3560	7728	40825.3	3660494
2009	1	3555465	5930495	6104452	4703955	1552880	6256835	2238488	1433488	1544970	253220	28047774
2011	1	5446659	7066368	7272274	4265258	1656875	5922133	2128522	1629319	1760914	401006	31627195

industrial products

- WO_2: Simultaneous training for workers (active forces) and citizens for development of mechanization and improved equipment.
- WO_3: Formation of regulations and guidelines for encouragement in the waste management sector, and employing private sector capital in this regard.

Quantitative Strategic Planning Matrix

Tables 6 and 7 show the WO strategies attractiveness score for each internal and external factor on the QSPM.

Discussion

Pollution resulting from the poor management of urban waste in the area of health and aesthetics imposes irreparable consequences upon society. Among them, the lack of waste management can lead to various diseases. The most important step in raising the level of understanding about the foundations of solid waste management is to have precise SWOT metrics.

In a study conducted in Tanzania, results suggested that the management plan in the city of Dar al-Salam acts stronger than a normal and ordinary plan; the comprehensive urban management plan for the city of Dar al-Salam is more general, and the city management plan is more specialized. Important factors in the stability and plan performance of this city were citizen participation in planning, coordinating groups working together, and

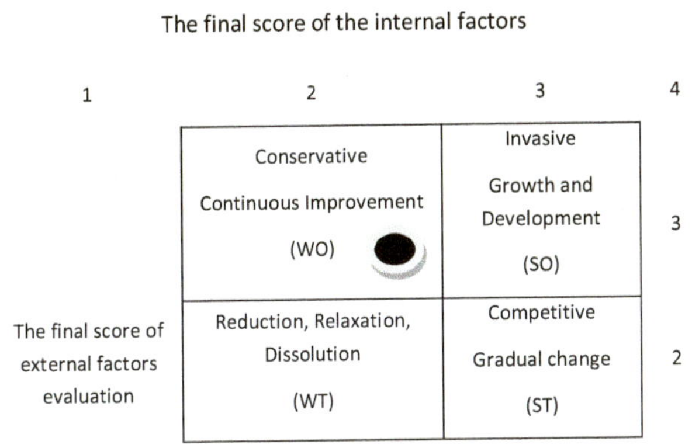

Figure 1. External and internal factors matrix.

providing equipment and resources for groups (4). Results of the evaluation matrix of internal and external factors in the city of Rasht indicate that waste management has weak internal factors. External factor evaluation points, however, show that in the current situation, strengthening opportunities and overcoming threats could achieve good results (2). Results obtained using quantitative strategic planning showed that implementing waste management law created the highest attractiveness, and education and proper method for pollutant reduction in burial sites created the least attractiveness (2).

Studies also indicate that Minab city's waste management strategy where WT strategies are based on weaknesses and threats is appropriate. Media and advertising strategies have the highest priority, and increasing the assignment of waste collection and recycling strategies to the private sector has the lowest priority (5). In this study, strategies were prioritized (Table 8) to determine the attractiveness of strategies using the QSPM.

In 2007, a study in Tehran ascertained that municipal solid waste comprised more than 97% of Tehran's solid waste, while 3 other types comprised less than 3%, namely hospital waste (1.0%), industrial waste (0.6%), and construction and demolition waste (0.5%). The contribution of household solid waste to total municipal solid waste was about 62.5% (6). The study also identified important challenges in solid waste management in Tehran including proper collection and management of hospital waste; public education aimed at reducing and separating household

Table 6. Quantitative strategic planning matrix (internal factors)

Internal Factors	Normalized Weight	WO_1		WO_2		WO_3	
		AS	TAS	AS	TAS	AS	TAS
Strengths							
S_1	0.05	3	0.15	4	0.16	3	0.12
S_2	0.05	1	0.05	3	0.15	1	0.05
S_3	0.04	2	0.08	3	0.12	3	0.12
S_4	0.04	1	0.04	2	0.08	1	0.04
S_5	0.04	2	0.08	3	0.12	2	0.08
S_6	0.07	3	0.21	4	0.28	3	0.21
S_7	0.06	4	0.24	3	0.18	4	0.24
S_8	0.06	4	0.24	3	0.18	3	0.18
S_9	0.07	4	0.28	4	0.28	4	0.28
S_{10}	0.04	2	0.08	2	0.08	2	0.08
Weaknesses							
W_1	0.05	1	0.05	3	0.15	3	0.15
W_2	0.05	3	0.15	3	0.15	3	0.15
W_3	0.04	2	0.08	2	0.08	2	0.08
W_4	0.06	3	0.18	3	0.18	3	0.18
W_5	0.04	2	0.08	3	0.12	2	0.08
W_6	0.04	1	0.04	3	0.12	2	0.08
W_7	0.06	4	0.21	3	0.18	4	0.24
W_8	0.04	1	0.04	1	0.04	1	0.04
W_9	0.07	3	0.21	4	0.28	3	0.21
W_{10}	0.04	1	0.04	2	0.08	2	0.08
Total Sum	1	2.53		3.01		2.69	

Abbreviations: WO, weakness, opportunity; AS, available score; TAS, total available score.

Table 7. Quantitative Strategic planning matrix (external factors)

External Factors	Normalized Weight	WO_1		WO_2		WO_3	
		AS	TAS	AS	TAS	AS	TAS
Opportunities							
O_1	0.05	2	0.1	2	0.1	4	0.2
O_2	0.04	1	0.04	1	0.04	3	0.12
O_3	0.04	1	0.04	2	0.08	2	0.08
O_4	0.06	3	0.18	3	0.18	3	0.18
O_5	0.05	3	0.15	3	0.15	3	0.15
O_6	0.05	4	0.2	4	0.2	3	0.15
O_7	0.04	4	0.16	3	0.12	3	0.12
O_8	0.06	4	0.24	4	0.24	4	0.24
O_9	0.07	3	0.21	4	0.28	3	0.21
O_{10}	0.5	3	0.15	3	0.15	2	0.1
Threats							
T_1	0.05	1	0.05	2	0.1	2	0.1
T_2	0.04	1	0.04	1	0.04	3	0.12
T_3	0.05	4	0.2	1	0.05	2	0.1
T_4	0.04	1	0.04	2	0.08	2	0.08
T_5	0.05	3	0.15	2	0.1	4	0.2
T_6	0.06	3	0.18	3	0.18	3	0.18
T_7	0.07	4	0.28	3	0.21	3	0.21
T_8	0.05	4	0.2	1	0.05	1	0.05
T_9	0.04	1	0.04	2	0.08	1	0.04
T_{10}	0.04	2	0.08	4	0.18	3	0.12
Total Sum	1	2.73		2.64		2.75	

Abbreviations: WO, weakness, opportunity; AS, available score; TAS, total available score.

Table 8. Prioritized WO strategies

Scores Sum	External Factors	Internal Factors	Strategy
5.65	2.64	3.01	WO_2: Simultaneous training of workers and citizens for the development of mechanization and improvement of municipal services equipment
5.44	2.75	2.69	WO_3: Formulation of regulations and guidelines in order to encourage participation in waste management and attract private sector investment
5.26	2.53	2.73	WO_1: Upgrading recycling industries through financial support for the development and promotion of industry and marketing of recycled products

waste; educating municipal workers in order to optimize the waste collection system; and the participation of other related organizations and the private sector in solid waste management (7). The results of that study correspond with those of the current study.

Various studies have revealed that about 90% of municipal solid waste (MSW) is disposed of unscientifically in open dumps and landfills, creating problems to public health and the environment (8).

In another study conducted in Sweden, selected potential emerging waste treatment technologies were analyzed based on SWOT analysis, and the technologies were evaluated with a qualitative evaluation method based on waste handling capacity, development stage, and waste management problem solving capacity (9).

Generally, some causes of the failure in Tehran's municipality waste management and recycling can be stated as follows:

- Lack of coordination between the municipalities of different regions;
- Frequent changes in management and decision-making units;
- Lack of purpose and sustainable long-term plans to achieve goals;
- Lack of support for providing the necessary facilities, equipment, and resources to do the job right;
- Lack of incentives for private sector investment that will lead to 1-year contracts;
- Lack of motivation and confidence among citizens due to poor performance, lack of continuing education programs, and lack of collection of dry waste plans;
- Emergent and short-term projects not conducted fundamentally due to lack of time and money;
- Low quality of recycled products because of poor technology and lack of proper segregation of waste materials at the source, and
- Fragmentation and high number of recycling units of multiplicity, lack of oversight on their activities, and unauthorized agent activities.

Generally, recommendations that can be made to improve waste management include (*a*) defining "Recycling Day" as a symbolic movement in the country, (*b*) creating recycling exchange and offering recycling products, (*c*) gradual reduction in frequency of manually collecting waste in neighborhoods, (*d*) preventing unauthorized activities and badgers, (*e*) providing facts and figures about the problem of recycling waste and creating incentives to encourage more people to participate in this plan, and (*f*) avoiding parallel activities between parties related to the issue of waste management and recycling in order to reduce costs.

Conclusion

Waste management systems are dependent upon socio-economic issues such as population growth and gross domestic product (GDP) (10,11). Six waste management development drivers are categorized by Wilson in his study: (*a*) public health, (*b*) environmental protection, (*c*) resource value of waste closing the loop, (*d*) institutional development, (*e*) responsible issues, and (*f*) public awareness overtime (12). Waste management systems are involved with different multidisciplinary factors; therefore, trends in the development of waste treatment technologies have been led by various social, economic and environmental drivers in Tehran.

Encouraging nongovernmental organizations (NGOs), associations, urban and rural councils, and schools, universities and establishing programs for women, youth, and people interested in this issue with the collaboration of local authorities, municipalities, environmental agencies in order to gain public support for recycling waste through group focused activities should be considered. An important consideration is that, in the field of waste management, only by using the synchronized and simultaneous "education and culture making," "applying law" and "employing superior technologies and promoting them" can we be hopeful that waste management laws will take the right step toward optimal management of waste materials (13). The development of waste technologies also involves other externalities, like shifting personal and social viewpoints on waste such as 'waste' to 'resource'. A number of studies have been conducted by different researchers on the 'zero waste' concept (14).

Competing interests

The authors declare that they have no competing interests.

Authors' contributions

Monireh Majlessi, Aida Vaezi, and Mohsen Mehdipour conceived and designed the study. Mohsen Mehdipour performed the literature search and wrote the manuscript. All authors participated in data acquisition, analysis and interpretation. All authors critically reviewed, refined, and approved the manuscript.

Acknowledgments

It is necessary to thank all those who participated in this research, especially the authorities of District 1 of Tehran Municipality.

References

1. Abbasvand M. Examining urban waste management process of Golestan province. In: 4th National Conference on Waste Management; 2008; Mashad, Iran.
2. Abedinzadeh N, Abedinzadeh F, Abedi T. Examining strategic factors in waste management of Rasht city using SWOT analysis and QSPM matrix. Journal of Ecology 2011; 37(57): 93-104.
3. David FR. Strategic Management. Parsaeiyan A, Arabi M, trans. 21st ed. Tehran: Culture and Management Publications; 2011. p. 687.
4. Halla F. A SWOT analysis of strategic urban development planning: the case of Dar al Salaam city in Tanzania. Habitat International 2007; 31(1): 130-42.
5. Zarei M, Raeisi A. Documenting a strategic management plan for Minab city's waste. In: 6th National Conference on Waste Management; 2012; Mashad, Iran.
6. Damghani AM, Savarypour G, Zand E, Deihimfard R. Municipal solid waste management in Tehran: Current practices, opportunities and challenges. Waste Manag 2008; 28(5): 929-34.
7. Karbasi A, Monavari M, Mogouyi R. Strategic Management in the Environment. Kavosh Ghalam Publications; 2007.
8. Sharholy M, Ahmad K, Mahmood G, Trivedi RC. Municipal solid waste management in Indian cities – A review. Waste Manag 2008; 28(2): 459-67.

9. Zaman AU. Identification of waste management development drivers and potential emerging waste treatment technologies. Int J Environ Sci Technol (Tehran) 2013; 10(3): 455-64.
10. Mazzanti M, Zoboli R. Waste generation, waste disposal and policy effectiveness: Evidence on decoupling from the European Union. Resources, Conservation and Recycling 2008; 52(10): 1221-34.
11. EEA indicator fact sheet. http://www.eea.europa.eu/data-and-maps/indicators. Accessed April 22, 2009. Published 2008.
12. Wilson DC. Development drivers for waste management. Waste Manag Res 2007; 25(3): 198-07.
13. Fallahi Gilani R, Darvish A. Awareness and importance of waste separation and environmental protection: case study from Tehran's 22 municipality regions. In: 5th National Conference of Environmental Engineering; 2011; Terhan, Iran.
14. Zaman AU, Lehmann S. Challenges and opportunities in transforming a city into a 'Zero Waste City'. Challenges 2011; 2(4): 73-93.

Efficiency of horizontal roughing filter in removing nitrate, phosphate and chemical oxygen demand from effluent of waste stabilization pond

Seyed Mostafa Khezri[1], Gharib Majidi[2], Hossein Jafari Mansoorian[3], Mohsen Ansari[2], Farideh Atabi[4], Taha Tohidi Mogaddam[5], Nahid Rashtchi[6*]

[1]Associate Professor, Department of Environmental Engineering, School of Environment and Energy, Science and Research Branch, Islamic Azad University, Tehran, Iran

[2]MSc in Environmental Health Engineering, School of Public Health, Qom University of Medical Sciences, Qom, Iran

[3]Lecturer, Environmental Health Engineering Research Center, Department of Environmental Health, Kerman University of Medical Sciences, Kerman, Iran

[4]Assistant Professor, Department of Environmental Engineering, School of Environment and Energy, Science and Research Branch, Islamic Azad University, Tehran, Iran

[5]MSc in Environmental Engineering, Science and Research Branch, Islamic Azad University, Tehran, Iran

[6]MSc in Environmental Engineering–Water and Wastewater, Islamic Azad University, Western Tehran Branch, Tehran, Iran

Abstract

Background: The effective size of the end grain of horizontal roughing filters (HRFs) is larger than 2 mm. This study aimed to examine the efficiency of HRFs in removing nitrate, phosphate, and chemical oxygen demand (COD) from effluent of a wastewater stabilization pond.

Methods: This experimental study was conducted in 2013. The pilot project was transferred to the Karaj wastewater treatment plant (stabilization pond), and the installation, equipping, and start-up of the system began using an effluent treatment plant. Sampling was done from March to August in 3 rates, 0.5, 1 and 1.5 m/h, and included simultaneous sampling from inlet and outlet filtering to determine the concentrations of nitrate, phosphate, and COD.

Results: At filtration rates of 0.5, 1, and 1.5 m/h, the average nitrate removal equaled 25%, 32%, and 34%, respectively, average phosphate removal equaled 29%, 26%, and 28%, respectively, and the average COD removal at filtration rates of 0.5, 1, and 1.5 m/h equaled 62%, 66%, and 68%, respectively. Outlet values of phosphate and nitrate were lower than the standards set by the Environmental Standards Organization (ESO) ($P < 0.05$).

Conclusion: According to the results of this study, the HRF function was approximately adequate in COD removal, but its efficiency in nitrate and phosphate removal was lower.

Keywords: Wastewater stabilization pond, Horizontal roughing filter, Nitrate, Phosphate, Chemical oxygen demand

***Correspondence to:**
Nahid Rashtchi
Email: nahidrashtchi1392@gmail.com

Introduction

The increasing demand for water and the limitation of water sources illustrate the importance of recycling wastewater more and more. The cost of treating wastewater is lower than other methods of increasing water supplies. Considering the necessary water quality, the reuse of wastewater is divided into 2 essential parts: potable water and nonpotable water. Nonpotable water is used for irrigational, industrial, and aquatic usages and in entertainment and environmental projects (1). The effluents from biological treatment plants are not able to reach the standards necessary for reuse. To make reusing wastewater feasible, an advanced treatment must be conducted on the effluent of biological treatment plants, the dominant process of which is based on separating solid and liquid, like chemical coagulation, focalization, filtration, and disinfection (2).

Some parameters in outlet effluent considered for evaluating the performance of wastewater treatment plants are: (*a*) chemical oxygen demand, (*b*) nitrate, and (*c*) phosphate. The biodegradable organic materials (proteins, carbohydrates, and fats) are measured in terms of biological and chemical oxygen demand. In case these materials enter the environment without treatment, their biological persistence leads to a reduction of oxygen sources, the creation of anaerobic conditions, and arising odor problems (3,4). The Environmental Protection Organization (EPO) standards for discharge and reuse of wastewater are shown in Table 1 (5).

From the late 1960s, determining the effects of nutritional compounds in aquatic environments (the creation of eutrophication and pollution of underground waters to nitrates) limited the concentration of nitrogen and phosphorus in inlet effluent into the environment and receptive water (6). Based on studies conducted by Wang, the eutrophication in surface waters was decreased by controlling the discharge of wastewaters containing nitrogen and phosphorus and by treating domestic and industrial wastewaters; the concentration of dissolved oxygen in the studied area surface waters was increased (7).

There are ways to increase the quality of stabilization pond effluent, sand bed filters and are example of ways. Horizontal roughing filters (HRFs) are filters with an effective end grain size of larger than 2 mm. The efficiency of roughing filters in removing solids is higher than that of a sedimentation tank (8). During the pass of flow through the bed, the suspended substances are gathered. Material size of the bed is about 4 mm to 25 mm. The roughing filters are generally formed with three layers. The size of the course at the beginning of the flow path is large and at the end is small. This kind of layering increases absorption capacity while the solids entering the bed–depth gradually separate because of the decline in the holes' diameters. Roughing filters are between 5 and 9 meters long, their width is about 2 to 5 meters, and their height is about 1.5 meters (9). Advantages of HRFs include a higher capacity for gathering silt and sediment matters, lack of length limitation, no use of mechanical mobile pieces, and simplicity of establishment and utilization (8). Due to the feasibility of much length, this kind of filter will have a resistance power up to about 500-1000 NTU against suspended solids and turbidity (for example, in time of flood-water) (10).

Table 1. EPO standards for discharge and reuse of wastewater

Parameter	Discharge into surface waters	Irrigation
TSS (mg/l)	40	100
pH	6.5-8.5	6-8.5
Turbidity (NTU)	50	50
Total coliform (MPN)	1000	1000
Fecal coliform (MPN)	400	400
COD (mg/l)	60	200
Nitrate (mg/l)	50	-
Phosphate in terms of phosphorus	6	-

Abbreviations: EPO, Environmental Protection Organization; TSS, total suspended solids.

The aim of this study was to examine the efficiency of HRFs in nitrate, phosphate, and chemical oxygen demand (COD) removal from the effluent of waste stabilization ponds.

Methods

This experimental study was performed in 2013 and used a HRF. The pilot was designed and developed based on Wegelin criteria approved by the World Health Organization (WHO) (11). After its construction, the pilot was transferred to the Karaj wastewater treatment plant, and installation, equipping, and start-up of the system began using treated outlet effluent. The wastewater treatment plant of Karaj works on a stabilization pond. The sampling period lasted from March to August.

The development and installation of pilot

This pilot was constructed of a sheet of nongalvanized iron 3 mm thick and 2 sheets with dimensions of 1.5 × 2 meters. After rolling, the sheets became incomplete cylinder shaped and were welded along their length. Both ends were covered by two circular sheets, and then welding and leakage detection were performed. The quad netted wall made of galvanized sheet was used to separate the bed layers. Holes 4 mm in diameter and 4 square cm in density were created in these 4 pieces using a turnery drill. The walls were welded to the body at a distance of 1.6 m and 1.3 m from the beginning of the filter. The distances between drainage pipes in the first, second, and third holes were 20 cm, 30 cm, and 40 cm, respectively. On these drain pipes, netted faults with holes 5 mm in diameter and a density of 7 holes per square cm were installed. In the third drainage, each hole of one piezometer was installed to determine the hydrological gradient of flow. The filter's exit was guided by a 1-inch diameter trunk-like pipe into the drainage of the pump room bottom. The filter bed was washed hydrologically. The exit faucet of the filter was closed, and the filter holes completely filled with effluent. Then, the arranged drainage pipe faults on the filter floor opened at the same time. As a result of this action, hydraulic cutting force will dislodge sediments from the surface of media and out of the floor drains. The washing strategy of the filter bed was based on change of pressure head lost. At the beginning of the filter start-up, the effluent level in the entrance area was 10 cm from the bed level. As sediment was gradually gathered in the bed, the height of effluent in the inlet area increased to the same level as the filter bed. At this time, the bed washing process was done.

Sampling and conducting experiments

The sampling period for nitrate and phosphate at filtration rates of 0.5, 1 and 1.5 m/h was 30 days, with samples taken every other day. The sampling period for COD at a filtration rate of 0.5 m/h was 60 days, with samples taken every other day. The sampling period for COD at filtration rates of 1 and 1.5 m/h was 26 days, on a daily basis with sampling performed every day. A total of 15 samples for nitrate and phosphate were taken at filtration rates of 0.5, 1, and 1.5 m/h . A total of 30 samples for COD were taken at the filtration rate of 0.5 m/hand at filtration rates of 1 and 1.5 m/h 26 samples were taken. All experiments were measured in accordance with "Sandard Methods for the Examination of Water and Wastewater" (12).

Results

In Table 2, the average amount, standard deviation, and slope of nitrate changes for inlet, outlet, and removal efficiency are presented according to filtration rates. In Table 3, the average amount, standard deviation, and range of phosphate changes for inlet, outlet, and removal efficiency are presented according to filtration rates. In Table 4, the average amount, standard deviation, and range of changes for COD for inlet, outlet, and removal efficiency are presented according to filtration rates. Figures 1 and 2 show the changes in efficiency of nitrate and phosphate removal, respectively, at 3 filtration rates. Figures 3 and 4 present the changes in efficiency of chemical oxygen demand removal at 3 filtration rates.

Discussion

The average nitrogen removal efficiency values at the studied filtration rates equaled 25%, 32%, and 34%, respectively. For phosphate, these figures were 29%, 26%, and 28%, respectively, and for COD at the studied filtration rates were 62%, 66%, and 68%, respectively. The average removal efficiency of nitrate, phosphate, and COD

Table 2. Average quantities of nitrate changes according to filtration rate

Zone	Quantities				
	Filtration rate (m/h)	Average (mg/l)	Standard deviation	Minimum (mg/l)	Maximum (mg/l)
Inlet					
	0.5	19.2467	4.10259	12.50	26.50
	1	44.2077	28.10156	8.80	100.80
	1.5	22.9643	9.02105	7.40	39.10
	Total[a]	28.2119	19.56063	7.40	100.80
Outlet					
	0.5	14.2200	2.93068	9.60	19.90
	1	30.4769	20.12632	4.80	74.60
	1.5	14.9643	5.62284	5.60	23.90
	Total[a]	19.5000	13.67273	4.80	74.60
Removal Efficiency (%)					
	0.5	25.400	9.2875	8.0	39.0
	1	32.000	8.6313	19.0	46.0
	1.5	34.000	5.6432	25.0	42.0
	Total[a]	30.310	8.7024	8.0	46.0

[a]Average of the 3 filtration rate.

Table 3. Average quantities of phosphate changes according to filtration rate

Zone	Quantities				
	Filtration rate (m/h)	Average (mg/l)	Standard deviation	Minimum (mg/l)	Maximum (mg/l)
Inlet					
	0.5	9.1867	3.84111	2.30	15.20
	1	11.4615	2.55556	6.50	14.60
	1.5	10.4857	2.42006	6.80	14.30
	Total	10.3238	3.11431	2.30	15.20
Outlet					
	0.5	6.3600	3.01492	2.00	12.80
	1	8.4769	1.97575	4.40	11.70
	1.5	7.5000	1.76940	4.40	11.30
	Total	7.3952	2.45068	2.00	12.80
Removal Efficiency (%)					
	0.5	29.733	12.0266	11.0	46.0
	1	26.000	6.2183	15.0	33.0
	1.5	28.214	7.6779	17.0	39.0
	Total	28.071	9.0430	11.0	46.0

Table 4. Average quantities of COD changes according to filtration rate

Zone	Quantities				
	Filtration rate (m/h)	**Average (mg/l)**	**Standard deviation**	**Minimum (mg/l)**	**Maximum (mg/l)**
Inlet					
	0.5	63.6333	41.25069	23.00	208.00
	1	64.7308	33.49096	11.00	125.00
	1.5	86.2593	22.11785	48.00	140.00
	Total	71.3373	34.75253	11.00	208.00
Outlet					
	0.5	21.0333	11.80439	3.00	45.00
	1	19.7692	8.58980	4.00	32.00
	1.5	27.0000	7.24834	12.00	40.00
	Total	22.5783	9.91195	3.00	45.00
Removal Efficiency (%)					
	0.5	62.200	22.1553	22.0	88.0
	1	66.577	10.8043	43.0	80.0
	1.5	68.407	5.9048	57.0	84.0
	Total	65.590	15.0787	22.0	88.0

Abbreviations: COD, chemical oxygen demand.

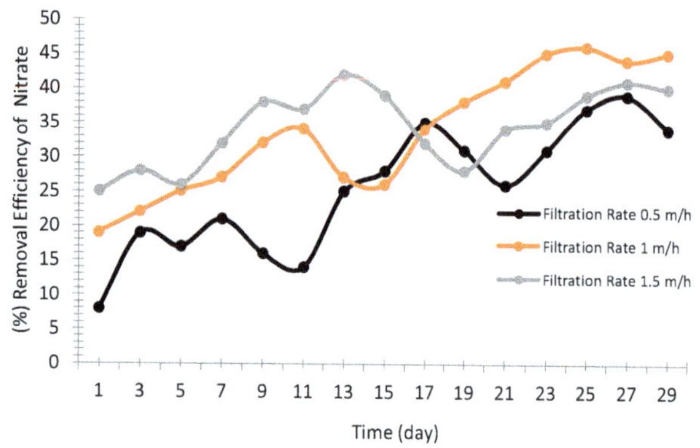

Figure 1. Changes of nitrogen removal efficiency at three filtration rates.

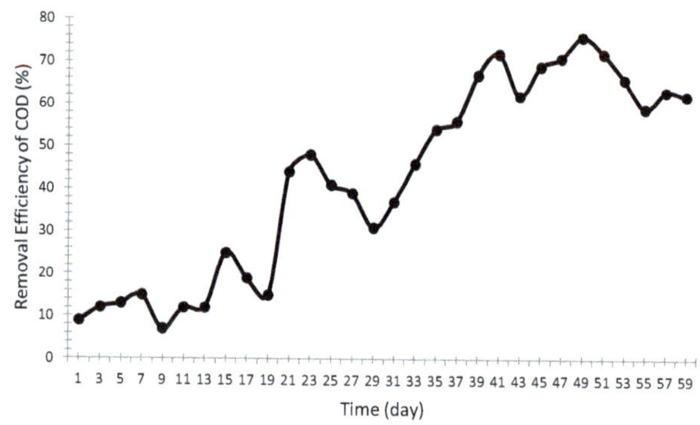

Figure 3. Changes of COD removal efficiency at filtration rate of 0.5 m/h.

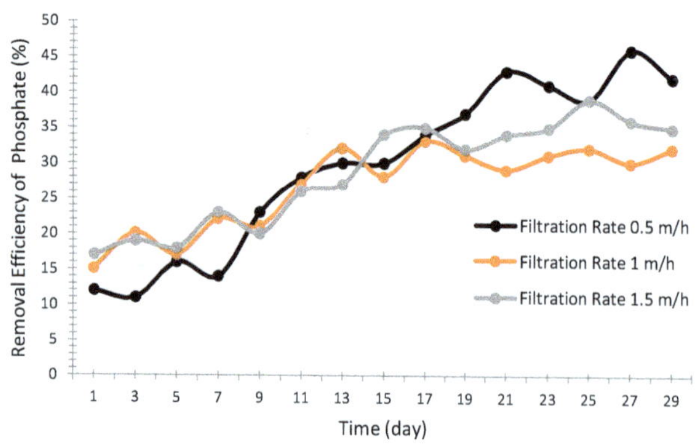

Figure 2. Changes of phosphate removal efficiency at three filtration rates.

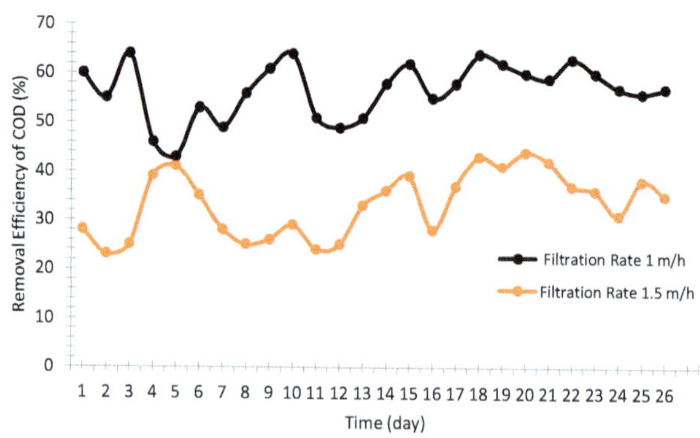

Figure 4. Changes of COD removal efficiency at filtration rates of 1 and 1.5 m/h.

at the studied filtration rates equaled 34%, 28.07%, and 65.59%, respectively.

Using the Scheffe test, the removal efficiency of nitrate and phosphate at different filtration rates were compared. The percentage of nitrate removal was higher at the filtration rate of 1.5 m/h than at 0.5 m/h ($P > 0.05$). Because the data for percentage of COD removed was abnormal, the Mann-Whitney test was used to compare the rates with each other. The COD removal rates at the three tested filtration rates had no significant differences ($P > 0.05$).

In a study conducted by Ehteshami et al, the average COD removal in constant performance statuses of the HRF at similar filtration rates equaled 60%, 51%, and 38%, respectively (13). The present study, however, showed no significant difference in COD removal efficiency. The results of the current study had no conformity with those of Ehteshami's study.

Sarvmeili examined the performance of the HRF with the filtration rate 2.5 m/h in improving effluent quality for urban purposes and obtained values of 63%, 22%, and 37% for removal turbidity, suspended solids, and COD, respectively (14). The average removal efficiency of COD in the present study was 65.5%, which was higher than that of Seromeli's study.

The changes in removal efficiency of nitrate, phosphate, and COD are shown in Figures 1 to 4. The highest nitrogen removal efficiency (46%) relates to filtration rate 1 m/h and occurred 42 days after the pilot study began. The least efficiency was 8% on the first day of filter work. The highest removal efficiency of phosphate (46%) related to the filtration rate of 0.5 and occurred 27 days after the pilot study began. The least efficiency was 11% on the fourth day of pilot study. The removal efficiency of phosphate at each rate increased and had no discernible fluctuation. The highest removal efficiency of COD (76%) related to the filtration rate of 0.5 m/h and occurred 49 days after the pilot work began. The least efficiency was 7% at the beginning of the pilot study. Within the first 6 days, COD removal efficiency equaled 15% at the filtration rate of 0.5 m/h. This increase over time can be related to the formation of a microbial film in the roughing filter bed, which led to a reduction in pore diameter, an increase in the substrate contact surface, and dominance of chemical and biological processes in removing elements and microbial load (15).

Based on the results of this study, the HRF in COD has an optimal performance, but its efficiency is low in removing nitrate and phosphate. The *t* test was used to compare the outlet values of COD and phosphate with the EPO standards. A significant difference was observed between outlet COD of HRF and the standard of the EPO for discharge into surface water and irrigation ($P<0.05$). There was also a significant difference between the outlet phosphate from HRF and the EPO standards for discharge surface waters ($P<0.05$). Due to the abnormality of the outlet nitrate data, the Wilcoxon test was used to compare outlet values with EPO standards. There was significant difference between outlet nitrate from HRF and the EPO standard for discharge into surface waters ($P<0.05$). Outlet values of COD, phosphate and nitrate were lower than EPO standards ($P<0.05$).

Conclusion

The study results showed that the efficiency of the HRF in removing nitrate, phosphate and COD from the effluent of a wastewater stabilization pond was affected by filtration rates. An increase in filtration rate enhanced the efficiency of the HRF. This result was in agreement with the above-mentioned studies. At the various filtration rates, nitrate and phosphate removal was more dependent than COD removal. This result was in agreement with studies by Khazayi (15), Ehteshami et al (13), and Wegelin et al (12). A biological oxygen demand (BOD) removal of 85% to 90% is not unusual for stabilization ponds, and the removal of viruses, bacteria, protozoa, and helminthes is also reported to be very high (16). Therefore, using the HRF after stabilization pond effluents can be an alternative to depth filtration as a pretreatment for membrane filtration. The filter media of the study pilot was 10-15 mm gravel for roughing filtration. This size was assessed in Mazumder et al study (16). Low removal rates of nitrate and phosphate may be caused by the filter media size. Stabilization pond effluent has an extremely high algal content, so caution should be exercised during use of the HRF. Horizontal roughing filtration plays a significant role in the treatment line, because a high COD removal and average nitrate and phosphate removal efficiency was achieved simultaneously and in one-step without requiring any sophisticated control of pH, redox potential, etc. According to the results, the best situation for better operation of the HRF is a filtration rate of 1 m/h for 5 days.

Competing interests

The authors declare that they have no competing interests.

Authors' contributions

Seyed Mostafa Khezri, Farideh Atabi, Taha Tohidi Mogaddam, and Nahid Rashtchi designed the study. Gharib Majidi, Mohsen Ansari, and Hossein Jafari Mansoorian performed the literature search and wrote the manuscript. All authors participated in data acquisition, analysis, and interpretation. All authors critically reviewed, refined, and approved the manuscript.

References

1. Torabian A, Motalebi M. Management plan of treated effluent reuse - case study: Ekbatan town. Journal of Environmental Studies 2004; 29(32): 57-62. [In Persian].
2. Mohamadi A, Naseri S, Mahvi AH, Roshani B, Firozmanesh M, Salehi R. The study of performance of multimedia filters to removal the bacteria in the municipal wastewater to reuse and chlorine reduction for disinfection. Journal of Kordestan University of Medical Sciences 2005; 8(4): 8-15. [In Persian].
3. Tchobanoglous G, Louis F, Burton H, Stensel D. Wastewater Engineering: Treatment and Reuse. 4th

ed. New York: McGraw-Hill; 2004.

4. Salvato JA, Nemerow NL, Agardy FJ. Environmental Engineering. 5th ed. New Jersey: Wiley & Sons; 2003.
5. Ghaneian M, Mesdaghinia A, Ehrampoush M. Principeles of Wastewater Reuse; Applications, Standards and Side Effectes. Tehran: Teb Gostar; 2001. [In persian]
6. Gerardi MH. Nitrification and Denitrification in the Activated Sludge Process. New Jersey: John Wiley & Sons; 2003.
7. Wang H, Wang H. Mitigation of lake eutrophication: Loosen nitrogen control and focus on phosphorus abatement. Progress in Natural Science 2009; 19(10): 1445-51.
8. Khazaei M, Nabizadeh R, Nadafi K, Nourieh N, Omidi Oskouei A. Elimination of suspended solids from aerated lagoon effluent by horizontal roughing filter. Journal of Qom University of Medical Sciences 2010; 4(1): 42-7. [In Persian]
9. Nabizadeh Noudehi R, Nadafi K, Vaezi F, Khazaei M, Safdari M. Efficiency of horizontal roughing filter (HRF) in coliform removal from aerated lagoon effluent. Water and Wastewater. 2008; 19(2): 2-9. [In Persian]
10. Fazeli M. Determination of design basic and development of DHRF. [Ph.D thesis] Tehran: Tehran University; 2003. [In Persian]
11. Wegelin M, Boller M, Schertenleib R. Particle removal by horizontal-flow roughing filtration. J Water Suppl Res Tech Aqua 1987; 36 (2): 80-90.
12. American Water Work Association. Standard Methods for the Examination of Water and Wastewater. 20th ed. American Water Work Association; 2005.
13. Ehteshami M, Takdastan A, Alavi N, Jafarzadeh Haghighifard N, Ahmadi Moghdam M, Khazayi M, et al. Efficacy of HRF in COD removal from secondary effluent of Yasuj municipal wastewater. Armaghane-danesh 2011; 16(4): 391-9. [In Persian]
14. Sarvmeili M. Upgrading of Wastewater Effluent Quality for Municipal Non-potable Applications by Horizontal Roughing Filter. Tehran; 2006. [In Persian]
15. Khazayi M. The study of performance of horizontal roughing filter (HRF) and hydrogen peroxide complex - a series of silver ions to reduce the bacterial load in the effluent, city of Qom [Thesis]. Tehran: Tehran University of Medical Sciences and Health Services; 2007. [In Persian]
16. Mazumder A, Kumar Roy P, Nath Barman R, Majumder M, Mukhopadhay B. Verification of filter efficiency of horizontal roughing filter by Weglin's design criteria and artificial neural network. Water Eng Sci 2008; 1(2): 117-33.

37

Feasibility of electrochemical oxidation process for treatment of saline wastewater

Kavoos Dindarloo[1], Hamza Ali Jamali[2*], Parvin Lakbala[1], Hamid Mahmoodi[3], Fatemeh Kazemi[4]

[1]Assistant Professor, Environmental Health Engineering Research Center, Instructor Department of Health, Hormozgan University of Medical Sciences, Bandar Abbas, Iran
[2]Assistant Professor, Department of Environmental Health Engineering, Qazvin University of Medical Sciences, Qazvin, Iran
[3]MSc, Environmental Health Engineering Research Center, Instructor Department of Health, Hormozgan University of Medical Sciences, Bandar Abbas, Iran
[4]MSc, Environmental Health Engineering Research Center, Hormozgan University of Medical Sciences, Bandar Abbas, Iran

Abstract
Background: High concentration of salt makes biological treatment impossible due to bacterial plasmolysis. The present research studies the process of electrochemical oxidation efficiency and optimal levels as important factors affecting pH, salt concentration, reaction time and applied voltage.
Methods: The sample included graphite electrodes with specifications of 2.5 cm diameter and 15 cm height using a reactor with an optimum capacity of 1 L. Sixty samples were obtained with the aid of the experiments carried out in triplicates for each factor at 5 different levels. The entire experiments were performed based on standard methods for water and waste water treatments.
Results: Analysis of variance carried out on effect of pH, salt concentration, reaction time and flow intensity in elimination of chemical oxygen demand (COD) showed that they are significant factors affecting this process and reduce COD with a coefficient interval of 95% and test power of 80%. Scheffe test showed that at optimal level, a reaction time of 1 hour, 10 g/L concentration, pH = 9 and 15 V electrical potential difference were obtained.
Conclusion: Waste waters containing salt may contribute to the electro-oxidation process due to its cations and anions. Therefore, the process of electrochemical oxidation with graphite electrodes could be a proper strategy for the treatment of saline wastewater where biological treatment is not possible.
Keywords: Saline wastewater, Graphite electrode, Salinity removal, Electrochemical oxidation.

***Correspondence to:**
Hamzah Ali Jamali
Email: jamalisadraei@yahoo.com

Introduction

Saline wastewater contains high amounts of organic compounds and soluble inorganic salts which are produced from industries such as fish processing, sea food packing, tanning and petrochemicals (1). In biological treatment of wastewaters with high salt concentrations especially in the of aerobic activated sludge phase process, the efficiency of decontamination would be very low due to bacterial plasmolysis in high concentration of salt (over 1%) (2,3). Desalination is required before treatment process. Therefore, to treat the waste waters containing total dissolved solids (TDS), other advanced treatment methods such as ultra-filtration (4), nano-filtration (5), reverse osmosis (6), electro-Fenton processes (7), and photochemical electrodialysis (8) have been studied.

In the methods of membrane filtration of saline wastewaters where some solution is used for demineralization, the influent organic matter to the membrane should be zero level (9). Waste waters containing high salt appeared to have high electrical conductivity due to high concentration of cations and anions. Hence, this seems to be an appropriate method in combination with electrochemical methods in the treatment of such waste waters (10).

Many studies have been conducted on electro oxidation of organic compounds where various materials are used as anode. This method has been successfully employed in the treatment of wastewaters from industries such as textile, tanning, distillation and leachate industries as well as urban wastewater. Different anodes have been employed for the treatment of industrial wastewaters. Recently, electrode graphite has been widely used for the decomposition of organic matter because it is economical. Graphite has a large surface area; this feature enables it to increase the rate of organic matter removal through adsorption and electro-oxidation. These electrodes are more efficient compared with other electrodes. Hydroxyl radicals are dominant because of the physical adsorption of oxygen on to the graphite electrode where they cause complete decomposition of organic materials. However, one of the considerable disadvantages of graphite electrode is its relative short life due to corrosion of the its surface especially when electric oxidation occurs in high potential difference (11).

Detoxification of tannery wastewater through electrolysis by the use of Ti/Pt anode and SS304 cathode was studied. The results showed a 52% decrease in chemical oxygen demand (COD) using electro oxidation process (11). In a study by Rao et al (12), using Ti/Pt electrode in the successful oxidation of tannery waste water, the study showed that the material of the electrode has an effect on COD removal. Kargi Dincer reported that biological treatment of saline wastewater by activated sludge resulted in low COD removal efficiencies as a result of plasmolysis of cells caused by high salt content (13). Szpyrkoicz et al suggested the electro oxidation process as a supplementary treatment after biological treatment as a more economical process of ammonium removal (14). In electrochemical oxidation, the organic pollutants are eliminated by chlorine and hypochlorite. During the oxidation process, the reaction of electrographite in the presence of sodium chloride produces chlorine (14).

Anode reactions:

$2Cl^- \rightarrow Cl_2 + 2e^-$ (1)

$4OH^- \rightarrow O_2 + 2H_2O + 4e^-$ (2)

Cathode reactions

$2H_2O + 2e^- \rightarrow H_2 + 2OH^-$ (3)

Reactions at the anode (Equations 1 and 2) and at the cathode (Equations 3) for man integrated cell at the anode. Hydroxide is produced at the cathode and reacts with chloride and hypochlorite. The compounds of hypochlorite and free chlorine are chemically reactive which decomposes organic pollutants into carbon dioxide and water, hence HOCl is produced:

HOCl decomposition reaction:

$Cl_2 + H_2O \rightarrow H^+ + Cl^- + HOCl$ (4)

$HOCl \leftrightarrow H^+ + OCl^-$ (5)

Hypochlorite is a leading organic matter. The final reaction in the electro oxidation process is expressed according to Equation 6 below:

Organic matter + $OCl^- \rightarrow$ interstitial material $\rightarrow CO_2 + Cl^- + H_2O$ (6)

The present study was carried out to find out the factors such as salt concentration, reaction time, the intensity of voltage and pH affecting the treatment of saline waste water through electrooxidation process and determination of optimal conditions for each of the factors.

Methods

This research was a descriptive-analytical study conducted in a cubic-rectangular batch reactor made of Plexiglas with an optimum capacity of 1/L with dimensions of 14 cm × 7 cm ×15 cm. Graphite columns with diameter of 2.5 cm and length of 15 cm were interconnected by pieces of wire and embedded in the reactor as 2 series of parallel electrode. Each series of graphite electrode connected to direct current was supplied by AC/DC convertor (PAYANIK, RN-3003D). The experimental setup for the electro-oxidation studies is shown in Figure 1.

2.5 g bovine albumin serum and hydrochloric acid were used to prepare synthetic wastewater as well as required salt in the process and concentration of COD at the required level of saline wastewater. To balance the pH level, caustic 1 N and hydrochloric acid solutions made by Merck Company were used. All experiments were performed according to the standard methods for the analysis of water and wastewater (15). Experimental design was carried out based on the book for experimental design (16). The optimal level of each factor – pH, primary concentration of salt, current intensity and time – was determined separately. Since the present study aimed at comparing the mean percent of COD removal at different levels of the factors, graphs were used for choosing sample size. The frequency of each test was selected at a confidence interval of 95% and a power of test of 80%. A mean difference of 20% or higher for COD removal between the 2 levels of each factor in the experiment showed that it was statistically significant (17).

To determine the frequency of each test and the level of each factor, the standard deviation estimated to be 10% was evaluated based on the formula 7:

$$Q = \frac{1}{\sigma}\sqrt{\frac{\Sigma T_j^2}{r}} = \frac{1}{10} \times \sqrt{\frac{5 \times 15^2}{5}} = 1.5 \quad (7)$$

Where:

r = Number of groups

σ = Equal to Q

T^2 = Mean difference between the two concentrations.

Using the following formula, Ω coefficient was calculated at 0.5 error levels and 80% power of test, and the ratio of the numbers of pH factor levels in the sample graphs. According to above mentioned book, 3 experiments were repeated for each level. As the results of the calculations, the total numbers of the experiments was estimated 60 samples (16).

After the experiments were conducted and laboratory data for the related parameters were collected, graphs were constructed using Excel and SPSS version 16. To identify optimal level of each variable, analysis of variance (ANOVA) and Scheffe test were used.

Results

Effects of pH

Tables 1 & 2 and Figure 2 show the results of wastewater COD changes (790 mg/L primary COD) at 10 g/L salt concentration, 1 hour reaction time, 15 V potential difference and different pH.

Also, ANOVA results for the effect of pH on COD removal at 10 g/L salt concentration,1 hour reaction time, and 15 V potential difference showed that pH had a significant ($F = 44.24$, $P < 0.001$) effect on the process.

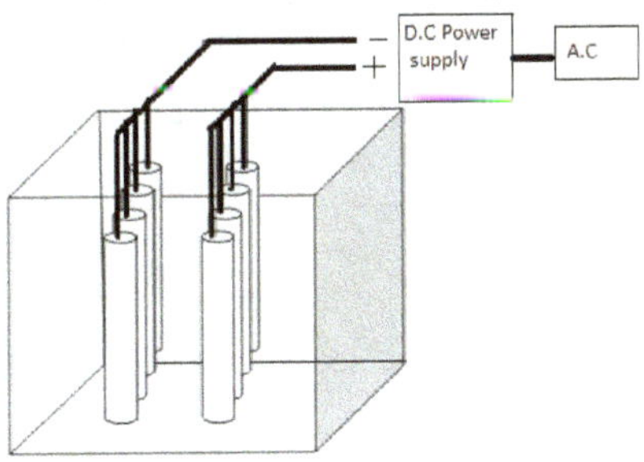

Figure 1. Schematic diagram of the reactor used in this study

Table 1. Data of reduction of COD at different pH levels with 10 g/L salt concentration, 1 hour reaction time, and 15 V difference

pH	No. of experiments	Mean	SD	SE	95% CI
3	3	42	3	1.7	34.54-49.45
5	3	52.3	6.6	3.8	35.79-68.87
7	3	63	6.5	3.7	46.71-79.28
9	3	80.33	4.5	2.6	69.13-91.53
11	3	87.33		2.3	77.29-97.37

Abbreviations: SD, standard deviation; SE, standard error.

Table 2. Comparison test for different levels of pH factor in reducing COD at 10 g/L salt concentration, 1 hour reaction time, and 15 V potential difference at 95% CI

pH level compared	Other pH levels	Mean difference	SD	*P*
	3	38.33 (SE)	4.2	<0.001
9	5	28 (SE)	4.2	<0.001
	7	17.33 (SE)	4.2	<0.029
	11	-7	4.2	<0.615

Abbreviation: SD, standard deviation.

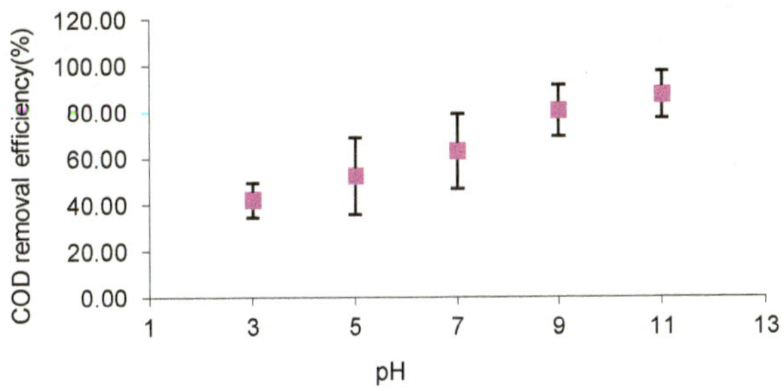

Figure 2. The graph of COD removal changes at different levels of pH at 10 g/L salt concentration, 1 hour reaction time, and 15 V potential difference.

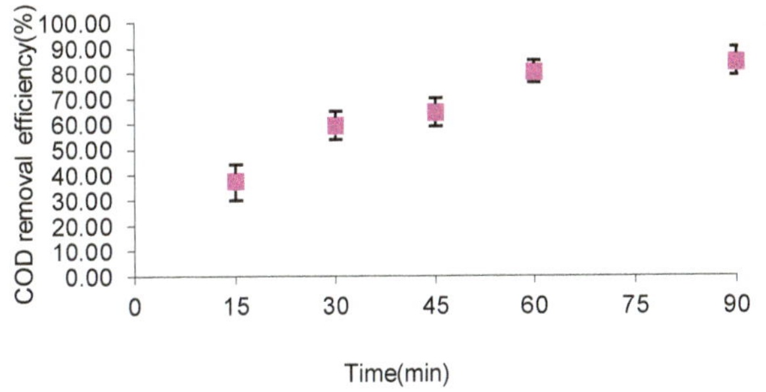

Figure 3. The graph of changes in COD removal at different levels of reaction time, 10 g/L salt concentration, pH = 9 and 15 V potential difference.

Table 3. Data description in reduction percent of COD at different reaction time with 10 g/L salt concentration, pH = 9 and 15 V difference

Time	No. of experiments	Mean	SD	SE	95% CI
15	3	37.23	2	1.2	30-44
30	3	59.33	5.5	3.17	54-65
45	3	64.33	5.5	3.17	59-70
60	3	80.33	4.5	2.6	76-85
90	3	84	1	0.57	79-90

Abbreviations: SD, standard deviation; SE, standard error.

Table 4. Comparisons of different levels of reaction time in reducing COD for the determination of optimal level at 95% CI

pH level compared	Other pH levels	Mean difference	SD	*P*
	15	43(SE)	3.39	<0.001
16	30	21 (SE)	3.39	<0.002
	45	16 (SE)	3.39	<0.013
	90	-3.66	3.39	<0.877

Abbreviation: SD, standard deviation.

Effect of reaction time

Tables 3 & 4 and Figure 3 show the results of wastewater COD changes in this study with 10 g/L salt concentration, pH=9 and 15 V potential difference at different reaction time.

ANOVA results for the effects of reaction time on COD removal at 10 g/L salt concentration, pH=9, and 15 V potential difference showed that reaction time had a significant (F=60.55, $P<0.001$) effect on this process.

Effect of salt concentration

Tables 5 & 6 and Figure 4 show the results of wastewater COD changes at 1 hour reaction time, pH=9 and 15 V potential difference time at different salt concentrations. ANOVA results for the effects of salt concentration on COD removal at 1 hour reaction time, pH=9, and 15 V potential difference showed that salt concentration had a significant effect on this process (F=0.4.72, $P<0.05$).

Influence of applied voltage

Tables 7 & 8 and Figure 5 show the results of wastewater COD changes at 1 hour reaction time, pH=9 and 10 g/L salt concentration, at different potential differences.

ANOVA results for the effects of potential differences on COD removal with a 1 hour reaction time, pH=9, and 10 gr/L salt concentration showed that potential difference had a significant effect on the process (F=8.75, $P<0.05$).

Table 5. Data description of percentage reduction of COD at different salt concentrations, 1 hour reaction time, pH = 9 and 15 V potential difference

Saline concentration (g/L)	No. of experiments	Mean	SD	SE	CI %95
10	3	80.33	4.5	2.6	69.13-91.53
15	3	83.66	3.2	1.8	75.68-91.65
20	3	84.66	3.7	2.18	75.26-94.07
25	3	88	3	1.73	80.54-95.45
30	3	91	1.5	0.88	87.53-95.12

Abbreviations: SD, standard deviation; SE, standard error.

Table 6. Comparison test for different levels of voltage percentage on COD reduction at different salt concentrations with 1 hour reaction time, pH = 9, and 15 V difference

Saline concentration level compared	Other time levels	Mean difference	SD	*P*
	15	-3.33	2.7	0.82
10	20	-4.33	2.7	0.65
	25	-7.66	2.7	0.17
	30	-11 (SE)	2.7	0.03

Abbreviation: SD, standard deviation.

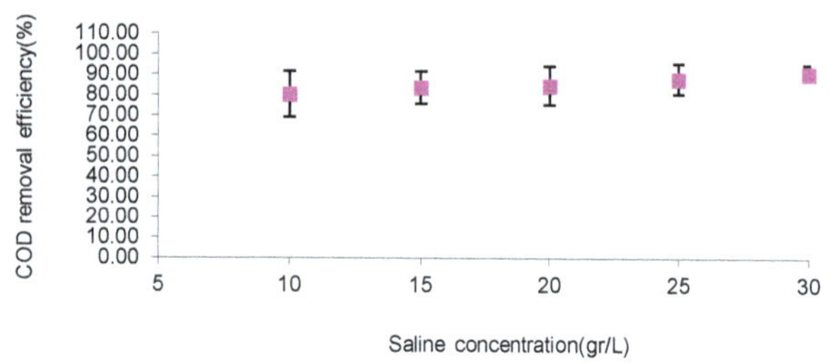

Figure 4. COD removal changes at different levels of salt concentration, with a 1 hour reaction time, pH = 9 and 15 V potential difference.

Table 7. Data description in COD reduction percentage at different potential differences, 1 hour reaction time, pH = 9 and 10 g/L salt concentration

Voltage	No. of experiments	Mean	SD	SE	CI 95%
2	3	64.66	4.5	2.6	53.46-75.8
5	3	70.66	3	1.7	63.7-78.25
8	3	73.66	3.21	1.8	65.68-81.65
10	3	77	1.7	1	72.69-81.3
15	3	80.33	4.5	2.6	69.13-91.53

Abbreviations: SD, standard deviation; SE, standard error.

Table 8. Comparison test for different levels of potential differences on COD reduction at 1 hour reaction time, pH = 9 and 10 g/L salt concentration

Voltage level compared	Other voltage levels	Mean difference	SD	*P*
	2	15.66 (SE)	2.9	0.005
15	5	6.66	2.9	0087
	8	3.33	2.9	0.329
	10	-11 (SE)	2.9	0.852

Abbreviation: SD, standard deviation.

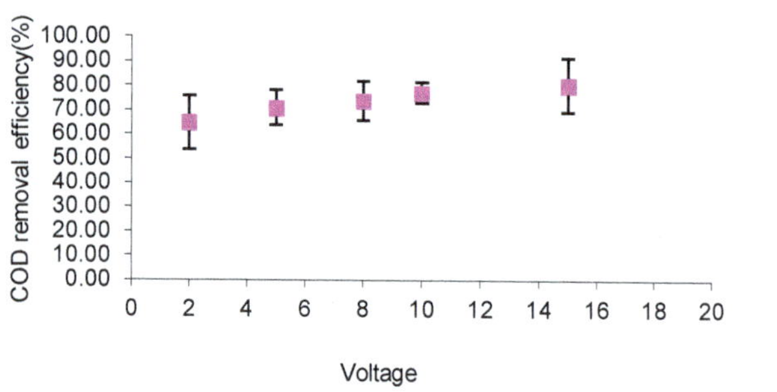

Figure 5. COD removal changes at different levels of potential difference, at 1 hour reaction time, pH = 9 and 15 potential difference.

Discussion

ANOVA results for the effects of pH on COD removal at 10 g/L salt concentration, 1 hour reaction time, and 15 V potential difference showed that pH had a significant effect on this process (F = 44.24, $P < 0.001$). The results showed that an increase in pH from 3 to 11, resulted in a COD decrease from 87% to 42%. Scheffe test for the comparison of different levels of pH factor was significant and showed that as pH increases, removal of COD increases as well which could be due to hydroxyl radical production in the electro-oxidation process. The findings of this study are in accordance with those of Sundarapandiyan et al (2) which showed that an increase in pH from 5 to 11, causes a COD decreases from 89% to 57%. According to Equations 1-5, the reason for this is that in acidosis state, hypochlorite ions, CLO^-, remain unstable and in combination with hydrogen ion tends to form HCLO. The hypochlorite which is formed in an alkaline state accounts for the most important factor inorganic matter oxidation. However, Yan et al (18) reported a higher removal of COD in acidic conditions using the Fenton process a sit is more efficient in acidic conditions.

ANOVA results for the effects of reaction time on COD removal at 10 g/L salt concentration, pH = 9, and 15 V difference showed that reaction time had a significant effect on this process (F = 60.55, $P < 0.001$). The mean COD removal of was 37.33% at a 95% CI and 80% power of test at 15 minutes reaction time (Table 3). Scheffe test for the comparison of different levels of reaction time factor was significant and showed that with increase in reaction time, COD removal also increases. In comparing different levels of time, it is observed that 60 minutes interval is significantly different from 15, 30, and 45 minutes intervals. There was, however, no significant difference at 90 minutes time interval where COD reduction rate increased by 3% which does not seem reasonable with the amount of energy consumed. Therefore, a reaction time of 60 minutes is suggested to be an optimal level. The finding of this study is in accordance with those of Zhang et al (19)and Yazdanbakhsh et al (20). However, Yan et al and Javid et al showed a higher time for COD decrease which could be due to the difference in potential difference used in the process (18,21).

ANOVA results for the effects of salt concentration on COD removal at 1 hour reaction time, pH=9, and 15 V potential difference showed that salt concentration had a significant effect on the process (F=4.72, $P<0.05$). The mean COD removal was 80.33% at 95% CI and 80% power of test at 10 g/L salt concentration (Table 5). The reason is likely due to an increase in the production of hypochlorite ions which occurs through the addition of NaCl. This is consistent with Sundarapandiyan et al study (2). Scheffe test for the comparison of different levels of salt concentration factor was only significant at 10 and 30 g/L, however it was insignificant at other levels. This shows that although salt acts as a facilitator, its increase in the environment has no effect on the efficiency of the process.

ANOVA results for the effects of potential differences on COD removal at 1 hour reaction time, pH=9, and 10 g/L salt concentration showed that it had a significant effect on the electrochemical oxidation process (F=8.75, $P<0.05$).The mean COD removal was 64.66% at 95% CI and 80% power of test at 15 minutes reaction time (Table 7). Seems that rendering increase of voltage results in hypochlorite ion increase; this is consistent with Sundarapandiyan study (2). Also, Al-Qaim et al (22) reported that with the increase of voltage the removal efficiency of caffeine by electrochemical oxidation increased to 95% at 10 V from 75% at 6 V and 10% at 3 V. Also, the study by Duan et al (23) showed that phenol removal efficiency is almost 100% at 3 V after 300 minutes of polarization, with only 40% and 83% of phenol removed at 1.5 and 2 V, respectively (23). Scheffe test was used for the comparison of different levels of reaction time which was significant; although potential difference is effective in the electrochemical oxidation process considering the useful capacity of the reactor, an 8-15 Voltage difference seems to be sufficient. An increase in potential differences with this capacity causes foam formation and discoloration due to destruction of graphite electrode. The study of Yan et al showed an increase in COD removal with an increase in voltage. It indicates that some organic compounds are decomposed following voltage increase (18,20).

Conclusion

ANOVA analysis showed that pH, salt concentration, reaction time, and flow intensity are significant in COD removal at a CI 95% and test power of 80%. Scheffe test showed the optimal levels for the factors thus; reaction time 1 hour,10 g/L concentration, pH=9 and 15 V electrical potential difference. The electrochemical oxidation process with graphite electrodes could be a proper strategy for the treatment of saline wastewater where biological treatment is not possible.

Acknowledgements

The authors appreciate the cooperation of the Vice chancellor of Research and Technology, Hormozgan University of Medical Sciences.

Competing interests

The authors declare that they have no competing interests.

Authors' contributions

All the authors contributed equally to this study and therefore reviewed and approved the final draft of the manuscript.

References

1. Lefebvre O, Moletta R. Treatment of organic pollutant in industrial saline wastewater: a literature review. Water Res 2006; 40(20): 3671-82.
2. Sundarapandiyan S, Chandrasekar R, Ramanaiah B, Krishnan S, Saravanan P. Electrochemical oxidation and reuse of tannery saline wastewater. J Hazard Mater 2010; 180(1-3): 197-203.
3. Kargi F, Dincer AR. Biological treatment of saline wastewater by bed batch operation. J Chem Technol Biotechnol 1997; 69(2): 167-72.
4. Brites Alves AM, Norberta de Pinho M. Ultrafiltration for colour removal of tannery dyeing wastewaters. Desalination 2000; 130(2): 147-54.
5. Aouni A, Fersi C, Ben Sik Ali M, Dhahbi M. Treatment of textile wastewater by a hybrid electrocoagulation/nanofiltration process. J Hazard Mater 2009; 168(2-3): 868-74.
6. Cassano A, Molinari R, Romano M, Drioli E. Treatment of aqueous effluents of the leather industry by membrane processes. J Memb Sci 2001; 181(1): 111-26.
7. Kurt U, Apaydin O, Gonullu MT. Reduction of COD in wastewater from an organized tannery industrial region by electro-Fenton process. J Hazard Mater 2007; 143(1-2): 33-40.
8. Rodrigues MA, Amado FD, Xavier JL, Streit KF, Bernardes AM, Ferreira JZ. Application of photoelectrochemical-electrodialysis treatment for the recovery and reuse of water from tannery effluents. J Clean Prod 2008; 16(5): 605-11.
9. Mänttäria M, Viitikkob K, Nyströma M. Nanofiltration of biologically treated effluents from the pulp and paper industry. J Memb Sci 2006; 272(1-2): 152-60.
10. Grimm J, Bessarabov D, Sanderson R. Review of electro-assisted methods for water purification. Desalination 1998; 115(3): 285-94.
11. Vlyssides AG, Israilides CJ. Detoxification of tannery waste liquors with an electrochemical system. Environ

Pollut 1997; 97(1-2): 147-52.
12. Rao NN, Somasekar KM, Kaul SN, Szpyrkowicz L. Electrochemical oxidation of tannery wastewater. J Chem Technol Biotechnol 2001;76(11): 1124-31.
13. Kargi F, Dincer AR. Use of halophilic bacteria in biological treatment of saline wastewater by fed-batch operation. Water Environ Res 2000; 72(2): 170-4.
14. Szpyrkowicz L, Kaul SN, Neti RN, Satyanarayan S. Influence of anode material on electrochemical oxidation for the treatment of tannery wastewater. Water Res 2005; 39(8): 1601-13.
15. APHA, AWWA, WPCF. Standard Methods for the Examination of Water and Wastewater. 21st ed. Washington, DC: American Public Health Association; 2005.
16. Douglas C. Montgomery, Design and Analysis of Experiments. 8th ed. Wily Publication; 2012.
17. Neter J, Wasserman W, Kutner M H. Applied linear statistical models: Regression, analysis of variance, and experimental designs. Homewood, IL: Irwin; 1974.
18. Yan L, Ma H, Wang B, Wang Y, Chen Y. Electrochemical treatment of petroleum refinery wastewater with three –dimensional multi-phase electrode. Desalination 2011; 276(1-3): 397-402.
19. Zhang J, Zhang Y, Quan X. Electricity assisted anaerobic treatment of salinity wastewater and its effects on microbial Communities. Water Res 2012; 46(11): 3535-43.
20. Yazdanbakhsh AR, Kermani M, Komasi S, Aghayani E, Sheikhmohammadi A. Humic acid removal from aqueous solutions by peroxi-electrocoagulation process. Environ Health Eng Manag J 2015; 2(2): 53-8.
21. Javid AH, Malakootian M, Mehdipour M. Investigation of ozone and coagulant material's (aluminum sulfate, ferric chloride, poly aluminum chloride and lime) efficiency in "Kerman Kork" industry wastewater treatment. Environ Health Eng Manag J 2015; 2(1): 1-6.
22. Al-Qaim FF, Mussa ZH, Othman MR, Abdullah MP. Removal of Caffeine from aqueous solution by indirect electrochemical oxidation using a graphite-PVC composite electrode: A role of hypochlorite ion as an oxidizing agent. J Hazard Mater 2015; 300: 387-97.
23. Duan F, Li Y, Cao H, Wang Y, Crittenden JC, Zhang Y. Activated carbon electrodes: electrochemical oxidation coupled with desalination for wastewater treatment. Chemosphere 2015; 125: 205-11.

PERMISSIONS

All chapters in this book were first published in EHEMJ, by Kerman University of Medical Sciences; hereby published with permission under the Creative Commons Attribution License or equivalent. Every chapter published in this book has been scrutinized by our experts. Their significance has been extensively debated. The topics covered herein carry significant findings which will fuel the growth of the discipline. They may even be implemented as practical applications or may be referred to as a beginning point for another development.

The contributors of this book come from diverse backgrounds, making this book a truly international effort. This book will bring forth new frontiers with its revolutionizing research information and detailed analysis of the nascent developments around the world.

We would like to thank all the contributing authors for lending their expertise to make the book truly unique. They have played a crucial role in the development of this book. Without their invaluable contributions this book wouldn't have been possible. They have made vital efforts to compile up to date information on the varied aspects of this subject to make this book a valuable addition to the collection of many professionals and students.

This book was conceptualized with the vision of imparting up-to-date information and advanced data in this field. To ensure the same, a matchless editorial board was set up. Every individual on the board went through rigorous rounds of assessment to prove their worth. After which they invested a large part of their time researching and compiling the most relevant data for our readers.

The editorial board has been involved in producing this book since its inception. They have spent rigorous hours researching and exploring the diverse topics which have resulted in the successful publishing of this book. They have passed on their knowledge of decades through this book. To expedite this challenging task, the publisher supported the team at every step. A small team of assistant editors was also appointed to further simplify the editing procedure and attain best results for the readers.

Apart from the editorial board, the designing team has also invested a significant amount of their time in understanding the subject and creating the most relevant covers. They scrutinized every image to scout for the most suitable representation of the subject and create an appropriate cover for the book.

The publishing team has been an ardent support to the editorial, designing and production team. Their endless efforts to recruit the best for this project, has resulted in the accomplishment of this book. They are a veteran in the field of academics and their pool of knowledge is as vast as their experience in printing. Their expertise and guidance has proved useful at every step. Their uncompromising quality standards have made this book an exceptional effort. Their encouragement from time to time has been an inspiration for everyone.

The publisher and the editorial board hope that this book will prove to be a valuable piece of knowledge for researchers, students, practitioners and scholars across the globe.

LIST OF CONTRIBUTORS

Mohammad Malakootian
Environmental Health Engineering Research Center, Department of Environmental Health, Kerman University of Medical Sciences, Kerman, Iran

Behnam Hatami
MSc, Department of Environmental Health, Kerman University of Medical Sciences, Kerman, Iran

Shidwash Dowlatshahi and Ahmad Rajabizadeh
Instructure, Environmental Health Engineering Research Center, Department of Environmental Health, Kerman University of Medical Sciences, Kerman, Iran

Ali Asghar Najafpoor and Hossein Alidadi
Associate Professor, Health Sciences Research Center, Department of Environmental Health Engineering, School of Health, Mashhad University of Medical Sciences, Mashhad, Iran

Abbas Sadeghi and Mojtaba Davoudi
Assistant Professor, Health Sciences Research Center, Department of Environmental Health Engineering, School of Health, Mashhad University of Medical Sciences, Mashhad, Iran

Batoul Mohebrad
Educated Student of Environmental Health Engineering, School of Health, Mashhad University of Medical Sciences, Mashhad, Iran

Ahmad Hosseinzadeh, Salman Jafarpour and Asma Zarei
Environmental Health Engineering, Student Research Committee, School of Health, Mashhad University of Medical Sciences. Mashhad, Iran

Mohammad Shakerkhatibi
Assistant Professor, Department of Environmental Health Engineering, School of Health, Tabriz University of Medical Sciences, Tabriz, Iran

Nahideh Mohammadi
MSc Student, Student Research Committee, Tabriz University of Medical Sciences, Tabriz, Iran

Khaled Zoroufchi Benis
Assistant Professor, Environmental Engineering Research Center, Faculty of Chemical Engineering, Sahand University of Technology, Tabriz, Iran

Alireza Behrooz Sarand
Assistant Professor, Department of Chemical Engineering, Urmia University of Technology, Urmia, Iran

Esmaeil Fatehifar
Professor, Environmental Engineering Research Center, Faculty of Chemical Engineering, Sahand University of Technology, Tabriz, Iran

Ahmad Asl Hashemi
Department of Environmental Health Engineering, School of Health, Tabriz University of Medical Sciences, Tabriz, Iran

Leila Rezaei
MSc, Bandar Abbas Health Center, Hormozgan University of Medical Sciences, Bandar Abbas, Iran

Vali Alipour
Assistant Professor, Environmental Health Engineering Department, School of Health, Hormozgan University of Medical Sciences, Bandar Abbas, Iran

Mohammad Taghi Ghaneian
Associate Professor, Department of Environmental Health, Faculty of Public Health, Shahid Sadoughi University of Medical Sciences, Yazd, Iran

Mohammad Hassan Ehrampoush
Professor, Department of Environmental Health, Faculty of Public Health, Shahid Sadoughi University of Medical Sciences, Yazd, Iran

Ali Jebali and Seyedhossein Hekmatimoghaddam
Assistant Professor, Department of Laboratory Sciences, School of Paramedicine, Shahid Sadoughi University of Medical Sciences, Yazd, Iran

Mohammad Mahmoudi
Department of Environmental Health, Faculty of Public Health, Shahid Sadoughi University of Medical Sciences, Yazd, Iran

Anooshiravan Mohseni Band-pay and Monireh Majlesi
Associate Professor, Department of Environmental Health Engineering, School of Public Health, Shahid Beheshti University of Medical Science, Tehran, Iran

Mona Tabrizi Azad
MSc in Environmental Health, Department of Environmental Health, Shahid Beheshti University of Medical Sciences, Tehran, Iran

Mohammad Miri
Ph.D Student of Environmental Health, Department of Environmental Health Engineering, School of Health, Shahid Sadoughi University of Medical Sciences, Yazd, Iran

Reza Ali Fallahzadeh
MSc of Environmental Health, Department of Environmental Health Engineering, School of Health, Shahid Sadoughi University of Medical Sciences, Yazd, Iran

Mohammad Hassan Ehrampoush
Professor of Environmental Health, Department of Environmental Health Engineering, School of Health, Shahid Sadoughi University of Medical Sciences, Yazd, Iran

Mohammad Hossien Salmani
Analytical Chemistry, Department of Environmental Health Engineering, School of Health, Shahid Sadoughi University of Medical Sciences, Yazd, Iran

Moyad Avazpoor
Faculty instructor, Department of Environmental Health Engineering, Ilam University of Medical Science, Ilam Iran

Mohammad Taqi Yousefipoor
BS of Environmental Health Engineering, Ilam University of Medical Science, Ilam, Iran

Majid Dusty
MSc, Department of Parasitology, Ilam University of Medical Science, Ilam, Iran

Mohsen Mehdipour
Environmental Health in SBMU, Member of Environmental Health Engineering Research Center, Kerman University of Medical Sciences, Kerman, Iran

Fariba Seifipour
MSc Department of Environmental Health Engineering, Ilam University of Medical Science, Ilam, Iran

Zeinab Gholami
Environmental Health, Tehran University of Medical Science, Tehran, Iran

Saeed Motesaddi
Associate Professor, Department of Environmental Health Engineering, School of Public Health, Shahid Beheshti University of Medical Sciences, Tehran, Iran

Parviz Nowrouz and Reza Nemati
Environmental Health Engineering, Department of Environmental Health Engineering, School of Public Health, Shahid Beheshti University of Medical Sciences, Tehran, Iran

Behrouz Alizadeh
PhD Student of Medical Informatics, Department of Medical Informatics, School of Allied Medical Sciences, Shahid Beheshti University of Medical Sciences, Tehran, Iran

Fariba Khalili
Ph.D Student of Environmental Health Engineering, Department of Environmental Health Engineering, School of Public Health, Tehran University of Medical Sciences, Tehran, Iran

Khalilullah Kazemi Khabiri
Department of Geography, School of Urban Planning, International Campus, Ferdowsi University, Mashhad, Iran

Mohammad Ajza Shokouhi and Omid Ali Kharazmi
Department of Geography, School of Urban Planning, Ferdowsi University, Mashhad, Iran

Mohammad Reza Bemanian
Department of Architecture, School of Art and Architecture, Tarbiat Modares University, Tehran, Iran

Akbar Eslami
Associate Professor of Environmental Health Engineering, Environmental and Occupational Hazards Control Research Center, Shahid Beheshti University of Medical Sciences, Tehran, Iran

Zeinab Gholami
MSc of Environmental Health Engineering, Student Research Committee, School of Public Health, Tehran University of Medical Sciences, Tehran, Iran

Shokofeh Nargesi and Bahareh Rostami
BSc in Environmental Health, Ilam University of Medical Sciences, Ilam, Iran

Mohammad Forouhar Vajargah
Department of Fisheries, School of Natural Resources, University of Guilan Sowmehsara, Sowmehsara, Iran

Moayed Avazpour
Research Office of Environmental Health, Department of Environmental Health Engineering, School of Public Health, Shahid Beheshti University of Medical Sciences, Tehran, Iran
Instructor of Environmental Health, Department of Environmental Health Engineering, Ilam University of Medical Science, Ilam, Iran

Ahmad Mohamadi Yalsuyi
Department of Aquaculture, School of Fisheries and Environment, Gorgan University of Agricultural Sciences and Natural Resources, Gorgan, Iran

Masoud Sattari
Department of Fisheries, School of Natural Resources, University of Guilan Sowmehsara, Sowmehsara, Iran
Department of Marine Sciences, Caspian Sea Basin Research Center, University of Guilan, Rasht, Iran

Aliakbar Hedayati
Department of Aquatic Production and Exploitation, School of Fisheries and Environment, Gorgan University of Agricultural Sciences and Natural Resources, Gorgan, Iran

Zabihollah Yousefi and Zeinab Tahernezhad
Department of Environmental Health Engineering, School of Public Health, Mazandaran University of Medical Sciences, Sari, Iran

Seyed Noroddin Mousavinasab
Department of Biostatistics, School of Public Health, Mazandaran University of Medical Sciences, Sari, Iran

Reza Safari
Iranian Fisheries Science Research Institute (IFSRI), Caspian Sea Ecology Research Center, Agricultural Research Education and Extension Organization (AREEO), Sari, Iran

Ahmadreza Bekhradnia
Department of Medicinal Chemistry, Pharmaceutical Sciences Research Center, Mazandaran University of Medical Sciences, Sari, Iran

Zahra Heidari and Mohsen Motevasel
Department of Chemical Engineering, Petroleum University of Technology, Abadan, Iran

Nematollah Jaafarzadeh
Environmental Technologies Research Center, Ahvaz Jundishapur University of Medical Sciences, Ahvaz, Iran

Amirreza Talaiekhozani
Assistant Professor, Department of Civil Engineering, Jami Institute of Technology, Isfahan, Iran

Mohammad Reza Talaei
Associate Professor, Department of Chemical Engineering, Faculty of Engineering, University of Isfahan, Isfahan, Iran

Mehdi Yazdan and Seyed Masoud Mir
Department of Chemical Engineering, Jami Institute of Technology, Isfahan, Iran

Shokufeh Delfi
Department of Environmental Health Engineering, School of Health, Tabriz University of Medical Sciences, Tabriz, Iran

Mohammad Mosaferi
Health and Environment Research Center, Tabriz University of Medical Sciences, Tabriz, Iran

Ali Khalafi
Department of Chemical Engineering, School of Chemical Engineering, University of Tehran, Tehran, Iran

Khaled Zoroufchi Benis
Department of Chemical Engineering, School of Chemical Engineering, Sahand University of Technology, Tabriz, Iran

Balal Oroji and Eisa Solgi
Department of Environmental Sciences, School of Natural Resources and Environmental Sciences, Malayer University, Malayer, Hamadan, Iran

Asghar Sadighzadeh
Nuclear Fuel Cycle Research School, Nuclear Science and Technology Research Institute, Tehran, Iran

Mehdi Ahmadi
Associate Professor, Environmental Technologies Research Center, Department of Environmental Health Engineering, School of Public Health, Ahvaz Jundishapur University of Medical Sciences, Ahvaz, Iran

Maedeh Rozkhosh
M.Sc. of Assessment and Land Use Planning, Science and Research Branch, Islamic Azad University of Khozestan, Faculty of Environment, Ahvaz, Iran

Nemat-allah Jaafarzadeh Haghighifard
Professor, Environmental Technologies Research Center, Department of Environmental Health Engineering, School of Public Health, Ahvaz Jundishapur University of Medical Sciences, Ahvaz, Iran

Bahram Kamarehie, Mansour Ghaderpoori, Ali Jafari and Mohammadamin Karami
Assistant Professor of Environmental Health, School of Health and Nutrition, Lorestan University of Medical Sciences, Khorramabad, Iran

Aliakbar Mohammadi
Lecturer, Department of Environmental Health Engineering, Neyshabur University of Medical Sciences, Neyshabur, Iran

Khaled Azarshab
MSc of Water and Wastewater, Faculty of Environment, Islamic Azad University, West Tehran Branch, Tehran, Iran

Afshin Ghaderpoury
MSc of Environmental Health Engineering, Students Research Committee, Shahid Beheshti University of Medical Sciences, Tehran, Iran

Najaf Noorizadeh
MSc of Occupational Health Engineering, Department of Occupational Health, School of Health, Shahid Beheshti University of Medical Sciences, Tehran, Iran

Majid Kermani
Associate Professor of Environmental Health Engineering, Research Center for Environmental Health Technology, School of Public Health, Iran University of Medical Sciences, Tehran, Iran
Associate Professor of Environmental Health Engineering, Department of Environmental Health Engineering, School of Public Health, Iran University of Medical Sciences, Tehran, Iran

Sevda Fallah Jokandan
MSc of Environmental Health Engineering, Department of Environmental Health Engineering, School of Public Health, Iran University of Medical Sciences, Tehran, Iran

Mohsen Dowlati
MSc of Environmental Health Engineering, Department of Environmental Health Engineering, School of Public Health, Iran University of Medical Sciences, Tehran, Iran
MSc of Environmental Health Engineering, Research Center for Environmental Health Technology, School of Public Health, Iran University of Medical Sciences, Tehran, Iran

Mina Aghaei
Environmental Health Engineering, Department of Environmental Health Engineering, School of Public Health, Tehran University of Medical Sciences, Tehran, Iran

Farshad Bahrami Asl
Environmental Health Engineering, Department of Environmental Health Engineering, School of Public Health, Hamadan University of Medical Sciences, Hamadan, Iran

Sima Karimzadeh
MSc of Environmental Health Engineering, Department of Environmental Health Engineering, School of Public Health, Urima University of Medical Sciences, Urima, Iran

Shahnaz Kushkbaghi
MSc of Environmental Health Engineering, Department of Environment, School of Agriculture and Natural Resource, Yazd Branch, Islamic Azad University, Yazd, Iran

Mohammad Hassan Ehrampoush
Professor of Environmental Health Engineering, Research Center for Environmental Health Technology, Department of Environmental Health, School of Health, Shahid Sadoghi University of Medical Sciences, Yazd, Iran

Seyed Abolghsem Mirhosseinidehabadi
Associate Professor, Department of Environment, School of Agriculture and Natural Resource, Yazd Branch, Islamic Azad University, Yazd, Iran

Asadollah Karimi
Environmental Engineering Research Center, Faculty of Chemical Engineering, Sahand University of Technology, Tabriz, Iran

Esmaeil Fatehifar
Professor, Environmental Engineering Research Center, Faculty of Chemical Engineering, Sahand University of Technology, Tabriz, Iran

Reza Alizadeh
Associate Professor, Environmental Engineering Research Center, Faculty of Chemical Engineering, Sahand University of Technology, Tabriz, Iran

Iraj Ahadzadeh
Assiatant Professor, Faculty of Chemistry, Tabriz University, Tabriz, Iran

Ali Asghar Najafpoor
Associate Professor, Health Sciences Research Center, Department of Environmental Health Engineering, School of Health, Mashhad University of Medical Sciences, Mashhad, Iran

Ahmad Hosseinzadeh and Somaye Allahyari
Health Sciences Research Center, Department of Environmental Health Engineering, School of Health, Mashhad University of Medical Sciences, Mashhad, Iran
Student Research Committee, Mashhad University of Medical Sciences, Mashhad, Iran

Allah Bakhsh Javid
Assistant Professor, Department of Environmental Health Engineering, School of Health, Tehran University of Medical Sciences, Tehran, Iran

Habibollah Esmaily
Associate Professor, Health Sciences Research Center, Department of Biostatistics, School of Health, Mashhad University of Medical Sciences, Mashhad, Iran

Amirreza Talaiekhozani
Assistant Professor, Department of Civil Engineering, Jami Institute of Technology, Isfahan, Iran

Somaye Bahrami
Environmental Engineering, School of Post Graduate, Islamic Azad University Branch of Bushehr, Bushehr, Iran

Seyed Mohammad Javad Hashemi
M.Sc, Department of Civil Engineering, Jami Institute of Technology, Isfahan, Iran

Sahand Jorfi
Assistant Professor, Environmental Technologies Research Center, Ahvaz Jundishapur University of Medical Sciences, Ahvaz, Iran
Assistant Professor, Department of Environmental Health Engineering, School of Health, Ahvaz Jundishapur University of Medical Sciences, Ahvaz, Iran

Gholamreza Goudarzi
Associate Professor of Environmental Health, Air Pollution and Respiratory Diseases Research Center, Ahvaz Jundishapur University of Medical Sciences, Ahvaz, Iran

Rajab Rashidi
Assistant Professor of Occupational Health, Department of Occupational Health, Nutrition Health Research Center, School of Health, Lorestan University of Medical Sciences, Khorramabad, Iran

Fariba Keishams
Department of Environmental Health, School of Health, Isfahan University of Medical Sciences, Isfahan, Iran

Mahsa Moradi
MSc of Environmental Health, Air Pollution and Respiratory Diseases Research Center, Ahvaz Jundishapur University of Medical Sciences, Ahvaz, Iran

Shahram Sadeghi
MSc of Environmental Health, Environmental Health Research Center, Kurdistan University of Medical Sciences, Sanandaj, Iran

Fereydoun Masihpour and Mojtaba Shegerd
BSc of Occupational Health, Health Center of East, Ahvaz Jundishapur University of Medical Sciences, Ahvaz, Iran

Ehsan Abouee Mehrizi
Department of Environmental Health Engineering, School of Public Health, North Khorasan University of Medical Sciences, Bojnurd, Iran

Mohammad Veysi Shikhrobat
BSc of Health Services Administration, Health Center of East, Ahvaz Jundishapur University of Medical Sciences, Ahvaz, Iran

Yusef Omidi Khaniabadi
MSc of Environmental Health, Air Pollution and Respiratory Diseases Research Center, Ahvaz Jundishapur University of Medical Sciences, Ahvaz, Iran
MSc of Environmental Health, Health Care System of Karoon, Ahvaz Jundishapur University of Medical Sciences, Ahvaz, Iran

Asiyeh Moteallemi
Department of Environmental Health Engineering, School of Nursing, Torbat Jam Faculty of Medical Sciences, Torbat Jam, Iran

Bijan Bina
Department of Environmental Health Engineering, School of Health, Isfahan University of Medical Sciences, Isfahan, Iran

Soheila Mortezaie
Department of Occupational Health Engineering, School of Health, Isfahan University of Medical Sciences, Isfahan, Iran

Sahar Akhavan, Soheila Ebrahimi and Alireza Movahedi Naeini
Department of Soil Sciences, Soil and Water Engineering School, Gorgan University of Agricultural Sciences and Natural Resources, Gorgan, Iran

Maryam Navabian
Department of Water Engineering, School of Agriculture, University of Guilan, Rasht, Iran

Mahmoud Shabanpour
Department of Soil Science, School of Agriculture, University of Guilan, Rasht, Iran

Ali Mojtahedi
Department of Microbiology, School of Medicine, Guilan University of Medical Sciences, Rasht, Iran

Sisay Derso
Environmental Health Research Team, Ethiopian Public Health Institute, Addis Ababa, Ethiopia

Girum Taye, Theodros Getachew, Atkure Defar, Habtamu Teklie, Kassahun Amenu, Terefe Gelibo and Abebe Bekele
Health System Research Directorate, Ethiopian Public Health Institute, Addis Ababa, Ethiopia

Hadi Negahdari and Faramarz Moattar
Department of Environmental Engineering, Faculty of Natural Resources and Environment, Science and Research Branch, Islamic Azad University, Tehran, Iran

Sirus Javadpour
Material Science and Engineering Department, School of Engineering, Shiraz University, Shiraz, Iran

Hashem Negahdari
Department of Civil Engineering, School of Engineering, Islamic Azad University, Shiraz Branch, Shiraz, Iran

Amir Zahedi
Committee Research, Department of Environmental Health Engineering, School of Health, Ahvaz Jundishapur University of Medical Sciences, Ahvaz, Iran

Sorour Ghodrati
Department of Environmental Assessment and Land Use Planning, School of Environment and Energy, Islamic Azad University, Science and Research Branch, Tehran, Iran

Mehdi Ahmadimoghaddam
Environmental Technologies Research Center, Department of Environmental Health Engineering, School of Health, Ahvaz Jundishapur University of Medical Sciences, Ahvaz, Iran

Nematollah Jaafarzadeh
Environmental Technologies Research Center, Department of Environmental Health Engineering, School of Health, Ahvaz Jundishapur University of Medical Sciences, Ahvaz, Iran

Balal Oroji and Eisa Solgi
Department of Environmental Sciences, School of Natural Resources and Environmental Sciences, Malayer University, Malayer, Hamadan, Iran

Mehdi Bibak and Javid Imanpour Namin
Department of Fisheries, School of Natural Resources, University of Guilan, Sowmehsara, Iran

Ali Agharokh
Research Center for Persian Gulf, School of Persian Gulf, University of Persian Gulf, Bushehr, Iran

Saeid Tahmasebi
Department of Statistics, School of Basic Sciences, University of Persian Gulf, Bushehr, Iran

Shidvash Dowlatshahi and Mahshid Loloei
Instructor, Environmental Health Engineering Research Center and Department of Environmental Health, School of Public Health, Kerman University of Medical Sciences, Kerman, Iran

Ahmad Reza Haratinezhad Torbati
Environmental Health Engineering, Department of Environmental Health, School of Public Health, Kerman University of Medical Sciences, Kerman, Iran

Yaser Sharifi
MSc, Department of Microbiology, Qom Branch, Islamic Azad University, Qom, Iran

Ahmad Ali Pourbabaei and Abbas Morovvati
Assistant Professor, Department of Soil Science, University of Tehran, Tehran, Iran

Ali Javadi
Department of Pathobiology, School of Public Health, Tehran University of Medical Sciences, Tehran, Iran

Mohammad Hossein Abdolmohammadi
Assistant Professor, Research Center for Environmental Pollutants, Qom University of Medical Sciences, Qom, Iran

Mehri Saffari
Associate Professor, Department of Agronomy and Plant Breeding, Faculty of Agriculture, Shahid Bahonar University, Kerman, Iran

Ahmad Reza Yazdanbakhsh
Associate Professor, Department of Environmental Health Engineering, Shahid Beheshti University of Medical Sciences, Tehran, Iran

Majid Kermani
Assistant Professor, Department of Environmental Health Engineering, Iran University of Medical Sciences, Tehran, Iran

Sanaz Komasi
MSc of Environmental Engineering, Department of Environmental Engineering, Islamic Azad University, West Tehran Branch, Tehran, Iran

Ehsan Aghayani
Department of Environmental Health Engineering, Tarbiat Modares University of Medical Sciences, Tehran, Iran

Amir Sheikhmohammadi
Department of Environmental Health Engineering, Shahid Beheshti University of Medical Sciences, Tehran, Iran

Monireh Majlessi
Associate Professor, Department of Environmental Health Engineering, School of Public Health, Shahid Beheshti University of Medical Science, Tehran, Iran

Aida Vaezi
MA of Environmental Science, Islamic Azad University, Science and Research Branch, Tehran, Iran

Mohsen Mehdipour Rabori
Environmental Health in SBMU, Member of Environmental Health Engineering Research Center, Kerman University of Medical Sciences, Kerman, Iran

Seyed Mostafa Khezri
Associate Professor, Department of Environmental Engineering, School of Environment and Energy, Science and Research Branch, Islamic Azad University, Tehran, Iran

Gharib Majidi and Mohsen Ansari
MSc in Environmental Health Engineering, School of Public Health, Qom University of Medical Sciences, Qom, Iran

Hossein Jafari Mansoorian
Lecturer, Environmental Health Engineering Research Center, Department of Environmental Health, Kerman University of Medical Sciences, Kerman, Iran

Farideh Atabi
Assistant Professor, Department of Environmental Engineering, School of Environment and Energy, Science and Research Branch, Islamic Azad University, Tehran, Iran

Taha Tohidi Mogaddam
MSc in Environmental Engineering, Science and Research Branch, Islamic Azad University, Tehran, Iran

Nahid Rashtchi
MSc in Environmental Engineering-Water and Wastewater, Islamic Azad University, Western Tehran Branch, Tehran, Iran

Kavoos Dindarloo and Parvin Lakbala
Assistant Professor, Environmental Health Engineering Research Center, Instructor Department of Health, Hormozgan University of Medical Sciences, Bandar Abbas, Iran

Hamza Ali Jamali
Assistant Professor, Department of Environmental Health Engineering, Qazvin University of Medical Sciences, Qazvin, Iran

Hamid Mahmoodi
MSc, Environmental Health Engineering Research Center, Instructor Department of Health, Hormozgan University of Medical Sciences, Bandar Abbas, Iran

Fatemeh Kazemi
MSc, Environmental Health Engineering Research Center, Hormozgan University of Medical Sciences, Bandar Abbas, Iran

Mohammad Malakootian
Professor, Environmental Health Engineering Research Center, Department of Environmental Health, Kerman University of Medical Sciences, Kerman, Iran

Behnam Hatami
MSc, Department of Environmental Health, Kerman University of Medical Sciences, Kerman, Iran

Shidwash Dowlatshahi and Ahmad Rajabizadeh
Instructure, Environmental Health Engineering Research Center, Department of Environmental Health, Kerman University of Medical Sciences, Kerman, Iran

Neamat Jaafarzadeh Haghighi Fard
Professor, Environmental Technologies Research Center, Ahvaz Jundishapur University of Medical Sciences, Ahvaz, Iran
Professor, Department of Environmental Health Engineering, School of Public Health, Ahvaz Jundishapur University of Medical Sciences, Ahvaz, Iran

Behnam Moradi
BSc, Department of Environmental Health Engineering, School of Public Health, Ahvaz Jundishapur University of Medical Sciences, Ahvaz, Iran
Student Research Committee, Ahvaz Jundishapur University of Medical Sciences, Ahvaz, Iran

Mokhtar Abbasi, Rahman Alivar Babadi, Hossein Bahrani and Azadeh Mirzaie
BSc, Department of Environmental Health Engineering, School of Public Health, Ahvaz Jundishapur University of Medical Sciences, Ahvaz, Iran

Ahmad Zare Javid
PhD, Nutrition and Metabolic Diseases Research Center, Ahvaz Jundishapur University of Medical Sciences, Ahvaz, Iran

Maryam Ravanbakhsh
Student Research Committee, Ahvaz Jundishapur University of Medical Sciences, Ahvaz, Iran
MSc, Department of Environmental Health Engineering, School of Public Health, Ahvaz Jundishapur University of Medical Sciences, Ahvaz, Iran

Index

www.ingramcontent.com/pod-product-compliance
Lightning Source LLC
LaVergne TN
LVHW081020210926
848485LV00004B/910